Craniofacial Anomalies

Rebecca A. Eder
Editor

Craniofacial Anomalies

Psychological Perspectives

With a Foreword by Jeffrey L. Marsh, M.D.

With 30 Illustrations

Springer-Verlag
New York Berlin Heidelberg London Paris
Tokyo Hong Kong Barcelona Budapest

Rebecca A. Eder
Department of Psychology
St. Louis Children's Hospital
St. Louis, MO 63110, USA
and
Department of Psychology
Washington University
St. Louis, MO 63130, USA

Library of Congress Cataloging in Publication Data
Eder, Rebecca A.
Craniofacial anomalies: psychological perspectives/Rebecca A. Eder.
p. cm.
Includes bibliographical references and index.

ISBN-13: 978-1-4612-7549-7 e-ISBN-13: 978-1-4612-2466-2
DOI: 10.1007/978-1-4612-2466-2

1. Face–Abnormalities. 2. Skull–Abnormalities. I. Title.
QM695.F32E34 1995
617.5′2043′019–dc20 93-31776

Printed on acid-free paper.

Softcover reprint of the hardcover 1st edition 1995

Production coordinated by Chernow Editorial Services and managed by Terry Kornak; manufacturing supervised by Jacqui Ashri.
Typeset by Best-set Typesetter Ltd., Hong Kong.

9 8 7 6 5 4 3 2 1

To Barbara

Foreword

The motivation for the first surgical reconstruction of a congenital facial deformity is unknown. Ancient medical writings and Renaissance woodcuts document attempts to repair cleft lip, the most frequently encountered and necessarily recognized of the craniofacial anomalies. It is probable that restoration of a "normal" appearance to destigmatize the affected individual was at least one, if not the only, objective of surgical intervention. While the psychosocial consequences of craniofacial deformity were and are appreciated by cultures less medically sophisticated than ours, the physiological consequences of craniofacial anomalies have only been defined over the past century. Emphasis on physiological rather than psychosocial function tended to dominate the medical literature on craniofacial anomalies from the mid-nineteenth to the mid-twentieth centuries. This probably reflects both the development and popularization of surgery based on pathophysiology and the paucity of tools and investigators for psychosocial research during that time period. The introduction of general anesthesia, antisepsis, diagnostic medical imaging, antibiotics, intravenous fluids, blood component therapy, and intensive care and specialized surgical facilities, along with the reorganization of medical education, have allowed surgery to be extended to every locus in the body no matter how remote or seemingly dangerous. While operations upon the face and skull allowed individuals affected with craniofacial anomalies to breathe, eat, see, hear, and speak more normally, normal psychosocial development and social integration did not necessarily follow. By the 1960s, some surgeons and pediatricians were questioning the efficacy of certain operations for craniosynostosis, that is, premature fusion of cranial sutures. It had been thought, for almost one hundred years, that fused sutures needed to be surgically "released" to prevent increased intracranial pressure, hydrocephalus, blindness, mental retardation, and even death. On critical examination, there was minimal evidence to support these assumptions. Reconstruction of craniofacial anomalies to facilitate the affected individual's psychosocial development and social integration had become an accepted indication for surgery by the 1970s. Normalization of psychosocial development by normalization of craniofacial appearance has remained both an important indication for and a major objective of surgery over the past quarter century.

Although it seems intuitively obvious that facial deformity negatively affects psychosocial development and that, conversely, surgical reconstruction of the deformity will positively affect psychosocial development, the validity of these assumptions is yet to be proven. Surgeons not only accept "psychosocial benefit" as an indication for an operation but also use similar reasoning to advise surgery prior to the individual's becoming aware of the implications of facial deformity, even if additional surgery will be necessary as the child grows. It is assumed that the psychological morbidity of repetitive operations is less than that of unreconstructed facial deformity throughout childhood followed by one operation upon maturity, provided that the surgery effectively destigmatizes the deformity.

What is the evidence to support these assumptions and medical behavior? In this text, Eder has edited an outstanding collection of contributions from leading authorities on craniofacial surgery and psychosocial development in an attempt to document current understanding and, more importantly, to provide stimulation and guidance for necessary further research.

Part 1 addresses appearance, expression, and perception. Munro provides a craniofacial surgeon's perspective regarding the methods and rationale of reconstruction of craniofacial anomalies. He questions: Whether craniofacial surgery avoids or diminishes psychosocial problems? Whether multiple surgeries are preferable to one definitive surgery with respect to psychosocial benefit? and How are the biological versus psychological needs of an individual with a craniofacial anomaly best met? His observation, that although the postoperative appearance may be less disfiguring than that preoperatively it often is not normal, raises the question of how much deviation from the norm is compatible with normal psychosocial acceptance. Langlois addresses three types of information which the facial appearance communicates that regulate social behavior and interaction: age, gender, and affect. She postulates that individuals with craniofacial anomalies appear older than their chronological age or of ambiguous age and gender. This confusion may yield misperception by others that results in inappropriate expectations about and reactions toward the affected individual. Berry introduces the concept of the event perception approach to facial perception. This approach recognizes that in addition to nondynamic structural characteristics, such as the anthropometric measurements recorded for facial harmonics, the dynamic characteristics of motion (e.g., emotion) and change (e.g., growth) affect facial perception. If alteration of facial form, that is, nondynamic characteristics, is achieved at the expense of diminution of expressive motion, one must ask whether the alteration is cost/benefit effective. Shepard and Magai note that socioemotional development contains both intra- and interpersonal aspects. They discuss the important role of caregivers in the socialization of emotional expression and in the affective, experiential development of their children. Furthermore in the context of infant–mother interaction, there is a two-way street between infant and mother facial expressivity. They question how the mother of an infant with limited or idiosyncratic facial display learns to interpret that infant's emotions and needs.

Attachment and parenting is the subject of Part 2. Field notes that a preference for physical attractiveness produces differential expectations based on that physical attractiveness. These, in turn, may yield differential behavior that is attractiveness driven. Unattractive children have been observed to be less competent in social development than physically attractive peers. With respect to infants with craniofacial anomalies, they seem to be less active and less responsive than normal infants. Similarly, their mothers seem less active and responsive than those of the unaffected infants. The morbidity of these unresponsive early interactions is unknown. Petersen, Pawl, and Lieberman further discuss attachment in infants with disabilities. They note that the maternal–infant relation tends to focus on negative rather than positive aspects for infants with craniofacial anomalies. The primary focus of studies of maternal–infant relations changes from the infant in studies of normals to the mother in studies of abnormal infants. Nonetheless no association between parental responsiveness and the degree of disability in the child has been shown: different forms and degrees of parental responsiveness are the norm. Attachment in infants and preschoolers who require hospitalization is discussed by Crowell, Waters, and Szanjnberg. They note that attachment can be formalized into the child's ability to use the parent as a base for exploration and a safe haven, as well as the child's confidence in parental availability and responsiveness. Parents need to be "present, predictable, and confident." Health care professionals should evaluate and use the "parents' potential as collaborators in treatment."

Eder introduces Part 3, which focuses on social cognition, self-concept, and social interaction. She explores the emotional basis of self-understanding to better understand development of the self-concepts of children with cleft lip/palate. Examination of the literature presents contradictory data as to whether being born with a cleft lip/palate results in adjustment problems. Resolution of this inconsistency may reside in considering the deformity in the context of the individual and family life cycles. Eder postulates that the child's emotionality develops out of the interaction between infant temperament, parental personality, and the caregiver–infant attachment. The effect or lack thereof of the cleft lip/palate on the affected individual's emotionality and subsequent self-concept may relate to whether or not one or more of these three variables is impacted as a consequence of the cleft. In a pilot study of preschoolers with clefts, she observed that both the affected children and their mothers rated them higher on feelings of aggression and stress than their peers or their peers' mothers. Rubin and Wilkinson explore peer rejection and social isolation in childhood. They note that peer interaction is necessary for normal social and emotional development. The pathway to rejection and isolation may begin with the parent–infant interaction: if the parent withdraws from the deformed infant, the infant will be stimulated less; the infant then may respond less and in turn induce less response from the parent, thereby perpetuating a vicious cycle that results in an insecure attachment relationship. In older children, the peer response to craniofacial anomalies may be bimodal: isolation may result from being ignored or excessive attention may be drawn through teasing. Since the behavioral correlates of unattractiveness and facial deformity seem to differ, research on unattractiveness may not be relevant for craniofacial anomalies. Reis and Hodgins conclude the discussions with concentration on the physical attractiveness and stigma literatures. They raise the question of whether beauty is a more positive attribute or ugliness a more negative one. They note that the research on unattractiveness focuses on the effects of physical attractiveness rather than those of unattractiveness. The impact of stigmatizing deformity can be evaluated with respect to concealability, course over time, disruptiveness, aesthetic factors, origin, and peril posed to others. While unattractiveness seems to induce only negative outcomes, facial disfigurement can have advantages as well as disadvantages for the affected individual. Others tend to both help and hinder stigmatized individuals to a degree greater than that for non-stigmatized persons.

In Part 4, authors Serofica, Tobiasen, Speltz, Galbreath, and Greenberg discuss investigations into the psychosocial consequences of uncorrected or incompletely corrected craniofacial deformity. Studies on this and of the timing of such reconstructive surgery, and of effective reconstruction are necessary to both validate, hopefully, the above-stated hypotheses, upon which current management is predicated, and to better understand the general issue of appearance and psychosocial function. Dr. Eder and her colleagues report such investigations in this text. While more questions are asked than answered, an excellent review of relevant attractiveness, caregiver–infant bonding, socioemotional development, event perception, and emotionality literature is provided for those unfamiliar with it. General aspects of psychosocial development and deviations are focused on data from studies of individuals with craniofacial anomalies when such studies exist. More importantly, in my opinion, are the recommendations of the various contributors for directions of further research. Enough time has elapsed since the popularization of major craniofacial reconstructive surgery that infants who received such operations have grown into adults. The lack of adequate prospective studies has limited the information that can be recovered from the experiences of these individuals. The challenge to readers of this book is to design such studies so that the infants and young children who are operated on in the near future may meaningfully contribute to our understanding of facial deformity and its reconstruction in the not too distant morrow.

Jeffrey L. Marsh, M.D.
Professor of Surgery, Plastic
and Reconstructive
Associate Professor of Pediatrics
in Surgery (Plastic and Reconstructive)
Professor of Radiology, Division
of Radiology Research
Washington University School of
Medicine and Medical Director
Cleft Palate and Craniofacial
Deformities Institute
St. Louis Children's Hospital
St. Louis, MO 63110

Preface

Craniofacial anomalies (CFAs) represent one of the most commonly occurring birth defects. Clefts of the lip and/or palate (CLP) alone occur in approximately 1.5 out of every 1,000 births. The prevalence of all the other anomalies is equal to or exceeds that of CLP (Day, 1985).

Recent diagnostic and surgical advances have resulted in substantial changes in the medical treatment of persons with craniofacial anomalies. However, relatively little has changed in the approach to psychological issues associated with CFAs. The prevailing assumption on the part of clinicians and researchers—that facial disfigurement must result in psychological problems—has remained unchallenged for nearly half a century (e.g., Macgregor, Abel, Byrt, Lauer, & Weissman, 1953; Pruzinsky, 1990). This book was undertaken to advance our understanding of the psychological impact of CFAs by reevaluating the prevailing view in light of the most current perspectives and findings in developmental psychology.

In a review of craniofacial birth defects, Day stated that, "Without regard to its severity or rarity, each CFA takes on additional significance because it affects the human face. No other portion of our body is invested with so much meaning, recognition, and importance" (1985, p. 344). Reviews such as these often describe specific psychological problems believed to be associated with these anomalies. For example, CFAs have been speculated to be associated with problems in mother–infant bonding, self-esteem, social acceptance, school performance and adjustment, and adult mental heath (e.g., Day, 1985; Kapp-Simon, 1981; Pruzinsky, 1990).

There is a considerable discrepancy between the perceived impact of CFAs on psychological functioning and conclusions derived from actual empirical research. For example, persons with CFAs have not been found to differ from the norm on measures of psychopathology (e.g., Richman & Eliason, 1982; Williams, 1982). Furthermore, few reliable differences are reported on measures of self-esteem and self-perception (e.g., Eder, *this volume*). What accounts for this discrepancy?

Previous investigators have attributed the preponderance of non-significant results to the use of unreliable measures and/or to the lack of appropriate control groups with which to compare individuals with CFAs (e.g., Clifford, 1987; Tobiasen, 1984). For example, few of these studies have systematically varied or examined the effect of degree of disfigurement and/or attractiveness in their subjects (see also Tobiasen, *this volume*).

The major complaint about past work—a complaint that is echoed throughout this volume—is that it lacks a general theoretical perspective (e.g., Berry, Speltz, Galbreath, & Greenberg; and Tobiasen, *this volume*). That is, the narrow focus on the role of disfigurement in psychological development makes the conclusions from research on the development of individuals with CFAs quite disconnected from current knowledge about *typical* psychological development. Given that CFAs occur in the context of normal development, it would be productive for investigators to consider developmental processes.

The central goal of *Craniofacial Anomalies: Psychological Perspectives* is to provide a theoretical framework for psychological research on craniofacial problems by applying a developmental perspective. Developmentalists are primarily interested in the extent to which individuals show normal developmental pathways. This approach thus emphasizes the competence or resilience of individuals with CFAs (even in the "face" of adversity). A developmental approach encourages researchers and practitioners first to define, follow, and understand normal pathways of development as a means of outlining how CFAs might interact with these pathways. In a developmental perspective, psychological disorders are viewed as developmental deviations (e.g., Sroufe, 1989; Rutter & Garmezy, 1983). Hence, developmentalists are also concerned with the extent to which factors associated with being born with a CFA result in developmental deviations.

To begin to address these questions, a group of distinguished scholars was asked to apply their expertise in social, emotional, and personality development to understand the psychological development of children with CFAs. Their contributions allow this volume to cover a wide range of topics in developmental psychology. Contributors were asked to discuss the central constructs and findings from their research domains in terms of the implications for the study and treatment of individuals with CFAs. Given that many of the contributors had never studied this specific population, this was a formidable task. It is clear from the high quality of the chapters that all the contributors put a great deal of thought into their work.

Part 1 focuses on several different aspects of the human face. It begins with a description of craniofacial anomalies by Ian R. Munro, a renowned maxillofacial surgeon. Judith H. Langlois then considers the role of the face in appearance-based stereotypes. Diane S. Berry provides a theoretical framework for understanding the many different types of information provided via one's face. Part 1 concludes with Beth Shepard and Carol Magai's discussion of the role of facial expressions of emotion in socioemotional development.

The chapters in Part 2 address the important role that parent–child interaction plays in development. Tiffany Field describes parent–infant interactions in children with CFAs. Two chapters are concerned with caregiver–infant attachment: Sandra H. Petersen, Jeree H. Pawl, and Alicia F. Lieberman discuss the development of caregiver–child attachment relationship in children with disabilities; and Judith A. Crowell, Everett Waters, and Nathan Szanjnberg examine the implications of attachment theory for children who require hospitalization.

Part 3 examines the implications of recent research findings on social cognition and social interaction for persons with CFAs. It begins with Rebecca A. Eder's discussion of the emergence of individual differences in young children's self-concept. In their chapter, Kenneth H. Rubin and Margaret Wilkinson discuss two types of disturbances in children's peer relations: peer rejection and social isolation. Part 3 concludes with a review by Harry T. Reis and Holley S. Hodgins of the physical attractiveness and stigma literatures. They propose that these two literatures lead to quite different expectations about the psychological, social, and developmental experiences of facially disfigured persons.

Part 4 presents current psychological research on children with craniofacial anomalies by investigators employing a developmental perspective. Felicisima C. Serafica discusses findings about the social and emotional development of persons with Down Syndrome. Joyce M. Tobiasen describes a model for understanding research on individuals with CFAs. Matthew L. Speltz, Holly Galbreath, and Mark T. Greenberg conclude this section and the volume by illustrating how a developmental framework is used in their program of research on the psychological correlates of craniofacial anomalies.

It is my hope that *Craniofacial Anomalies: Psychological Perspectives* will not only be a valuable resource for anyone involved in the care of persons with craniofacial anomalies but will also encourage more developmental psychologists to study individuals with CFA. By providing a theoretical context, the book will be useful to researchers interested in the psychological correlates of CFAs and their treatment. In addition, many of the contributors to this volume have suggested that an investigation of children and adults with CFAs will broaden our understanding of typical developmental processes. For example, the occurrence and repair of malformations of the face provide a context for examining how alterations in the face affect psychological processes. Shepard and Magai (*this volume*) suggest that malformations of the face (or the surgical treatment of these malformations) result in restrictions of facial musculature for children with CFAs. The facial feedback hypothesis states that infants acquire emotional understanding by making an association between the feedback of their facial musculature and their internal states. Given this hypothesis, children with CFAs should demonstrate less emotional understanding than other children. If this is not the case, it may be that facial feedback is not central to the emergence of emotional understanding, as previous researchers have suggested.

There are several ways in which the material in *Craniofacial Anomalies: Psychological Perspectives* can be used to provide more comprehensive care of patients with CFAs. First, physicians are encouraged to evaluate their implicit (and perhaps inaccurate) beliefs regarding the psychosocial issues associated with CFAs and to rely instead on empirical evidence rather when making decisions about the timing, number, and types of surgical interventions. Berry's chapter indicates that facial appearance provides others with information about a person's traits (e.g., dominance, intelligence). According to Berry, changing one's appearance via surgery may also change some of this information. One implication is that modifications of the facial characteristics typical of Down Syndrome children (via cosmetic surgery) may result in the (unwanted) consequence that parents and others develop higher, unrealistic expectations for these retarded children (Serafica, *this volume*).

Second, this volume will enable health care professionals to understand and reduce the amount of distress that children and their families experience during medical procedures and hospitalization. For example, Crowell, Waters, and Szanjnberg (*this volume*) describe how the caregiver–infant attachment relationship is useful for helping a family cope with a child's hospitalization.

Finally, it will enable mental health professionals to maximize their impact by focusing on clearly defined psychological problems that are typically associated with CFAs. For example, most cleft lip and palate teams have been concerned about their patients' self-esteem (e.g., Lefebvre & Arndt, 1988), despite the fact that researchers have failed to establish any differences in the self-esteem of children with CLP compared to noncleft peers. Although the self-concepts of children with CLP do not differ from noncleft children on the dimension of self-esteem, recent research indicates that there are reliable differences on other self-concept dimensions. Using a new self-concept measure (Eder, 1990), I found that 5-year-olds with CLP report more feelings of anger, aggression, and being out of control compared with noncleft peers (Eder, *this volume*). Clearly, such children would benefit from professionals' attention to these feelings.

In summary, this book provides a developmental perspective to psychological research on craniofacial anomalies. How successful this perspective will be in advancing our understanding of psychological issues associated with CFAs cannot be predicted. The early indications, as exemplified by the chapters in this volume, are very encouraging.

References

Clifford, E. (1987). *The Cleft Palate Experience*. Springfield, IL: Charles C Thomas.

Day, D.W. (1985). Craniofacial birth defects. In N. Hobbs, & J.M. Perrin (Eds.), *Issues in the care of children with chronic illness*. San Francisco: Jossey-Bass.

Eder, R.A. (1990). Uncovering young children's psychological selves: Individual and developmental differences. *Child Development, 61,* 849–863.

Kapp-Simon, K. (1981). Psychological adaptation of patients with craniofacial malformations. In G.W. Lucker, J.A. Ribbens, & J.A. MacNamara (Eds.), *Psychological aspects of facial form.* Ann Arbor: University of Michigan Press.

Lefebvre, A.M., & Arndt, E.M. (1988). Working with facially disfigured children: A challenge in prevention. *Canadian Journal of Psychiatry, 33,* 453–458.

Macgregor, F.C., Abel, T.M., Byrt, A., Lauer, E., & Weissman, S. (1953). *Facial deformities and plastic surgery: A psychosocial study.* Springfield, IL: Charles C Thomas.

Pruzinsky, T. (1990). Collaboration of plastic surgeon and medical psychotherapist: Reconstructive surgery for congenital craniofacial deformities. *Medical Psychotherapy, 3,* 103–116.

Richman, L.C., & Eliason, M. (1982). Psychological characteristics of children with cleft lip and palate: Intellectual, achievement, behavioral, and personality variables. *Cleft Palate Journal, 19,* 251–257.

Rutter, M., & Garmezy, N. (1983). Developmental psychopathology. In E.M. Hetherington (Ed.), *Carmichael's manual of child psychology: Vol. 4. Social and personality development* (pp. 775–912). New York: Wiley.

Sroufe, L.A. (1989). Pathways to adaptation and maladaptation: Psychopathology as a developmental deviation. In D. Cicchetti (Ed.), *The emergence of a discipline: Vol. 1. Rochester symposium on developmental psychopathology* (pp. 13–40). Hillsdale, NJ: Erlbaum.

Tobiasen, J.M. (1984). Psychosocial correlates of congenital facial clefts: Conceptualization and model. *Cleft Palate Journal, 21,* 131–139.

Williams, B.J. (1982). Social and psychological problems associated with cleft palate. *Clinics in Plastic Surgery, 9,* 317–326.

Acknowledgments

This book began with the idea that a developmental perspective would be especially productive in understanding the psychological impact of craniofacial anomalies and their treatment. This idea was first tested in a conference entitled "Psychological Aspects of Craniofacial Problems: Surgery Is Not Enough," which was organized by myself and Ian Munro and was sponsored by the Craniofacial Institute at the Humana Advanced Surgical Institutes (Ian Munro, M.D., director; Kenneth Salyer, M.D., president), with additional funding from the Foundation for Craniofacial Deformities (Marcy Rogers-Salyer, director). About half the contributors to *Craniofacial Anomalies* also participated in this conference. The remaining contributors to the book were invited to address issues that emerged from the discussions during both conference presentations and informal meetings.

The preparation of this book has been aided by a number of colleagues. The authors of these chapters have been exceptional on many counts. As a group, the contributors have shown courage in being willing to think and write about the implications of findings from their research areas for understanding individuals with craniofacial anomalies. The quality of their contributions reveals that I was lucky to have selected a group of thoughtful and creative scholars. These authors have also been cooperative and patient in bearing with revisions and the publication process. Finally, many of them were generous with their advice and help about which topics and scholars to include, the editorial process, and numerous other issues. Special thanks are expressed to Diane Berry and Ken Rubin for their advice in the early stages of this book and to Harry Reis for helping see this book through to the end.

Leigh Berry helped me through many phases of this project, from its nascence. Kim Harkins' editorial assistance in keeping track of old manuscripts and revisions is gratefully acknowledged. The patience, good advice, and support of my colleagues Debra Long and Robert Emmons at the University of California at Davis is especially appreciated. Finally, many thanks go to Peter and Betsy for the countless hours that they played quietly together to allow me to work on "the book."

Contents

Part 3: Social Cognition, Self-Concept, and Social Interaction

Part 4: Current Research on Craniofacial Anomalies

Contributors

Diane S. Berry
Department of Psychology, Southern Methodist University, Dallas, TX 75275, USA

Judith A. Crowell
Department of Psychiatry, State University of New York at Stony Brook, Stony Brook, NY 11794, USA

Rebecca A. Eder
Department of Psychology, St. Louis Children's Hospital, St. Louis, MO 63110, USA, and Department of Psychology, Washington University, St. Louis, MO 63130, USA

Tiffany Field
Mailman Center for Child Development, University of Miami Medical School, Miami, FL 33101, USA

Holly Galbreath
Department of Psychiatry, University of Washington School of Medicine, Seattle, WA 98195, USA

Mark T. Greenberg
Department of Psychology, University of Washington, Seattle, WA 98195, USA

Holley S. Hodgins
Department of Psychology, University of Rochester, Rochester, NY 14627, USA

Judith H. Langlois
Department of Psychology, University of Texas at Austin, Austin, TX 78712, USA

Alicia F. Lieberman
Infant–Parent Program, San Francisco General Hospital, University of California at San Francisco, San Francisco, CA 94941, USA

Carol Magai
Department of Psychology, Long Island University, Brooklyn, NY 11201, USA

Jeffrey L. Marsh
Washington University School of Medicine, and Cleft Palate and Craniofacial Deformities Institute, St. Louis Children's Hospital, St. Louis, MO 63110, USA

Ian R. Munro
Craniofacial Institute, Humana Advanced Surgical Institutes, Dallas, TX 75230, USA

Jeree H. Pawl
Infant–Parent Program, San Francisco General Hospital, University of California at San Francisco, San Francisco, CA 94941, USA

Sandra H. Petersen
Department of Education, Special Education Services Unit, Denver, CO 80203, USA

Harry T. Reis
Department of Psychology, University of Rochester, Rochester, NY 14627, USA

Kenneth H. Rubin
Department of Psychology, University of Waterloo, Waterloo, Ontario N2L 3G1, Canada

Felicisima C. Serafica
Department of Psychology, The Ohio State University, Columbus, OH 43210, USA

Beth Shepard
Department of Psychology, Trinity University, San Antonio, TX 78212, USA

Matthew L. Speltz
Department of Psychiatry, University of Washington School of Medicine, Seattle, WA 98195, USA

Nathan Szajnberg
Department of Child and Adolescent Psychiatry, Hartford Hospital, Hartford, CT 06115, USA

Joyce M. Tobiasen
Behavioral Medicine and Psychological Services, Sutherland Institute, University of Kansas Medical Center, Kansas City, KS 66160, USA

Everett Waters
Department of Psychology, State University of New York at Stony Brook, Stony Brook, NY 11733, USA

Margaret Wilkinson
Department of Psychology, University of Waterloo, Waterloo, Ontario N2L 3G1, Canada

Part 1
Appearance, Expression, and Perception

1
A Description of Craniofacial Anomalies: The Mechanism and Rationale of Surgery

IAN R. MUNRO

A craniofacial anomaly is a visible deformity affecting part of the face or skull. The deformity can be due to a variation in the skin or underlying soft tissues. Alternatively, the deformity can be due to irregularity in size or contour of the underlying skeleton. Craniofacial anomalies can also be divided between those that are due to congenital origin and those that are acquired. The acquired deformities can be further divided among those due to trauma and those due to tumors.

In the last 20 years there has been a significant increase in interest regarding management of craniofacial anomalies because of the enormous breakthroughs that have occurred in surgeons' technical ability to correct many of the more severe deformities that hitherto were considered untreatable. This is particularly true of many of the congenital abnormalities and those acquired abnormalities related to problems of the bony skeleton. Improvements have also occurred, although to a lesser degree, in the ability of plastic surgeons to manage soft tissue anomalies. However, the results of the treatment of the most devastating of all acquired deformities—that due to burns—remain frustrating, as the major stigmata of the skin injury can never be significantly removed.

Correction of craniofacial anomalies is not new. The earliest records of reconstructive facial surgery are from India, where women found to be committing adultery would be subjected to amputation of the nose. Susruta, in approximately 1500 B.C., developed a technique, subsequently known as the Indian rhinoplasty, that rotated skin from the forehead down onto the middle of the face, in order to reconstruct the semblance of a nose and thus remove the devastating social stigmatization.

For the next 3,000 years, there are few reports of reconstructive surgery for the face. Both the Egyptians and Incas carried out successful trephinations of the skull, presumably for reasons other than reconstructive. However, some skulls have been found in Peru that have segments

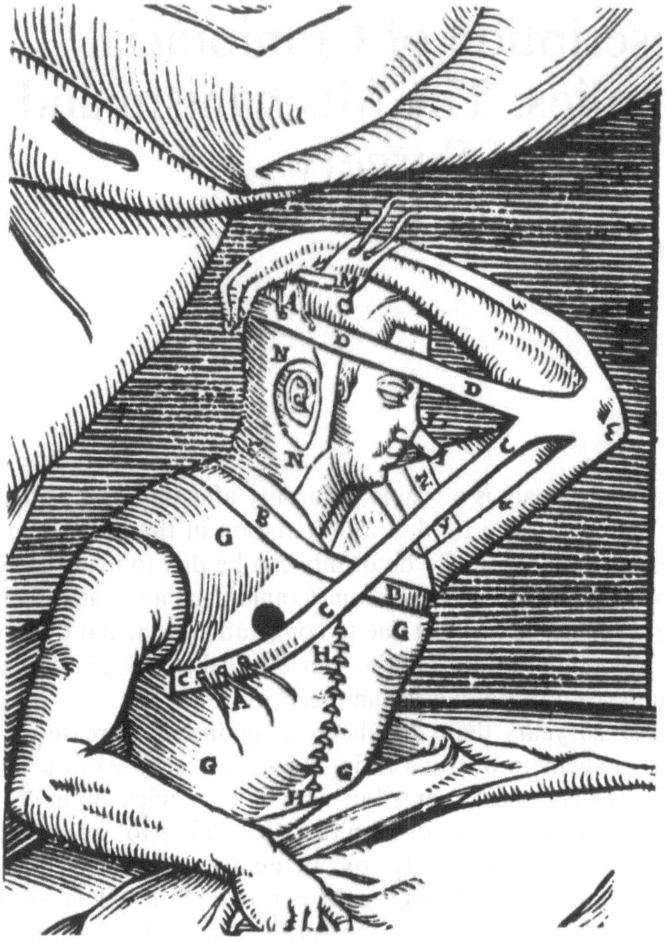

FIGURE 1.1. Illustration of the Tagliacotti technique of reconstructing a nose using a pedicle tube of skin from the arm. (Taken from Gasparis Tagliacotti-Edicion Facsimilar. Editor Fernando Ortiz Monasterio—Libreria de Manuel Porrua, S.A., Mexico, 1949.)

of bone replaced by gold sheets; it is assumed that these sheets were inserted to correct defects.

During the sixteenth century, in Italy, Tagliacotti (1597) developed a technique to reconstruct a nose that entailed lifting a pedicle of skin from the inner arm, attaching it to the face, and binding the arm over the head for 3 to 4 weeks to allow a new blood supply to be gained into the pedicle from the face (see Figure 1.1). The arm could then be separated from the face and shaped to form a nose.

It was not until the middle of the nineteenth century that the first recorded attempts were made to repair the defects of a cleft lip and a cleft palate.

World War I provided a tremendous stimulus for the development of techniques to correct deformities of the face due to trauma. The peculiarities of trench warfare resulted in an extremely high number of devastating injuries to the face. In England, Gillies was one of the pioneers in developing techniques to correct or at least ameliorate some of these deformities. Many of these deformities, however, were due to the combined loss of both soft tissue and bone, and the technical limitations at that time confined the reconstruction to that of soft tissue only. In the 1930s, Kazanjian and Converse as well as Longacre (1968, 1973), in thc United States, were particularly prominent in beginning to address the skeletal problems of craniofacial anomalies. Basically, they used the principles of adding on substances to the skeleton.

The first attempt to correct a major congenital deformity—that of Crouzons Syndrome—was made by Gillies in 1942, although he did not report this operation until 1950. He moved the entire middle part of the face forward but stated that he felt that the operation was so difficult and dangerous that it should not be attempted again. This managed to delay the onset of modern craniofacial surgery until the middle 1960s.

At that time, Paul Tessier, working in France, developed techniques for the correction of skeletal craniofacial deformities that were revolutionary in nature, extremely dangerous, and against all known surgical principles. Tessier demonstrated that it was possible to take very large segments of the bones of the skull and face, strip off their soft tissue attachments—and therefore their blood supply, cut and move these large bony segments, and place them into the correct anatomical position to produce a normal appearance. The most radical development by Tessier (Tessier et al., 1981), however, was the realization and demonstration that it was possible to move an eye, either vertically or horizontally, without jeopardizing the eyesight and thus allowing correction of some of the more grotesque craniofacial abnormalities.

People trained in Tessier's techniques have been able to raise the standard of reconstruction that is possible after the severe types of facial smashes seen in high-speed motor vehicle accidents. Hitherto, these severely disrupted craniofacial skeletons could not be completely repositioned, and the subjects of such an injury were always left with a major deformity. However, through the skill of a trained craniofacial surgeon, it is now possible for all the bones of the face and skull to be repositioned or rebuilt immediately, thus producing minimum late deformity.

Craniofacial techniques have also enabled the treatment of some tumors that previously were unapproachable. A particular problem is that of fibrous dysplasia, causing massive overgrowth of the craniofacial skeleton with distortion of the eye. It is now possible to remove large segments of bone and reconstruct them with normal bone from another part of the body, thus preventing spread of the disease and restoring the person to normal appearance. A more recent breakthrough has been in the management of some of the more unusual malignant tumors. Previously, these were either untreatable or, if resected, they left grotesque deformities. Nowadays, certain techniques allow the access to tumors that were once considered unresectable and permit immediate reconstruction of the bony skeleton, improving the quality of life for these people.

Many of these major craniofacial problems, whether congenital or acquired, are extremely rare, and considerable advances have been made in decreasing the morbidity attached to both the condition and the results of surgery by the development of centers with surgeons specializing in just these techniques (see, for example, Caronni, 1985; Marchac, 1987). Some of the advances are psychological as well as physiological. It was always believed that any operation entailing the skull necessitated having the patient's hair shaved and completely removed. This was found to be unnecessary and thus, after even the most major intracranial procedure, the patient can be looking normal within 2 weeks. A further and more recent development is the use of small metal plates and screws, which allow the rigid fixation of large segments of the facial skeleton, thus permitting, in particular, segments of the jaw to be repositioned without the necessity of having the patient's jaws wired together after surgery. These simple improvements have been of enormous psychological benefit.

Types of Congenital Craniofacial Problems

The correction of congenital craniofacial problems is more complex than that of acquired problems because the surgeon is either attempting to reposition the face or to reconstruct the face into a position in which it has never been beforehand (see, for example, Arndt, Travis, Lefebvre, & Munro, 1987; Munro & Lauritzen, 1985; Munro, 1989).

Patients with cleft lip and palate problems are the most common craniofacial deformities. The ideal timing for repair of the cleft lip is at 3 months of age. Physiologically, the child usually tolerates the operation well. The child can be out of the hospital within 6 to 24 hours of surgery, and nowadays many experienced surgeons allow breastfeeding to recommence the day of surgery. It is also technically easier to produce an accurate repair at 3 months of age rather than when the child is 1 or 2 days old.

Psychologically, there are two arguments regarding the timing of the surgery. If the child has the repair within 1 to 2 days of birth, the mother does not have to take a deformed child home. However, some surgeons believe that the parents then have an unrealistic expectation of the quality of result that can be achieved. But if the family members live with the deformed child for 3 months, they have a much better appreciation of the difficulties associated with repair.

Currently, the majority of surgeons around the world who treat many of these children prefer to operate around 3 months of age for physiological and technical reasons. A 0.25 mm error in alignment in a 1-day-old child will show as a noticeable 1 to 2 mm malalignment by age 1 year. The cleft palate is repaired best at around age 12 months. This is a compromise. Earlier repair may be an advantage for speech, but it is a disadvantage to subsequent facial growth. Late repair has an opposite effect. It is subsequently easier today to correct an underdeveloped midface in the 10% to 20% of patients in whom it may occur, rather than trying to correct bad speech in nearly all patients so treated by late palate closure.

Cleft lip and palate need no longer be the devastating deformity that it was 30 years ago. If treated by an experienced team (which needs to see at least 40 new patients a year), the child should be expected to have normal speech, a symmetrical lip with a fine scar, a nose close to normal in appearance, and a full set of well-fitting teeth. To achieve this requires good patient and parent cooperation. In most cases, further surgery will be required by age 5 years to improve the nose shape. The wearing of orthodontic braces is almost inevitable but should be limited to 1 session in early adolescence. With good psychosocial support and good parenting, such children should grow into normal well-adjusted adults. However, if the quality of the surgery is bad and repeated operations are carried out, the speech and hearing are ignored and the teeth are not treated, then a very different psychological outcome will be present. Unfortunately, this still occurs even in the most advanced countries, if children are treated by either inexperienced or inadequately trained people, or without the benefits of a team approach, or where the team does not have a big enough population load to maintain its expertise.

These problems of maltreatment are more likely to occur in the craniofacial deformities that are much rarer than those of cleft lip and palate and are even more complex to treat. Craniofacial conditions may be progressive and the timing for surgery varies for each type of deformity. In infancy, craniostenosis, or a fusion of the bones of the skull, is a relatively common problem. Plagiocephaly, or unilateral frontal bone asymmetry, is due to fusion of one coronal suture and the adjacent sutures in the base of the skull. Figure 1.2 demonstrates how the skeleton can be cut and repositioned to produce a normal shape, allowing ongoing normal development.

Another type of infant craniostenosis, called trigoncephaly, is due to fusion of the metopic suture between the frontal bones and produces a triangular-shaped head. This is corrected by removing the frontal bones, realigning them into the normal shape and repositioning them (Figures

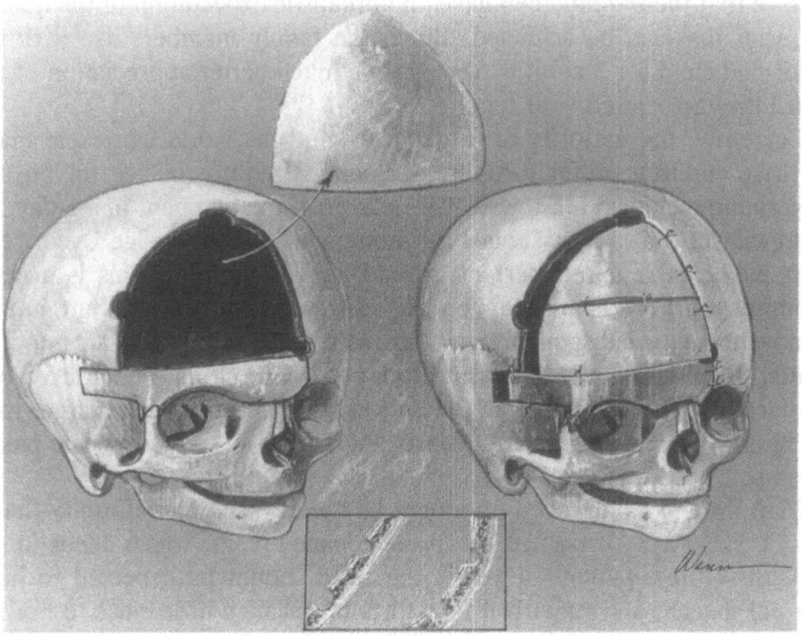

FIGURE 1.2. The correction of plagiocephaly. Left: The frontal bone and superior orbital rim are removed. Inset: The superior orbital rim is weakened on the inner cortex and bent to a convex shape to match the opposite uninvolved site. The frontal bone is cut, rotated, and replaced to match the opposite side of the skull.

1.3A,B). If this is done correctly it is an extrememly successful operation, rarely requiring further intervention. The operation for craniostenosis is ideally performed between ages 3 to 6 months. Before this time, the bones are very thin and difficult to work with. During the first year of life, the brain reaches 80% of its adult size, and this rapid growth can help to remodel the deformed skull once it has been released and repositioned. Small infants tolerate the surgery well if treated by experts. They are out of the hospital within 3 to 4 days of the operation and grow up without the knowledge of ever having been deformed. The only sequel is a scar on the top of the head. If these deformities are left untreated they will affect the adjacent bones of the skull and face.

The correction of orbital hypertelorism is certainly one of Tessier's biggest contributions to modern surgery (Tessier et al., 1981). Prior to Tessier's developments, this condition was untreatable. Surgery required for this condition is drastic but extremely effective. The bone cuts and repositioning are demonstrated in Figure 1.4.

The principle of the correction of orbital hypertelorism is that of considering the eye as being in a box. Once the box of bony skeleton has been cut and freed up, it can be moved in any direction, thus reposition-

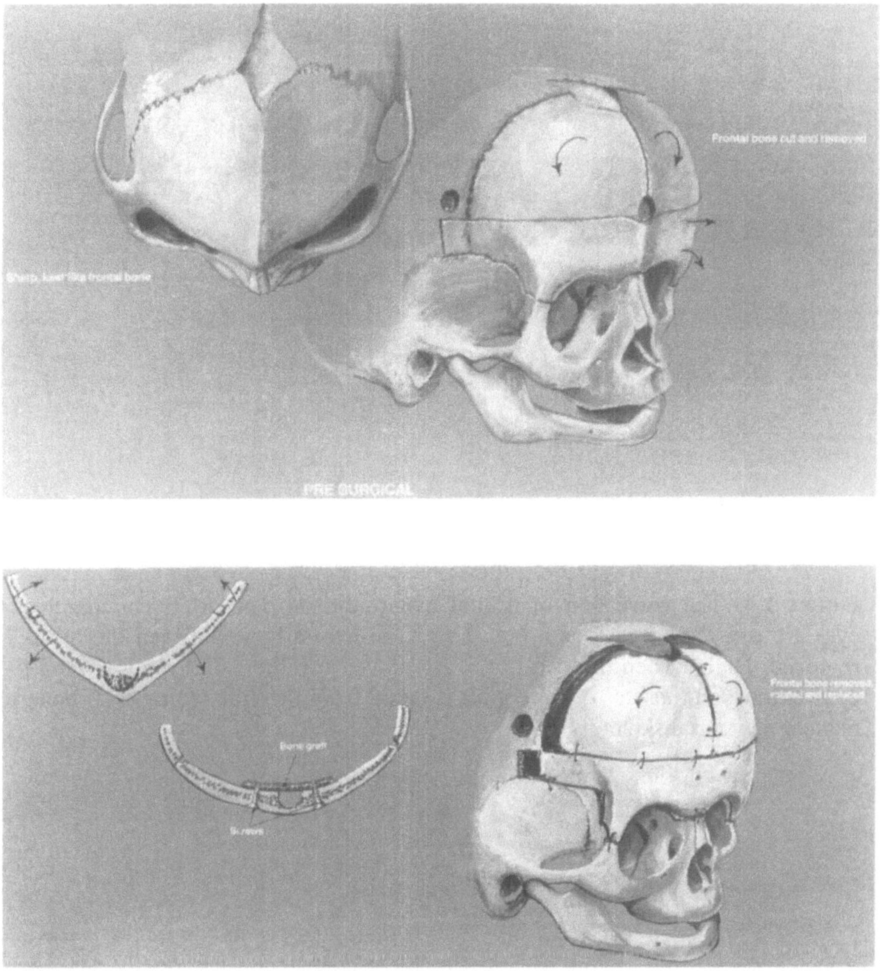

A

B

FIGURE 1.3. A: A skull with trigoncephaly due to fusion of the metopic suture between the frontal bones. The correction of trigoncephaly. B: The supraorbital bar is removed and reshaped into a normal rounded contour and then replaced as shown. The frontal bone is split, rotated, and replaced, leaving a gap posteriorly to allow for brain growth.

ing the eye as necessary. Figure 1.5 illustrates the technique for moving an orbit vertically. The eye and its immediately adjacent soft tissue attachments of the eyelids and canthi are the most critical features in the face. The untrained layperson's eye will pick up a deformity of as little as 1 mm in this region of the face. Thus, malposition of the eye can be considered one of the most stigmatizing of facial deformities. Ideally, patients with hypertelorism have the major first operation around the age of 2 to 3 years. At younger ages, the bones of the face are more fragile

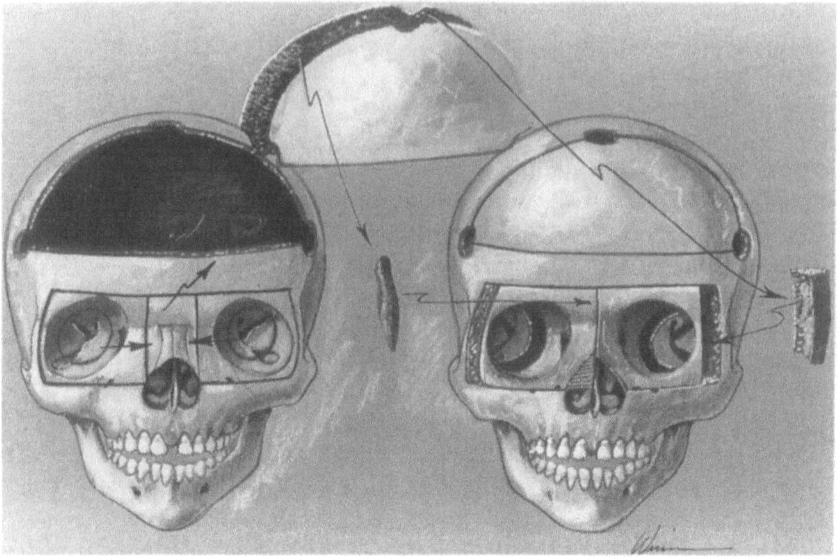

FIGURE 1.4. The correction of orbital hypertelorism. The orbits containing the eyes are considered each as a box. Left: The excess bone between the orbits is removed. Right: Then the two boxes are moved together, thus repositioning the eyes. Above and insets: A bone graft is taken from the craniotomy skull bone to make a new nasal skeleton.

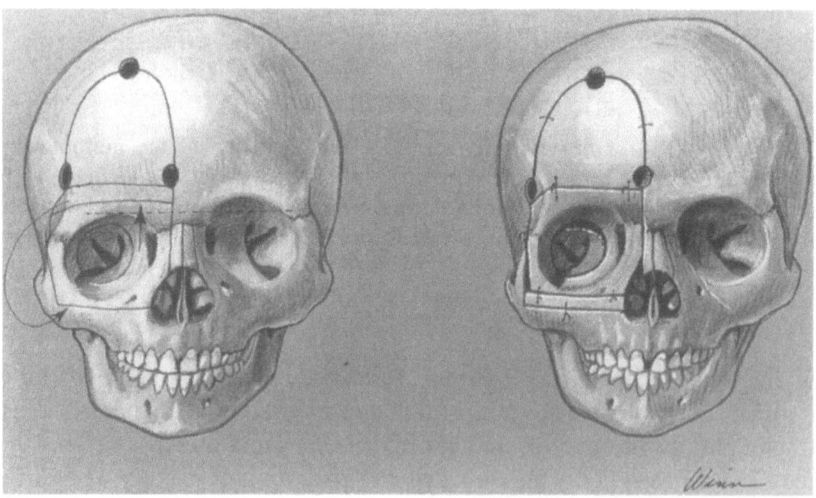

FIGURE 1.5. The correction of orbital hypertelorism. Left: When one eye is too low, the orbit is cut as a box to contain the eye. Right: The orbit and eye have been raised, and the bone removed from above the orbit has been placed below.

and difficult to work with. The children should be in the hospital for only 4 to 5 days, and their only recollection is of a visit to the hospital and a scar on the head, but never one of significant deformity nor of being stared at. Subsequently these children may need further but more minor surgery to compensate for changes as a result of growth.

Crouzons Syndrome consists of fusion of the skull bones (craniostenosis) that usually affects the anterior half of the skull and is combined with underdevelopment of the middle of the face. As the eye development is normal, the eyes literally grow out of the facial skeleton. The only part of the face that remains normal is that of the mandible. Ideally, children with this condition have a release of the craniostenosis between the ages of 3 to 6 months. If a child has not had correction of the craniostenosis in infancy, the bulging to the eyes becomes an urgent situation, with risk of blindness. Exorbitism exists when the eyes are completely outside the orbit. The correction of this deformity entails moving the adjacent bones forward around the eye, as seen in Figure 1.6.

Aperts Syndrome has certain features similar to those of Crouzons, with craniosynostosis and underdevelopment of the middle of the face. Children with Aperts Syndrome have more widely spaced eyes than those with Crouzons. The main difference, however, is that the fingers and toes are fused together (syndactyly). Aperts Syndrome children, therefore, need an operation in the first 3 to 6 months of age to release the

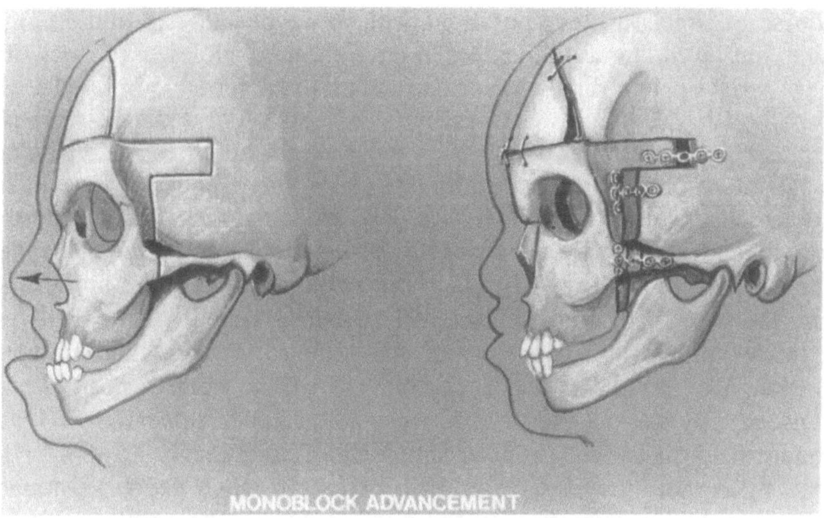

FIGURE 1.6. The correction of exorbitism. Left: The underdeveloped anterior skull and midface are cut as a single block. Right: The entire monoblock of the skeleton is advanced forward, enlarging the socket for the eyes and correcting the underbite.

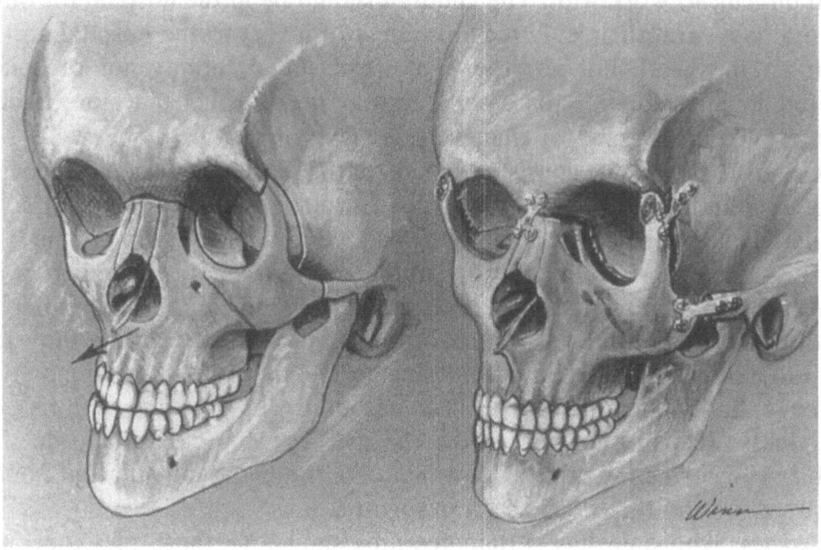

FIGURE 1.7. The correction of craniosynostosis associated with Apects or Crouzons Syndrome. Left: The midface is cut free from the base of the skull and beneath the eyes. Right: The skeleton is advanced and fixed with metal plates and screws.

craniosynostosis and allow a normal skull development. They then need two operations to release the fusion of all the fingers and toes. Over the course of time, further operations will be needed on the middle of the face, but by the time these children have reached adolescence, they often have a relatively normal-appearing face that is acceptable in public.

Although the fingers and toes have been separated, they are still limited both functionally and, even more significantly, cosmetically. It is most interesting that the biggest complaint these patients have in late adolescence is that their fingers are ugly. Nowadays, the craniosynostosis associated with Crouzons or Aperts Syndrome is usually corrected between the age of 3 to 6 months. In many cases, the skull will develop normally but the growth of the midface will remain affected, resulting in progressive flatness and concavity of the midface, with significant malocclusion. The forehead and mandible are in the correct position, and consequently these children are most abnormal in appearance. I have found that when these children enter school, and particularly when they start first grade, they are teased unmercifully by their peers. Although it is known that an operation on the midface will not be permanent due to subsequent growth differentials, it is still better to correct these problems before they enter first grade to allow a more integrated development. In those patients who have had a successful correction of their forehead in infancy, a lesser procedure can be utilized. Figure 1.7 shows the

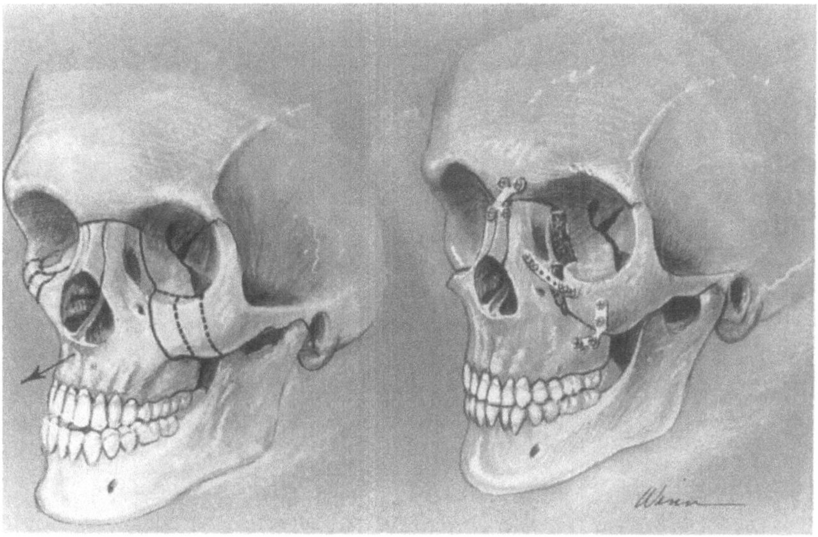

FIGURE 1.8. Correction of maxillonasal dysplasia (Binders Syndrome). Left: The nose is released from the skull at the frontonasal suture. An osteotomy is made across the orbital floor and then through the maxilla. The lateral positioning of this depends upon the area of midface flatness needing correction. Right: The face is advanced and fixed with metal plates and screws and bone grafts.

technique of just moving the midface forward with a Le Fort III maxillary osteotomy. This can now be done without shaving the patient's hair and without using postoperative intermaxillary fixation to wire the jaws together (previously, wiring was necessary for 6 to 8 weeks).

Maxillonasal dysplasia (Binders Syndrome) produces a facial anomaly that is not so grotesque as some of the previously described problems. However, it provides interesting insights into the psychological effects of facial deformities. This syndrome consists of a small nose with lack of support to the nasal tip and absence of the anterior nasal spine, and as the patients reach adolescence, they tend to develop a marked underbite or Class III malocclusion. Figure 1.8 shows the operation utilized to move the middle of the face and the nose forward. These patients, as in most craniofacial patients, show a tremendous improvement in self-confidence if the surgery has indeed been effective in improving the facial appearance.

When children with Binders Syndrome are small, they have a very underdeveloped nose, which is the main part of the syndrome, but without developing an underbite. Typically, these children do not present in a surgeon's office until they have reached first grade, at which time they start to be unmercifully teased at school. At that age, the nose can be augmented by adding bone. The bone graft does not grow with age, however, and by the time the child is nine or ten, the stigma of the

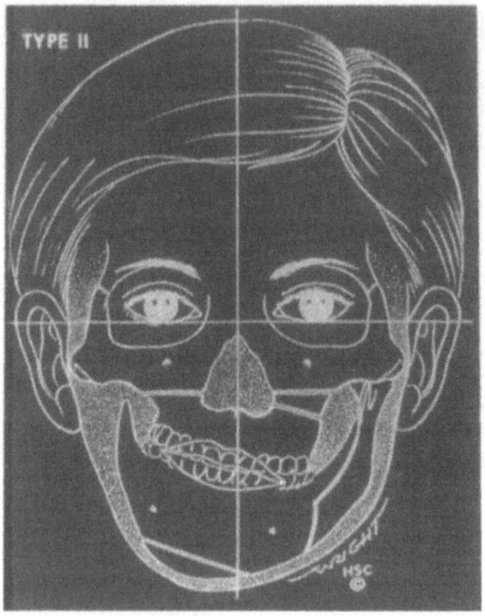

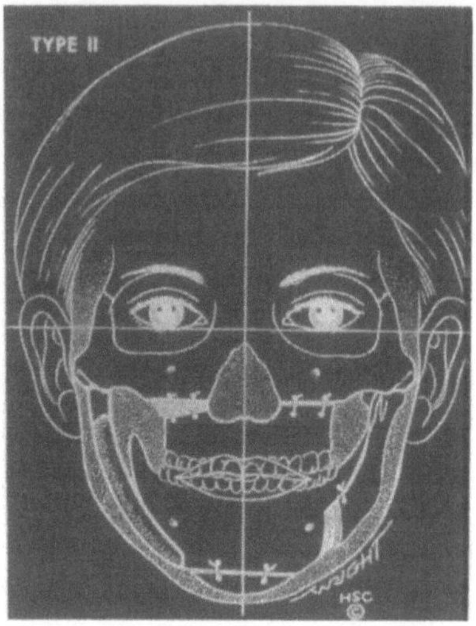

FIGURE 1.9. Correction of hemifacial microsomia. Left: Bone cuts shown in the maxilla and mandible to rotate the skeleton into the facial midline. Right: After the skeleton has been realigned and fixed with wires, costochondral graft from the opposite chest wall is used to construct the absent bone and mandibular condyle.

underdeveloped nose is again apparent. However, it has been our experience that at that time, although the children have been made aware that they can have further augmentation to the nose should they wish it, these children have said almost universally that they are quite prepared to wait until they are more fully grown before undergoing further surgery.

Hemifacial microsomia is the second most common craniofacial deformity after cleft lip and palate. It consists of underdevelopment of one side of the face and is frequently associated with absence of part of the mandible with its associated condyle. Figure 1.9 shows the operation used to level both the upper and lower jaw, to bring the chin into the midline, and to reconstruct the absent mandible and condyle with a segment of rib and cartilage taken from the opposite chest wall. Because of the psychological disadvantage of this deformity, we treated many patients during childhood, ranging from 7 to 11 years of age. When this surgery was developed, it was anticipated that the rib graft would not grow and that there would be a recurrence of the deformity as a child entered adolescence. Both the parents and the children were thus counseled that further surgery would probably be necessary after the adolescent growth spurt. However, rather unexpectedly, this has not occurred. In fact, the face tends to stay symmetrical during growth if the correct form has been achieved at the initial operation. As these patients now can be expected to grow normally, there is an even stronger indication to correct the facial deformity at a much earlier age. The children can be treated around age 5 or 6 years, thus preventing the teasing in first grade.

Orthognathic surgery is a branch of craniofacial surgery and is primarily associated with correcting malocclusion. However, the input of plastic surgery and craniofacial principles into orthognathic surgery has changed the emphasis of the surgery from just producing a normal bite to one of producing a normal face—with, incidentally, a normal bite. This has been particularly true and beneficial in patients who have had a cleft lip and palate. In at least 10% to 20% of these patients, there will be the development of a Class III underbite due to underdevelopment of the maxilla in adolescence. This is corrected by moving the lower part of the upper jaw forward, using what is known as the Le Fort I osteotomy (see Figure 1.10A,B). This has considerably raised the standard of final results that should be expected for a patient who has had a cleft lip and palate. The correction of patients with very large lower jaws has been achieved by a multiplicity of techniques since the 1930s. However, it was not until the early 1960s that a satisfactory technique was developed to easily correct the patient with a small lower jaw. Figure 1.11 shows the technique known as a sagittal mandibular osteotomy. This is an operation carried out from inside the mouth, leaving no external scars and can be used to enlarge, shorten or rotate the mandible. The operations of the Le Fort I and sagittal mandibular osteotomy can be combined to produce better facial corrections in many more people than would otherwise have been achieved by moving one jaw only. This is particularly true in people with an anterior open bite, whose teeth meet at the back but are unable to bite upon food in the front. Figure 1.12 shows the combined operation of moving the upper and lower jaw.

Initially, as mentioned earlier, when all these orthognathic procedures were developed, it was necessary for the patient to have the jaws wired together for a period of 6 to 8 weeks after surgery. However, the development of very small plates and screws has enabled us to eliminate intermaxillary fixation, which has improved the safety of the operation, decreased the swelling seen in the face postoperatively, and, of course, returned the patient to a normal, active life more quickly.

The techniques described above have shown that any part of the facial skeleton malpositioned or absent due to congenital origin can be reconstructed or repositioned to produce a normal face. These techniques have now been expanded to correct other problems more effectively. Temporomandibular ankylosis is fusion of the jaw joint, resulting in patients being unable to open the jaw. In the past, techniques were utilized to release the fusion and allow patients to open the jaw satisfactorily. Many of the early techniques had a significant failure rate with refusion of the joint. Therefore, the emphasis on development of new techniques has always been toward an effective and permanent release of

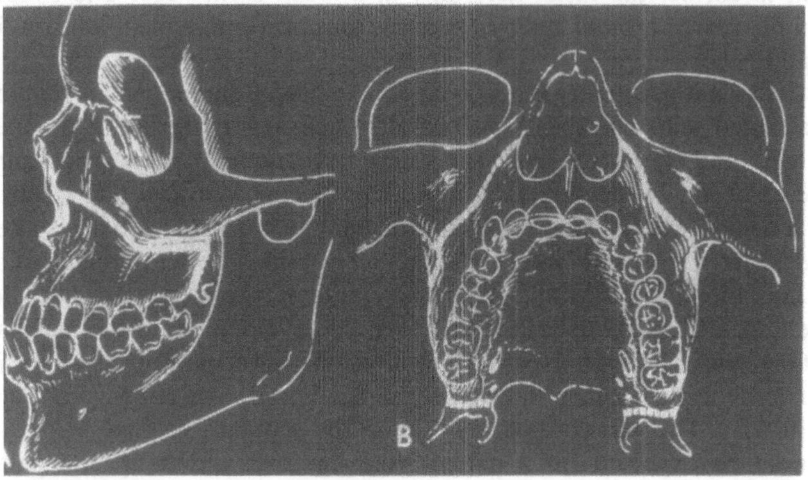

A

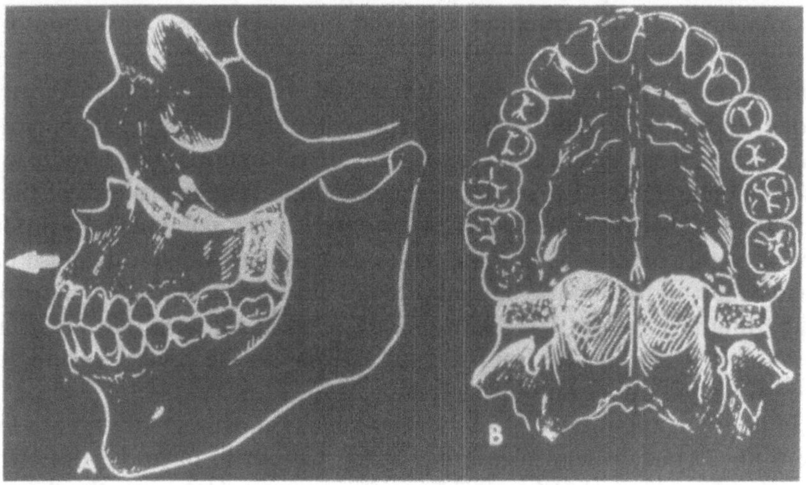

B

FIGURE 1.10. A: Bone cuts across the maxilla for a Le Fort I maxillary advancement. B: The maxilla is advanced to the correct occlusion and bone grafts are inserted.

the fusion. To ensure the successful release, early postoperative jaw exercises and movement were essential and no measures were taken to correct the associated facial deformity. If the temporomandibular ankylosis occurs in a child and is left untreated, there is an associated progressive deformity of the face. The degree of deformity depends upon the age of onset and is more severe if it occurs in a younger patient. As well as the inability to open the mouth, there is a deformity very similar in appearance to that seen with hemifacial microsomia. Thus, the tech-

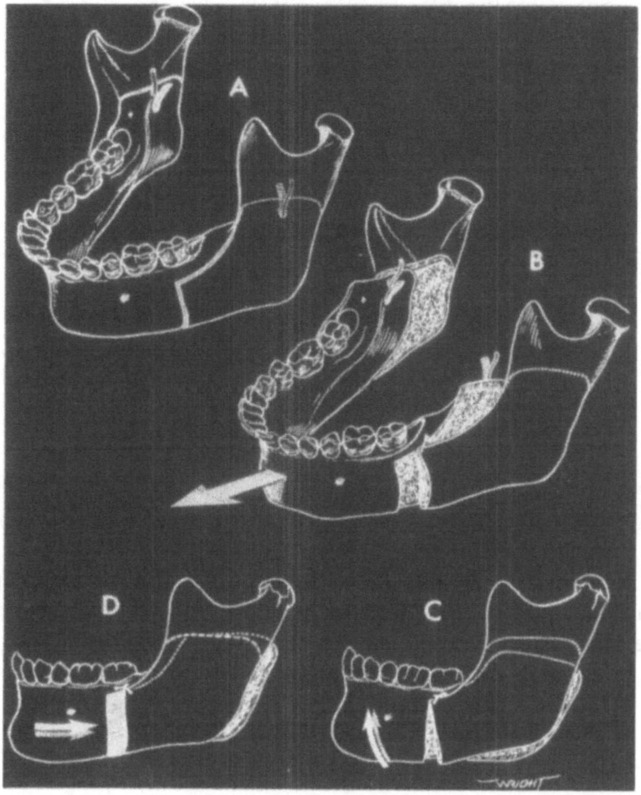

FIGURE 1.11. A: Osteotomy lines for a sagittal split of the mandible. B: The mandible can be lengthened without the need to add bone. C: The mandible can be rotated. D: The mandible can be set backwards.

niques used to correct hemifacial microsomia are now being successfully applied to a one-stage correction of the temporomandibular ankylosis, with the release of the jaw allowing for full and permanent mouth opening as well as correcting the facial asymmetry and deformity (see Figure 1.13).

Summary

The development of craniofacial principles in the last 20 years has led to a dramatic rethinking of patients with facial deformities, whether from soft tissue or skeletal abnormalities. It has been demonstrated that there is no bone in the head and face that cannot be either repositioned or removed and reconstructed. The technology was initially developed for congenital problems. However, it has been expanded for the use of acute trauma

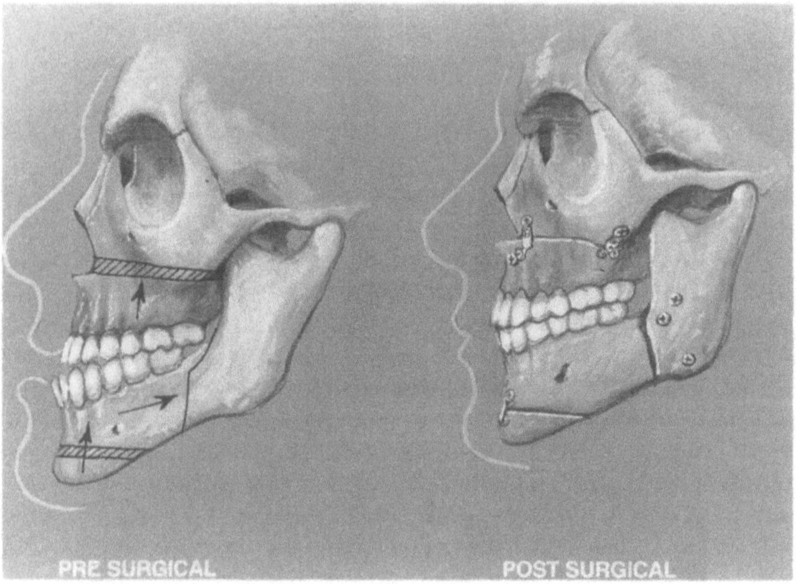

FIGURE 1.12. Correcting an anterior open bite. Left: The combined operation to raise the maxilla, recess, and rotate the mandible and vertically reduce the chin. Right: The bite has been closed and the osteotomized segments fixed with metal plates and screws to avoid wiring the jaws together.

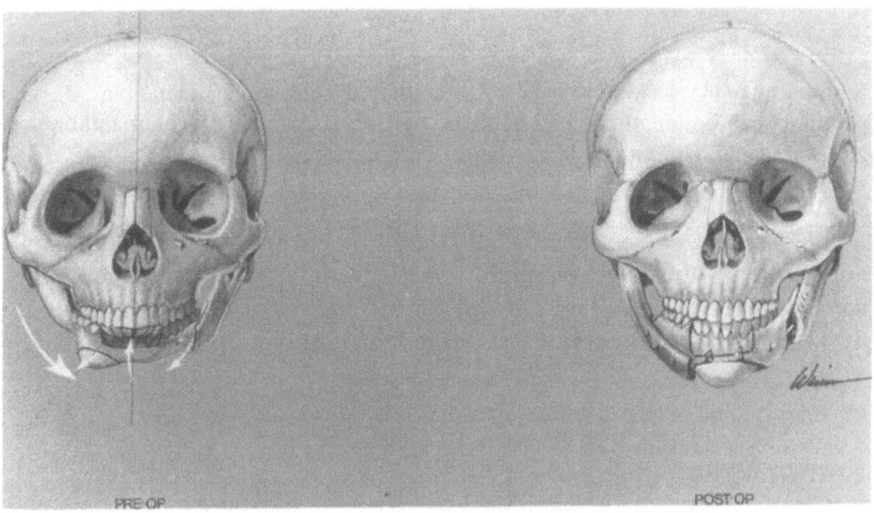

FIGURE 1.13. Correction of the temporomandibular ankylosis. Left: The right temporomandibular joint is fused together with bone: The lower jaw is underdeveloped, the chin is deviated to the side of the deformity, and the lower teeth are angulated forward almost horizontally. Right: The bone fusion is removed, the mandible advanced with a sagittal split, the teeth realigned, the chin placed in the facial midline, and a new temporomandibular joint built with a costochondral graft.

and more effective treatment of the late results of trauma when the correct initial techniques have not been utilized. Craniofacial surgery has now also been applied to expand the capabilities of surgeons to remove tumors, particularly in the base of the skull, that hitherto were inaccessible. Similarly, patients who have had to have large segments of the skeleton resected because of malignant tumors can have an immediate reconstruction, thus preventing the devastation of a facial deformity. The correction of these deformities crosses many disciplines, and in order to do it safely, it is necessary to develop a comprehensive craniofacial team. This includes the use of speech pathologists, dentists and orthodontists, anthropologists to measure the face, neurosurgeons, ophthalmologists to measure the eyes, otolaryngologists, and special anesthesia techniques, as well as dedicated intensive care units.

The most fascinating part of this type of surgery, however, is the psychosocial effect upon the patients and their families. It is necessary that these patients be comprehensively tested prior to surgery by a social worker, psychologist, and psychiatrist. It is important that the patients have a realistic expectation from the surgery and a proper understanding of its limitations prior to surgery. The psychosocial team plays a critical role from two points of view. First, there are still patients with grotesque craniofacial anomalies who, unfortunately, have been labeled mentally retarded but who, in fact, may have a normal intelligence. And second, conversely, some parents with a retarded and deformed child may have an unrealistic hope that correction of the face will produce better intellectual functioning.

The true incidence of craniofacial problems is difficult to determine. Cleft lip and palate occurs in 1 out of 750 live births. Hemifacial microsomia, the second most common deformity, occurs in 1 out of 1,500 live births. Because these deformities are so rare, the average doctor may see only one such case in his or her career. Even in North America these patients are often undiagnosed or misdiagnosed for several years. More frequently, though, the doctor is either not aware that treatment is possible or the degree of sophisticated treatment possible in a few regional centers. The patient may be referred to a local specialist, who may feel that correction is not possible and so counsels the parents or attempts treatment without experience, knowledge, or a proper team. Every time there is media publicity about craniofacial surgery, a flood of patients arrive at the regional centers who have either been untreated or, more frequently, mistreated.

In countries with more static populations than North America and where there is more inbreeding, the incidence and severity of craniofacial deformities seem to be greater.

For the severe congenital craniofacial deformities, a regional team for every 20 million people is sufficient. However, in societies where even minor deformities have to be treated and where the spin-off technology is applied to trauma and tumors, 1 team for every 6 to 10 million people will receive enough patients to maintain competence. The team should treat at least 2 new patients a week.

Successful treatment is also causing problems. Some patients are genetically autosomal dominant, such as with Apert, Crouzon, or Treacher Collins Syndrome. Untreated, these people tended not to marry and reproduce. This is no longer true. Now that these patients can look normal—and especially that it can be achieved at an early age—they are marrying, and even with genetic counseling are reproducing the same deformity. This does not seem to vary with social class.

Among patients with severe craniofacial abnormalities, a variety of situations can arise. The presence of a facial deformity, whether mild or severe, is a devastating event both for the parents and the child. The severity of the effect on the family is often out of proportion to the degree of the deformity. The active intervention of a good psychosocial group can help the family to adjust, but the knowledge of the possibility of active surgical intervention, even though it is recognized that the results may be less than ideal, is the most encouraging support that the parents and child can be given. Although lip service is given to the statement that beauty is only skin deep, in our society it is not possible socially to integrate successfully a person with a craniofacial abnormality, particularly some of the more severe ones. It seems that prevention of awareness of the deformity is more important than correction of the deformity at a later age when it may be technically easier and safer. If the person remains untreated until late adolescence or even later, even though there is tremendous anatomical change and associated psychological uplift, the psychological scarring that has occurred in earlier years seems to be permanent. It is devastating for children to be told that they have to live with a significant deformity until they reach adolescence before anything can be done to correct it. We have found that it is indeed better to correct these children as early as possible, even with the full realization that further surgery may be necessary as growth occurs, rather than condemning them during the critical years of social development to a craniofacial deformity. The most overriding problem all these children have in common is that the deformity of the face can never be covered up, and the initial reaction of any newcomer to the deformed face is a constant reminder to a child of his or her problem.

There is great difficulty in trying psychologically to assess the effect of deformity upon a particular patient or family (see Arndt, Travis, Lefebvre, et al., 1985; Lefebvre & Munro, 1978; Munro, 1981). There is tremendous variation among reactions in different families to the same problem, as well as within the family over different time periods. Studies made on one-time interviews or assessments are unreliable, particularly when not related to the presence or absence of association with an experienced and empathetic team. There is both euphoria and fear in knowing that treatment is possible. Inevitably, there is euphoria after the first surgery by an experienced team. However, disillusionment may start when it is realized that the patient is still stared at (albeit less so) and that complete normality may never be achieved. In assessing long-term results, the patients are certainly better off than if not treated, even though the initial euphoria is not maintained. But probably as much or more benefit comes from empathy, understanding, encouragement, and support from the surgeon and team as it does from the actual surgery.

References

Arndt, E.M., Travis, F., Lefebvre, A., & Munro, I.R. (1987). Psychosocial adjustment of 20 patients with Treacher Collins Syndrome before and after reconstructive surgery. *British Journal of Plastic Surgery, 40,* 605–609.

Arndt, E.M., Travis, F., Lefebvre, A., Niec, A., & Munro, I.R. (1985). Beauty and the eye of the beholder: Social consequences and personal adjustment for facial patients. *British Journal of Plastic Surgery, 39(1),* 81–84.

Caronni, E.P. (1985). *Craniofacial surgery.* Boston: Little, Brown and Co.

Lefebvre, A., & Munro, I.R. (1978). The role of psychiatry in a craniofacial team, *Plastic and Reconstructive Surgery, 61,* 564–569.

Longacre, J.J. (1968). *Craniofacial anomalies pathogenesis and repair.* Philadelphia: J.B. Lippincott.

Longacre, J.J. (1973). *Rehabilitation of the facially disfigured.* Springfield, IL: Charles C. Thomas.

Marchac, D. (1987). Craniofacial surgery. *Proceedings of the First International Congress of the International Society of Craniomaxillofacial Surgery.* Heidelberg: Springer-Verlag.

Munro, I.R. (1981). The psychological effect of surgical treatment of facial deformity. In G.W. Luker, K.A. Ribbens, & J.A. McNamara, Jr. (Eds.), *Psychological aspects of facial form* (pp. 171–199). Ann Arbor: Center for Human Growth and Development, University of Michigan.

Munro I.P. (1989). Rigid fixation and bone grafts for craniofacial surgery. *Clinics in Plastic Surgery, 16,* 1. P.N. Manson (Ed.). Philadelphia: Saunders.

Munro I.R., & Lauritzen, C.G. (1985). Classification and treatment of hemifacial microsomia. In E.P. Caronni (Ed.), *Craniofacial surgery* (pp. 391–400). Boston: Little, Brown.

Tagliacotti, G. (1597). *De curtorum chirurgia per insitionem.* Venice.

Tessier, P., Hervouet, F., Rougier, J., et al. (1981). *Plastic surgery of the orbits and eyelids* (S.A. Wolfe, Trans.). New York: Masson Publishing.

2
The Origins and Functions of Appearance-Based Stereotypes: Theoretical and Applied Implications

JUDITH H. LANGLOIS

The research literature in developmental and social psychology is replete with evidence documenting the importance of facial attractiveness in social behavior and social relations. Both adults and children prefer attractive over unattractive individuals. They attribute positive qualities and abilities to attractive individuals, negative qualities and abilities to unattractive individuals; and they behave differently toward attractive from how they behave toward unattractive persons (for reviews, see Adams, 1977; Berscheid & Walster, 1974; Langlois, 1986; Langlois & Stephan, 1981). Both adults and children use similar standards in evaluating the attractiveness of others (Langlois, 1986; Langlois & Stephan, 1977; Maruyama & Miller, 1981; Sorell & Nowak, 1981); different racial groups show substantial agreement in their attractiveness judgments (e.g., Cunningham, 1986; Kleck, Richardson, & Ronald, 1974; Stephan & Langlois, 1984); and even infants show preferences for attractive faces (Langlois et al., 1987). The preference for attractive persons, therefore, extends beyond single racial and age groups and is evident very early in life.

In this chapter, we will discuss the origins and functional significance of these pervasive preferences for facially attractive individuals. We will examine why attractiveness is so highly preferred by perceivers and what it is that infants, children, and adults perceive when looking at faces that vary in attractiveness. In particular, the degree to which faces convey information signaling age, gender, and affect, and the degree to which age, gender, and affective information are related to perceived attractiveness will be considered. Finally, the implications of the potential causes, origins, and functions of facially based stereotypes for both the surgical and psychosocial treatment of children and adults with craniofacial abnormalities and other disorders, such as Down Syndrome, will be discussed.

The Origins of Appearance-Based Stereotypes

A question of considerable importance to both the research literature and to the lives of children and adults with craniofacial abnormalities concerns the origins of preferences for attractive individuals. From where do such preferences come, and by what processes are they acquired? These questions are important to individuals with craniofacial problems because modifying the biases held by perceivers could improve the social relations of those who are negatively affected by them. Before such bias can be modified, however, its source must be understood. Similarly, questions concerning the origins of preferences for attractive faces are important to basic research in this area because answers to them could lead to new and unanticipated research directions and to new theories about the role and significance of physical attractiveness in social relationships and behavior.

Despite the significance of such questions, few studies have seriously examined the origins of appearance-based stereotypes. The lack of empirical work on the origins of attractiveness-based preferences seems to be due to two prevailing assumptions firmly held by both basic researchers and the lay public. The first such assumption is that standards of attractiveness vary from one historical period to another, from one cohort of individuals to another, and from one culture to another (e.g., Darwin, 1859). Thus, since the beginning of systematic research investigating the social psychological implications of facial appearance (e.g., Berscheid, Dion, Walster, & Walster, 1971; Dion, 1972; Dion, Berscheid, & Walster, 1972; Walster, Aronson, Abrahams, & Rottmann, 1966), standards of attractiveness and preferences shown for attractive over unattractive persons have been thought to originate from the cultural transmission of contemporary standards, definitions, and stereotypes: Beauty was assumed to reside in the eye of the beholder and only in the eye of the beholder.

The second such firmly held assumption is derived from the first: Standards, preferences, and stereotypes associated with attractiveness are learned gradually by children during years of exposure to them through the media and socialization agents. Preferences for and stereotypes about attractive and unattractive persons are assumed by most researchers to require extensive cultural input in the early years of life and are not thought to become evident until 3, 4, or 5 years of age (Adams & Crane, 1980; Berscheid & Walster, 1974; Dion, 1972, 1973; Dion & Berscheid, 1974; Langlois & Stephan, 1981), or even later (Cavior & Lombardi,

1973; Cross & Cross, 1971). In the next section of this chapter, we will present work in two diverse areas of inquiry that seriously challenge these commonly heard and firmly held assumptions.

Similarity of Attractiveness Judgments

If standards of attractiveness can be shown to vary arbitrarily, attractiveness (and, indeed, research on its effects) can be dismissed as a trivial, inconsequential aspect of Madison Avenue advertising. There is, however, evidence accumulating to suggest that our long-held assumptions may very well be incorrect and that there may be some universal standards of attractiveness that transcend time, age, and culture.

Within-Culture Agreement

If attractiveness were arbitrarily defined and merely in the eye of the beholder, judgments of it would show little consistency among raters and would yield low reliability coefficients. The data, however, are generally quite consistent in showing impressively high reliabilities.[1] Although a specific attractiveness judgment of a particular individual may not correlate highly with that of another particular individual, the reliability of group judgments of the attractiveness of most targets is consistently high. As an example, Iliffe (1960) reported a study in which attractiveness judgments were collected from more than 4,000 raters. The raters were both male and female and ranged in age from 15 to 55 and older. The reliability coefficients were in the very high .90s for raters of the same age and sex and in the high .80s and low .90s for dissimilar raters (e.g., 15-year-old girls and 55+-year-old men). In our laboratory, we typically find reliability coefficients in the high .90s when we ask Introductory Psychology students to rate young infants. Similarly, 3-year-olds, when given a simple-enough rating task, agree significantly with adults about the attractiveness of peers (e.g., Styczynski & Langlois, 1977).

Cross-Ethnic and Cross-Cultural Agreement

We (Langlois & Stephan, 1977; Stephan & Langlois, 1984) and others (e.g., Kleck et al., 1974) have examined the similarity of attractiveness judgments of Blacks, Hispanics, and Caucasians rating Black, Hispanic, and Caucasian infants and children. In general, high levels of agreement

---

[1] The absolute value of the particular coefficient of agreement in specific studies will vary depending on the type of statistic chosen to estimate reliability. Intraclass and alpha coefficients are typically in the high .80s and .90s. Other estimates may be lower but are typically significant and appropriately high for the particular statistic.

are found among these three ethnic groups, regardless of whether they are rating targets from their own group or from the other groups. Caucasian raters agree quite well with Blacks about which Black infants are attractive and which are not, and vice versa. Because, however, all raters live in the same culture, it is possible that they may have assimilated a Caucasian standard of beauty and applied it to all infants.

Cross-cultural studies, however, do not suffer from this objection. A few cross-cultural investigations addressing this issue have begun to appear in the literature. Attractiveness judgments have been collected from Asian raters judging Caucasians and vice versa; from Chinese, Indian, and English females judging Greek males; and from South African and American males and females judging each other (Bernstein, Lin, & McClellan, 1982; Cunningham, 1986; Johnson, Dannenbring, Anderson, & Villa, 1983; Maret, 1983; Maret & Harling, 1985; Richardson, Goodman, Hastorf, & Dornbusch, 1961; Thakerar & Iwawaki, 1979; Weisfeld, Weisfeld, & Callaghan, 1984). Although agreement is not as high as that obtained from within culture judgments, it is still impressively high (e.g., .66–.93).

In a particularly interesting cross-cultural study, Cunningham (1986) assembled an international sample of photographs of 50 female faces. Precise measurements were taken of 24 facial features, and the photos were rated for attractiveness. Cunningham found that although Black and Asian faces possessed ethnically distinct features, they also displayed most of the facial features associated with attractiveness in Caucasians. McArthur and Berry (1987) have similarly found near perfect agreement between ratings of the facial characteristics of adults by both U.S. and Korean students. Thus, ethnically diverse faces possess both distinct *and* similar, perhaps even universal, structural features. These features seem to be perceived as attractive, regardless of the racial and cultural background of the perceiver.

Infant Preferences for Attractive Faces

Recall that a second assumption about attractiveness is that an extensive learning process is required for children to be inculcated with society's standards and preferences for attractiveness. Contrary to this assumption, however, research is now available showing that even young infants seem to prefer more attractive faces as compared to less attractive faces. Across several sets of experiments, we and others have shown that infants as young as 3 months of age can discriminate between attractive and unattractive faces and that, in general, they seem to prefer attractive as compared to unattractive faces.

In the first set of studies we conducted, 3- and 6-month-old infants were shown slides of faces of adult women (Langlois et al., 1987). The faces had been reliably rated for attractiveness by undergraduates; 8 faces of relatively attractive women were matched on the basis of hair length, color, and facial expression with 8 faces of relatively unattractive women. The 16 faces were shown to infants in pairs. In one condition, attractive faces were paired with unattractive faces within trials; in a second condition, faces of the same level of attractiveness were paired, producing a situation in which infant preferences for attractive vs. unattractive faces could be examined across trials. Observers recorded infant looking time and gaze direction from a television monitor connected to a video camera focused on the infant's eyes and face. The observer and monitor were positioned so that the observer could not see either the screen nor the slides being projected, to ensure that scoring was not biased by knowledge of the attractiveness of the faces projected to the infants. Finally, to determine whether the mother's appearance influenced the infant's preferences, her attractiveness was rated by the research staff and her hair color and length noted.

The study found that both the older and the younger infants looked longer at the attractive female faces than at the unattractive ones when the faces were presented in contrasting pairs. Thus, when attractive and unattractive faces were presented simultaneously, by 3 months of age infants were capable of discriminating between the faces of female adults on the basis of adult-rated attractiveness, and they showed a preference for the attractive faces. When infants had to compare faces across trials, however, the older, but not the younger, infants looked significantly longer at attractive faces. The failure of the younger infants to look longer at attractive faces in the across-trial comparison condition is not surprising, given the greater difficulty of this condition for young babies. Neither the sex of the infants nor the attractiveness of the mother were found to influence the preferences of the infants. The preferences of the infants were not strong in terms of the length of time spent looking at the attractive and unattractive faces, but they were quite reliable and were typical of the strength of preferences often found in the infant visual preference literature (e.g., Caron, Caron, Caldwell, & Weiss, 1973; Haaf, 1974; Sherrod, 1979). Indeed, refusing to look at unattractive faces would not be an adaptive strategy for young infants because they are not able to choose the attractiveness of their caregivers.

These results, showing that infants can discriminate between and that they prefer attractive as compared to unattractive female faces, have been also obtained in 3- and 6-month-old infants by Samuels and Ewy (1985) and in 5-month-old infants by Shapiro, Eppler, Haith, and Reis (1987). A second study (Langlois, Ritter, Roggman, & Vaughn, 1991) found that 6-month-old infants also prefer the faces of adult caucasian males, adult black females, and other infants rated by adults as being more rather than less attractive.

That infants can discriminate attractive from unattractive faces is an important and startling discovery. However, to infer from longer looking times that infants have a preference for attractive faces is an assumption. Although such an assumption is commonly made in the infant perception literature (e.g., Banks & Salapatek, 1983; Fantz, 1965; Fantz & Fagan, 1975), at best these studies have demonstrated a visual but not necessarily an affective preference for some kinds of attractive faces. The visual preference studies with infants do not demonstrate that infants prefer attractive faces in a way that is consistent with the demonstrated behavioral preferences available in the literature with older children and adults (e.g., Berscheid et al., 1971; Dion, 1973; Kleck et al., 1974; Langlois & Stephan, 1977).

To support or refute the preference interpretation of the differential looking data, we performed two studies (Langlois, Roggman, & Rieser-Danner, 1990). The first study examined the social behaviors of 12-month-old infants with an attractive or an unattractive stranger. Twelve-month-olds rather than younger infants were selected because they are mobile and can engage in social behaviors such as approach and withdrawal. Because infant responses could be influenced by behavioral differences between attractive and unattractive adults, we had a single adult female (the "stranger") interact with 60 infants according to a strict, rehearsed script. Attractiveness was manipulated by having latex theater masks constructed by a professional mask maker to be either attractive or unattractive. Features differentiating the two masks were based on previous research on the relationship between facial measurements and judgments of attractiveness (e.g., Cunningham, 1986). The masks were extremely thin and lifelike; they moved with the stranger's face, allowing normal facial expressions. The stranger was kept "blind" at all times to the appearance of the mask she was wearing; all mirrors and other shiny surfaces in the laboratory were occluded to prevent the inadvertent discovery of the attractiveness condition.

The infants played in a laboratory room with their mothers. The observation sessions were videotaped and included a series of episodes in which the mother and infant played alone, the stranger entered and conversed with the mother, talked to the infant, approached and played with the infant, and then picked up the infant. The results of the study revealed that infants' preferences for attractiveness do in fact extend beyond mere visual preferences. Infants showed significantly more resistance to and withdrawal from the stranger in the unattractive condition; and more positive affect and play involvement with the stranger in the attractive condition. As in the visual preference work, infants looked longer at the stranger in the attractive condition, although the difference fell short of attaining conventional levels of significance.

In the second study (Langlois et al., 1990) 12-month-old infants played with attractive and unattractive dolls. Twelve-month-olds were selected because this is about the earliest age at which infants will play for any extended length of time. The faces of attractive and unattractive (as determined by undergraduate ratings) 9-month-old infants were traced from photographs onto a piece of cloth. Two dolls were then constructed, identical except for the stylized faces. Observers recorded the duration of play with each doll. Consistent with the visual preference studies and the mask study, the infants, especially girls, played longer with the attractive than with the unattractive doll.

These two studies show that the visual preferences of infants demonstrated in our previous research also were expressed in their social behaviors toward others and toward objects. These results are important because they show that there are important social consequences of attractiveness when infants interact with strangers. Indeed, these 12-month-old infants exhibited many of the same preferential behaviors for attractive individuals seen in older children and adults (e.g., Langlois & Stephan, 1977; Langlois & Downs, 1979).

Taken together, the results of all these studies with young infants suggest that preferences for attractiveness are either learned much earlier than previously assumed or are innate. These very early differential responses to facial attractiveness and the cross-cultural similarity of attractiveness judgments seriously call into question assumptions that attractiveness is merely "in the eye of the beholder" and that standards of attractiveness must be learned through gradual exposure to current cultural norms. These results also show, as any craniofacial patient already knows, the power of the face in influencing the social reactions of adults, children, and even of young infants to faces varying in levels of attractiveness. Thus, in stark contrast to our long and tenaciously held assumptions, beauty does not seem to be merely in the eye of the beholder but, rather, influences reactions to individuals based on their facial appearance in consistent and pervasive ways.

We turn now to a discussion of what attractiveness is, what functions it serves, and why preferences for it are so pervasive and early appearing.

The Functional Significance of Facial Attractiveness

Beauty. . . . Derived from the Latin word, bonus, or good. The quality or aggregate of qualities in a person or thing that gives pleasure to the senses or pleasurably exalts the mind or spirit; a brilliant . . . example or instance. (*Webster's New Collegiate Dictionary*, 1977, p. 98.)

Beauty. . . . The quality attributed to whatever pleases or satisfies the senses or mind, as by line, color, form, texture, proportion, rhythmic, motion, tone, etc., or by behavior, attitude, etc. (*Webster's New World Dictionary*, 1986, p. 124.)

What *is* attractiveness, and why is it so consistently preferred by adults, children, and infants alike? Neither edition of *Webster's Dictionary* is helpful in answering this question; both editions (as well as other dictionaries) merely provide definitions of beauty that are circular and unilluminating. This is so despite the fact that attempts to define and measure beauty and facial attractiveness have a long history. The Greeks, for example, tried (unsuccessfully) to define beauty in terms of proportion and symmetry (the width of the perfect face was two-thirds its height, according to the Greek definition, Liggett, 1974).

The attempt to define attractiveness in terms of measurements of facial features and proportions continues today (e.g., Cunningham, 1986; Hildebrandt & Fitzgerald, 1979; Lucker, 1981). A measurement approach to attractiveness can, however—at least under one set of circumstances—be demonstrated to fail categorically at predicting judgments of attractiveness. The so-called Thatcher Illusion (Thompson, 1980) demonstrates this phenomenon well. When viewed upside-down, as shown in Figure 2.1, the two photographs of former British prime minister Margaret Thatcher look relatively normal. If, however, the page is inverted so that the two photographs are viewed right-side-up, the face that now appears on the left is grossly distorted. The illusion is accomplished by inverting Thatcher's eyes and mouth in the left-hand photograph. However, because the eyes and mouth are still those of Thatcher, their measurements remain the same despite dramatic changes in the perception of the face. The Thatcher effect is consistent with the findings of Farkas, Munro, and Kolar (1987), who noted that aesthetic differences were visually evident in a sample of female faces even though most of the anthropometric measurements of the faces did not differ significantly. Even if measurements of facial features and proportions predict judgments of attractiveness, they still beg the question of *why* these features and proportions

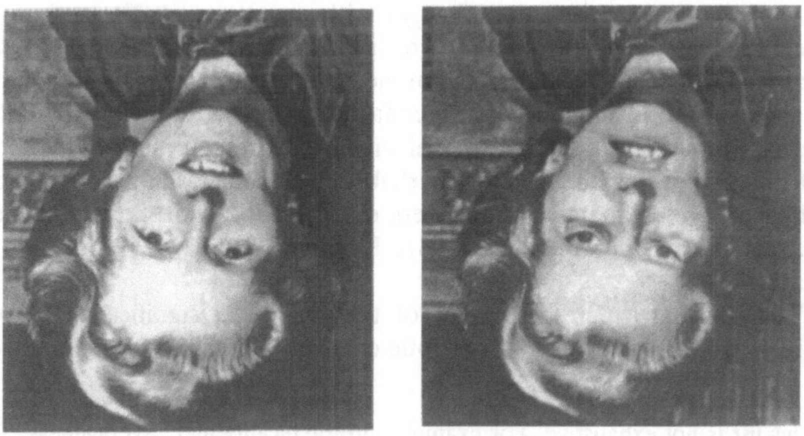

FIGURE 2.1. The Thatcher effect. (From "Margaret Thatcher: A new illusion," by P. Thompson, 1980, *Perception*, *9*, 483–484. By permission of Pion, London.)

are so consistently perceived as attractive. Thus, a functional approach to defining attractiveness may be more useful than a measurement approach in understanding the pervasive preferences exhibited for attractive faces.

Facial features and proportions convey not only information about attractiveness but also functional information about an individual's age, gender, affective state, behavioral and mental competence, strength, health, and propensity to interact in particular ways (e.g., Bradshaw, 1969; Buss & Barnes, 1986; Cunningham, 1986; Dion, 1974; Enlow, 1982; Maier, Holmes, Slaymaker, & Reich, 1984; Napoleon, Chassin, & Young, 1980; O'Grady, 1982; Richardson, Koller, & Katz, 1985). Such functional information facilitates efficient interpersonal interactions and functioning; therefore, the ability to perceive such information in faces should be present early in life and should be robust across ethnic variations in facial features. Indeed, such early and robust specialization by the nervous system for face perception is thought to be as important for the requirements of meaningful social relationships as are other specializations, such as speech (Kendrick & Baldwin, 1987; McArthur & Baron, 1983; Perrett, Rolls, & Caan, 1982; Yin, 1978). It is proposed here that attractiveness is a higher-order variable composed of information specifying age or maturity, gender, and affective state, among others.[2] To the extent that attractiveness judgments overlap with the perception and identification of level of maturity, gender, and affective state, it is not difficult to understand why the ability to discriminate faces based on these judgments is evident so early in life and is so similar across cultures.

Age Information

There is already considerable evidence showing that facial features and proportions convey information about age. It is well known, for example, that cranial/facial proportion changes with development: Facial features are raised as the face matures, which changes the relative sizes of the forehead and chin. Changes in forehead and chin size, in turn, create changes in the prominence of other facial features (Enlow, 1968, 1982). Perhaps not coincidentally, perceivers are extremely sensitive to this information in the face. Even remarkably small changes in proportion can influence age estimates of perceivers in systematic and predictable ways (e.g., Mark, Todd, & Shaw, 1981; Pittenger & Shaw, 1975; Todd & Mark, 1981).

The most articulate statement of the functional significance of perceivers' abilities to detect these subtle changes in craniofacial features and

[2] This list is not exhaustive. For example, prototypicality and "averageness" (see Langlois et al., 1987 and Langlois & Roggman, 1990) are other defining features of attractive faces, but they are beyond the scope of this chapter and will not be elaborated upon here.

proportions comes from McArthur and her colleagues (e.g., Berry & McArthur, 1986; McArthur & Baron, 1983). They propose an ecological approach to social perception in which facial (and other) characteristics will influence the perceptions and expectations of perceivers when these characteristics reveal information that is relevant to social interactions and adaptive functioning. They further suggest that age-related facial characteristics that identify immaturity should strongly influence perceivers because of the adaptive significance of the ability to differentiate appropriate interaction strategies to be employed with infants (e.g., caregiving and nurturance) vs. adults (e.g., sexual behavior). Finally, their ecological approach suggests that perceiver reactions to mature and immature facial characteristics will be overgeneralized, so that even adults with immature facial characteristics may be perceived as more childlike than those with mature facial characteristics (and vice versa). The overgeneralization occurs because it is presumably more adaptive, at least in the case of infant survival, to overgeneralize than to undergeneralize.

There is quite a bit of research that supports McArthur's ecological perspective and that suggests that age appearance, like attractiveness, elicits consistent differential expectations of behavioral and cognitive competence from perceivers (e.g., Bradshaw, 1969; Maier et al., 1984; O'Grady, 1982; Richardson et al., 1985). For example, adults with "babyish" cranial/facial proportions are judged as likely to be more friendly and agreeable, but less strong (Berry & McArthur, 1985, 1986; McArthur & Apatow, 1983–1984). Similarly, faces with babyish features elicit increased caregiving, protection, and assistance and are rated as more pleasant to observe (e.g., Alley, 1980, 1981, 1983; Lorenz, 1943). In contrast, children who appear older than their actual age seem to elicit dysfunctional expectations and behaviors from others. For example Brackbill and Nevill (1981) have found that perceptual cues (perceived height) overwhelm cognitive ones (knowledge of age) in determining adult expectations for children's achievement: Taller children were assigned inappropriately difficult tasks by adults, but same-age shorter children were assigned more reasonable tasks in this study.

In a particularly provocative example of the way in which facial characteristics may inform perceivers about age, maturity, and competence, McCabe (1984) showed in two different samples that physically abused children have cranial/facial proportions that appear older than those of same-age, matched, nonabused children. McCabe suggests that adults have unrealistic expectations for children perceived to be older and that a child's inability to meet these expectations may be one factor in abuse. Indeed, Lorenz long maintained that such affective responses to facially specified age cues (i.e., babyishness) are innate, a view that is consistent with McArthur's ecological approach (Berry & McArthur, 1985, 1986; McArthur & Baron, 1983). Age-related aspects of facial attractiveness, therefore, seem to convey important social information that is readily extracted by perceivers and used to form expectations of and behavioral responses toward others.

Moreover, these important age-related facial features have been shown in several studies to be related to attractiveness. In two studies, we have found that attractiveness and age-appearance were related (r = −.64) in a sample of infants: Less attractive infants were judged to be older than their attractive age-mates (Ritter, Langlois, & Casey, 1988). We have also found that when parents examined photographs of infants who varied in attractiveness, they overestimated both the age and the developmental competence of unattractive as compared to attractive infants. In addition, as compared to normative judgments of the abilities of this age group, judgments of the abilities of unattractive infants represented unrealistic rather than appropriate expectations. Thus, attractive and unattractive faces of infants seem to differ in the age or developmental status cues they convey to perceivers, and perceivers reliably extract such information from faces. Youthful characteristics in general seem to be preferred across numerous species and cultures (e.g., Eibl-Eibesfeldt, 1975; Symons, 1979).

Our finding that unattractive infants were expected to be capable of more behaviors than attractive infants may at first seem counter to other work showing that attractive individuals, even infants, are generally assumed to be more competent than unattractive individuals (e.g., Stephan & Langlois, 1984). However, unlike research in which perceivers are asked to make evaluations of competence in general or to indicate affective preferences for attractive vs. unattractive infants, *competence* was defined in our study as the number of specific behaviors and abilities (e.g., puts small objects in container) individually checked by adults. Thus, the parents were not asked to make global judgments of general competence but of whether or not the infant should, for example, be capable of putting a small object in a container. Indeed, older-appearing, unattractive infants and children may receive global evaluations indicating that they are viewed as less competent *because* they cannot meet the higher expectations for specific developmental abilities that adults seem to hold for them.

The results of these studies suggest several important implications for adult–child interactions and relationships. First, adults who do not have explicit age information are likely to use appearance information to evaluate the developmental abilities of children. Most adults do not have explicit age information about the children with whom they interact, even on a regular basis. For example, teachers may have a general idea of a particular child's age, but they probably are not constantly aware of the birthdays of all their students. Teachers may expect more mature behavior and competence from less attractive, older-appearing children than these children are capable of producing. Such unfulfilled expectations for specific age-appropriate abilities may in turn lead to evaluations of these children as generally less competent than their more attractive and youthful-looking peers. Indeed, in the Brackbill and Nevill (1981) study, adults, one group of whom were elementary school teachers, were susceptible to the biasing effect of height, even though they had been given explicit knowledge of the age of the children serving as target stimuli. A similar phenomenon may account for the results of the McCabe (1984) study in which abused children were found to look older than same-age, nonabused children. One factor in the abuse of these children may be that their parents held unrealistically high expectations for their behavior and maturity because of their appearance.

Implications

What are the implications of this body of information for individuals with craniofacial abnormalities and for those working with them? One implication is that negative reactions to craniofacial deformities may be due in part to the deformity itself and in part to violations of expected age information in faces. Children with many craniofacial syndromes either look older than their actual age or their age is difficult to judge from their appearance. In either case, a simple but potentially useful psychosocial intervention would be to regularly discuss age-appropriate expectations for both the cognitive and social behavior of these children with caregivers, teachers, and even peers and siblings.

Surgeons charged with facial reconstruction need to consider seriously the effect of the reconstruction on the age appearance of the patient. A case in point is the facial reconstruction of Down Syndrome children and adults. Many Down Syndrome children have a facial structure that is quite babyish in appearance. Although often surgery is performed to improve functional aspects of the craniofacial morphology of Down Syndrome patients, other surgical practices include procedures to alter the distinctive babyish appearance of these children (e.g., Lemperle & Radu, 1980).

Proponents of this practice argue, on the one hand, that these nonfunctional reconstructions change the appearance of the child so that he or she is no longer identified as having Down Syndrome. It is further argued that a Down Syndrome appearance leads to prejudice and unrealistically low expectations for the social and cognitive development of the child. On the other hand, these conclusions are debatable (e.g., Pueschel, Monteiro, & Erickson, 1986) and, in addition, the research on age or maturity appearance suggests that the babyish features of many Down Syndrome children may in fact lead to positive rather than negative affective reactions to them. Indeed, changing the appearance of Down Syndrome children may, at least under some circumstances, lead to the very reactions that the surgery is intended to avoid: The appearance of an older, cognitively advanced individual may elicit expectations for the behavior and performance of the Down Syndrome child that are then violated, sometimes seriously. The violation of these expectations may then lead to negative affective reactions and treatment (e.g., Shears & Jensema, 1969).

There are many ethical issues to be considered in the decision to perform nonfunctional facial reconstruction on Down Syndrome patients (e.g., Mearig, 1985). Most of these issues are ones of values and philosophy and cannot be resolved easily. The issue of how surgery affects age information signaled by the face and how this information is used by others to form expectations and behavior toward Down Syndrome children, however, could be resolved by research. For example, following the rationale of the study we conducted utilizing realistic theater masks to evoke reactions from infants exposed to attractive or unattractive faces, masks could be constructed from Down Syndrome patients before and after surgery. These masks could then be used in carefully controlled experimental situations that could reveal the effects of facial reconstruction on different types of perceivers (e.g., strangers, teachers, peers) under different situations.

Gender Information

Youthful features may influence judgments of attractiveness in both male and female infants and young children in similar ways, but not in older males and females. Rather, youthful features may be differentially related to attractiveness in adult males and females because of anatomical differences in their faces and because of stereotyped beliefs about the appropriate behavior and roles for males and females.

Although most of us are not aware of the anatomic differences between male and female faces, the differences are, nevertheless, considerable (e.g., Enlow, 1968, 1982; Farkas & Munro, 1987). The larger overall body size of males has significant morphological implications for the face. Male lungs are correspondingly larger, to provide for the larger male muscles and body organs; larger lungs require a larger airway beginning with the nose, which in turn leads to differences in other topographic structures of the face. Because of the larger, more protuberant character of the male nose, the contiguous part of the forehead also grows into a more protrusive position yielding a male forehead that tends to be more sloping in contrast to the more upright forehead of the female. Similarly, the supraorbital part of the male forehead tends to be very protrusive as compared to the female forehead (Enlow, 1982).

Because of the protrusive male forehead, the eyes of males appear more deep-set as compared to those of females, whose eyes appear to be closer to the front of the face. Female cheekbones appear much more prominent because the nose and forehead are less prominent. These

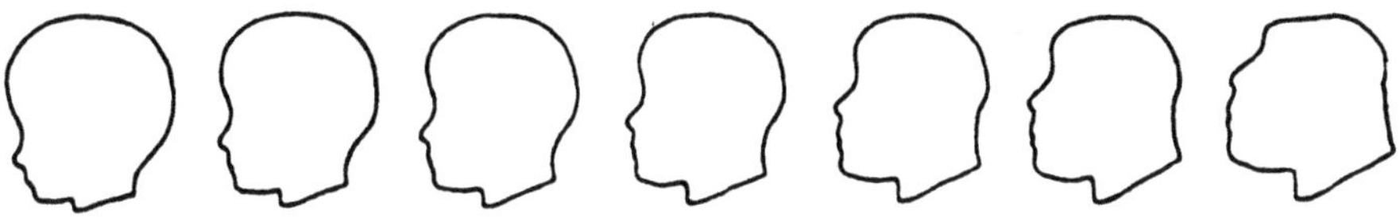

FIGURE 2.2. Age and gender communicated by profile shape. (From "Aging faces as viscal-elastic events: Implications for a theory of nonrigid shape perception" by J.B. Pittenger and R.E. Shaw, 1975, *Journal of Experimental Psychology: Human Perception and Performance, 1*, p. 376. Copyright (1975) by the American Psychological Association. Reprinted by permission.)

characteristics of the adult female face, in turn, form a facial structure that is much more juvenilelike than that of the adult male (Enlow, 1982). As we have seen, youthful features such as wide eyes and prominent cheeks are related to judgments of attractiveness in women (Cunningham, 1986), suggesting that attractive and unattractive female faces may differ in the extent to which they display information conveying gender. Figure 2.2 illustrates the more youthful or juvenile profile of female as compared to male faces: To most perceivers, the profiles change in appearance from that of an infant to that of a female to that of a male.

Thus, youthful features may signal not only information about age and behavioral maturity but also information about gender: Faces with larger nasal passages, deep-set eyes, and more protrusive and sloping foreheads are identified as male, whereas faces with less prominent noses and foreheads and more prominent cheeks and eyes are identified as female. Indeed, perceivers are as adept at identifying gender information in faces as they are at identifying age: Both adults and infants can readily discriminate gender in faces of all ages, even two-dimensional ones depicted by photographs (e.g., Fagan & Singer, 1979; Gewirtz & Hernandez, 1985; Hildebrandt & Fitzgerald, 1979; Karraker, 1986; Lasky, Klein, & Martinez, 1974).

In addition to youthful features, other features of the face are associated more with one gender than with another. Keating and her colleagues (Keating, 1985; Keating & Bai, 1986; Keating, Mazur, & Segall, 1977) have demonstrated that features proposed to panculturally signal dominance, strength, and maturity are differentially associated with attractiveness in males and females. Dominance signals in the face include wide faces and square jaws and bushy, thick eyebrows. Wide faces and square jaws are viewed as signaling dominance because jaw growth is associated with mature dentition and because fully developed teeth are used to threaten conspecifics among primates (Guthrie, 1970; Keating, 1985). Bushy or thick eyebrows reflect the increase in facial hair following puberty in males and are therefore thought to signal more strength and dominance relative to the thinner brows of children and females.

Keating et al. (1981) found that, in males, square jaws, wide faces, smaller eyes, and thinner lips were in fact perceived as more attractive and more dominant. Females with these facial characteristics were also perceived as more dominant but as less attractive. In contrast, females perceived as attractive were those with more facial characteristics such as larger eyes, rounder jaws, and thinner brows. Keating (1985) suggests that feminine or nondominant facial characteristics cause males to appear weak and unappealing because these facial cues are inconsistent with gender expectations for males. Conversely, dominance cues in the face are appealing in males and unappealing in females because they are consistent with gender expectations for males but inconsistent for females. Female faces with dominance cues and male faces with nondominant cues violate gender and status expectations and are therefore viewed as less attractive. Keating further speculates that physiognomic cues of dominance and strength are a product of primate evolution and therefore should be universal and in place early in life (Keating, 1985; Keating & Bai, 1986). Facial configuration, then, may provide a physiognomic basis of sex stereotyping.

The preceding argument suggests that, in addition to sex differences in the prominence of mature and immature facial features, there also should be within sex individual differences in the degree to which males and females possess these characteristics. We have already seen that this is the case in Berry and McArthur's (1985, 1986) work on babyish characteristics in male faces: Males with babyish faces are consistently viewed as less strong and dominant and more naive and kind than males with more mature faces. Other research also points toward the role of facial cues in influencing gender expectations and behaviors. Langlois and Downs (1979), in a study of preschoolers interacting with one another, found that attractiveness was associated with sex-stereotyped play behaviors. Specifically, the highly attractive boys in this study more often played with dolls and engaged in traditionally feminine sex-stereotyped play behaviors than did less attractive boys. Conversely, the less attractive girls engaged in more masculine sex-stereotyped play than did their more attractive female peers. Consistent findings are reported by LaVoie and Andrews (1976), who found that teachers judged unattractive children as exhibiting more masculine play behavior than attractive children.

More recently, Roberts, Green, Williams, and Goodman (1987) have reported on a sample of boys with extensive cross-gender behavior and a matched comparison group of boys with more masculine behavior. One of the most powerful, although serendipitous, findings obtained in this study was that parental perceptions of their sons' appearance were significantly related to feminine behavior. Parents of the feminine boys rated them as more pretty and likely to be mistaken for a girl, even as very young infants, than did parents of the comparison-group boys. The feminine boys were rated also as smaller in size than were the comparison-group boys. Within the comparison group, feminine appearance and feminine behavior also were correlated: More feminine-appearing boys expressed more feminine behaviors than did larger, more masculine-appearing boys. These results are consistent with those of Stoller (1968) as well as with those of Langlois and Downs (1979) and LaVoie and Andrews (1976) and suggest either biological differences between feminine- and masculine-appearing children or that appearance influences the socialization of these children and, ultimately perhaps, their gender identity. The feminine facial characteristics of these boys may cause adults and peers to react to and treat them more similarly to girls. In the same way, less attractive girls, who may appear more masculine in appearance (Keating, 1985), may be treated in a manner consistent with their appearance.

Implications

Several implications for the craniofacial child or adult can be derived from this section on facially based gender cues. First, as we found in the previous section on age information, negative reactions to adults and children with craniofacial deformities may be due to the violation or confusion of appropriate gender signals in the face as well as to the deformity itself. Aamot (1978), for example, found that perceivers had significantly greater difficulty in determining the gender of individuals with craniofacial deformities than that of individuals without deformities in reaction-time experiments. The effect was especially pronounced for females with craniofacial deformities. The reconstructive surgeon, then, needs to consult carefully the available craniofacial norms that have been developed separately for males and females (e.g., Farkas, 1987). Facial reconstructions, whenever possible, should preserve or establish facial configurations appropriate for males and females. When this is not possible, the implications of the violation of or the lack of facially based gender cues should be discussed with the patient and/or his or her parents: Knowledge of the reasons behind inappropriate or negative reactions from others could be important to the self-understanding of the craniofacial patient.

Affective Information

Affective cues and expressions are an obvious influence on attractiveness. For example, photographers the world over attempt to pose their subjects with smiles. This intuition on the part of photographers is mimicked by the intuition of researchers: In almost all research on physical attractiveness, targets are required to pose with a neutral facial expression to ensure that ratings of attractiveness are not confounded with emotional expression. The intuitions of both photographers and researchers are supported by empirical data. Several studies have shown that smiling faces are rated as more attractive than nonsmilling faces (e.g., Hildebrandt, 1983; Mueser, Grau, Sussman, & Rosen, 1984; Power, Hildebrandt, & Fitzgerald, 1982). However, although expression can affect mean attractiveness ratings with smiling groups rated higher than nonsmiling groups, the within-group rank order of attractiveness ratings remained essentially the same in these studies regardless of the expression posed. Thus, facial configuration seems to be a more powerful determinant of attractiveness than expression (e.g., Hildebrandt, 1983).

There has been almost no research conducted, however, on other aspects of the face that communicate affective information yet are independent of emotional state or expression. Faces can signal different affective states, not only through the facial affect system (e.g., Ekman, 1976; Izard, 1977) but also through the shape and physical structure of features of the face (Aronoff, Barclay, & Stevenson, 1988; Cunningham, 1986; Keating et al., 1981; Ohman, 1986). That mere shape of a facial feature can communicate affective information has been demonstrated by Aronoff et al. (1988). They showed that the spatial orientation of a facial feature (e.g., down-turned eyebrows) was perceived as threatening, even though no information was present in the face to reveal affective state such as muscle movement. The two faces drawn in Figure 2.3 illustrate how spatial orientation alone can influence the perception of affect.

The two faces are identical except for the eyebrows. Because the faces are schematics, they obviously do not possess real emotion cues. Nevertheless, most adults perceive one face as threatening and the other as sad, even though no alterations have been made to any feature other than the angle of the eyebrows. It is likely that other facial features would induce other reactions from perceivers. Mouths that, in repose, curve upward

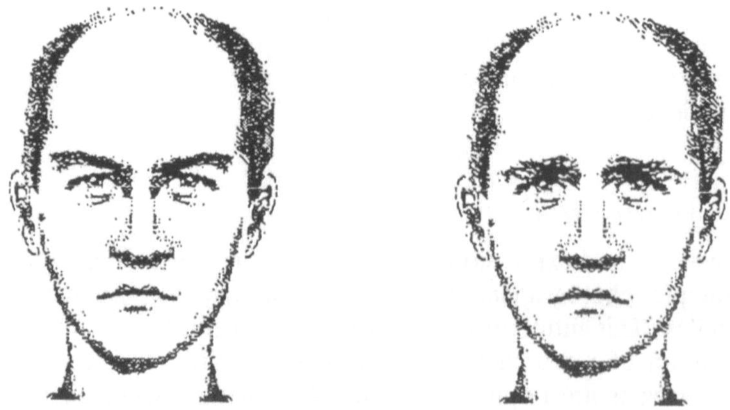

FIGURE 2.3. Identical faces except for shape of eyebrows.

rather than downward are likely to communicate positive as opposed to negative affective state and perhaps behavioral intention. Furthermore, faces in which mouths curve upward rather than downward may well be perceived as more attractive.

Why are perceivers so sensitive to the spatial orientation of facial features? Both the communication and perception of emotion information are critical social skills; the ability to perceive emotional information is an adaptive one, likely therefore to be present early in life. Indeed, infants are well known to have relatively sophisticated abilities to detect emotional cues in faces (Caron, Caron, & Myers, 1982, 1985; Nelson, 1987) and to prefer positive over angry emotional expressions (LaBarbera, Izard, Vietze, & Parisi, 1976; Schwartz, Izard, & Ansul, 1985). Thus, sensitivity to information signaling such emotional states as anger, rage, and submission may be built into the nervous system of the human (Nelson, 1987; Ohman, 1986). The ability to detect affective as well as gender and age information in faces may be part of the nervous system's early specialization for face perception (e.g., Perrett et al., 1982; Rinn, 1984; Yin, 1978). The sensitivity to spatial orientation of facial features may reflect this nervous system specialization; sensitivity to the static spatial orientation of eyebrows on schematic faces may in part be an overgeneralized reaction, such as those discussed earlier, in the section on age information (e.g., McArthur & Baron, 1983).

Implications

As we have noted for age and gender information, it may be that affective information is harder to determine or is perceived as negative affective state in the craniofacial patient, although there are no pertinent empirical data available to evaluate this claim. Cleft lip–palate individuals, for example, may have mouths that are less effective in signaling positive emotion. Thus, negative reactions to these individuals may be due in part to the inscrutableness of the face. If perceivers cannot "read" the face for affective state, they cannot empathize or sympathize with the craniofacial child or adult under sad or unhappy affective conditions, nor share laughter and joy under happy ones. More problematic may be the establishment of positive attachments and social responsiveness between parents and infants born with craniofacial abnormalities that interfere with the expression of affect (e.g., Field & Vega-Lahr, 1984). Until the emergence of language, facial signals are the primary means of communication between infants and their caregivers. The absence or occlusion of these signals due to a craniofacial abnormality may place these infants and their caregivers at risk for forming in secure attachments (see the chapter by Petersen, Paul, & Lieberman). Parents and other caregivers interacting with cleft lip–palate and other craniofacial patients need to be taught to compensate for the lack of cues in one or more areas of the face by using alternate or multiple cues to determine and react to affective expression. For example, for some craniofacial individuals, the crinkling of the eyes may be a better affective cue than downward or upward curved mouths; for others, especially infants, vocal cues such as positive coos and negative cries may be the most appropriate channel of affective communication.

Summary

In this chapter, we have suggested that faces communicate at least three different types of information that are important in regulating social behavior and social interaction: age, gender, and affect. It also has been argued that these facially based signals are related to judgments of attractiveness and that sensitivity to these aspects of facial appearance may be a wired-in component of the human nervous system. If these reactions reflect, at least in part, nervous system-level functioning, what optimism can be held for the possibility of changing negative reactions to the facially disfigured person? Although surgery can profoundly improve the appearance of craniofacial patients, many will nevertheless not be considered "attractive" even after surgery. Are they forever to experience discrimination and unpleasantness from others? To be honest, the craniofacial patient is likely to face more discrimination and negative social reactions than individuals with other disabilities because of the supreme importance of the face in human functioning and relations (e.g., Goldberg, 1974). However, humans are not creatures solely of biology and instincts; they also are products of an evolutionary process in which the capacity to learn and change has evolved. Attitudes toward the facially unattractive or disfigured, like those toward women and minorities, can be changed, albeit with considerable effort and time.

Many, if not most, individuals are not even aware that they posses negative attitudes toward the unattractive (e.g., Richardson et al., 1961). Indeed, most categorically deny that they behave differently toward attractive and unattractive children and adults. This lack of awareness lies at the heart of both unfavorable reactions toward the unattractive and disfigured and at interventions designed to change such reactions. We all should be aware of these largely unconscious attitudes and behaviors and their consequences to those to whom they are directed. Providing information about the existence and origins of these attitudes and stereotypes to both craniofacial patients and to those who interact with them could be useful in enhancing the self-concept of those receiving negative reactions and in changing the behavior of those engaged in differential treatment. Craniofacial patients need to know that they are not the "final" cause of negative reactions to them: Nature is. Perceivers need to know that they are not reacting unusually or maliciously by intent. And both perceivers and craniofacial patients need to know that these reactions can be at least partially brought under conscious awareness and control. Some studies have shown, for example, that bias can be effectively eliminated in observers when they are made aware of their bias (Langlois & Prestholdt, 1977). Other studies have shown that not all individuals react unfavorably to unattractive people (Dion & Dion, 1987; Snyder, Berscheid, & Matwychuk, 1988).

It is the responsibility of future research to determine how best to educate the general public about biases and prejudices that they may have toward the craniofacial patient. The hope is that one day this research will provide the means to change societal attitudes toward craniofacial patients so that they will not have to endure the double burden of considerable social as well as surgical pain.

References

Aamot, S. (1978). Reactions to facial deformities: Autonomic and social psychological. *European Journal of Social Psychology, 8,* 315–333.

Adams, G.R. (1977). Physical attractiveness research: Toward a developmental social psychology of beauty. *Human Development, 20,* 217–239.

Adams, G.R., & Crane, P. (1980). An assessment of parents' and teachers' expectations of preschool children's preference for attractive or unattractive children and adults. *Child Development, 51,* 224–231.

Alley, T.R. (1980). Infantile colouration as an elicitor of caretaking behavior in Old World primates. *Primates, 21,* 416–429.

Alley, T.R. (1981). Head shape and the perception of cuteness. *Developmental Psychology, 17,* 650–654.

Alley, T.R. (1983). Age-related changes in body proportions, body size, and perceived cuteness. *Perceptual & Motor Skills, 56,* 615–622.

Aronoff, J., Barclay, A.M., & Stevenson, L.A. (1988). The recognition of threatening facial stimuli. *Journal of Personality and Social Psychology, 54,* 647–655.

Banks, M.S., & Salapatek, P. (1983). Infant visual perception. In M.M. Haith & J.J. Campos (Vol. Eds.), Infancy and developmental psychobiology (pp. 435–571). In P.H. Mussen (Ed.), *Handbook of child psychology.* New York: Wiley.

Bernstein, I.H., Lin, T., & McClellan, P. (1982). Cross- vs. within-racial judgments of attractiveness. *Perception & Psychophysics, 32,* 495–503.

Berry, D.S., & McArthur, L.Z. (1985). Some components and consequences of a babyface. *Journal of Personality and Social Psychology, 48,* 312–323.

Berry, D.S., & McArthur, L.Z. (1986). Perceiving character in faces: The impact of age-related craniofacial changes on social perception. *Psychological Bulletin, 100,* 3–18.

Berscheid, E., & Walster, E. (1974). Physical attractiveness. In L. Berkowitz (Ed.), *Advances in experimental social psychology* (pp. 157–215). New York: Academic Press.

Berscheid, E., Dion, K.K., Walster, E., & Walster, G.W. (1971). Physical attractiveness and dating choice: A test of the matching hypothesis. *Journal of Experimental Social Psychology, 7,* 173–189.

Brackbill, Y., & Nevill, D.D. (1981). Parental expectations of achievement as affected by children's height. *Merrill-Palmer Quarterly, 27,* 429–441.

Bradshaw, J.L. (1969). The information conveyed by varying the dimensions of features in human outline faces. *Perception & Psychophysics, 6,* 5–9.

Buss, D.M., & Barnes, M. (1986). Preferences in human mate selection. *Journal of Personality and Social Psychology, 50,* 559–570.

Caron, R.F., Caron, A.J., & Myers, R.S. (1982). Abstraction of invariant face expressions in infancy. *Child Development, 53,* 1008–1015.

Caron, R.F., Caron, A.J., & Myers, R.S. (1985). Do infants see emotional expression in static faces? *Child Development, 56,* 1552–1560.

Caron, A.J., Caron, R.F., Caldwell, R.C., & Weiss, S.J. (1973). Infant perception of the structural properties of the face. *Developmental Psychology, 9,* 385–399.

Cavior, N., & Lombardi, P.A. (1973). Developmental aspects of judgments of physical attractiveness in children. *Developmental Psychology, 8,* 67–71.

Cross, J.F., & Cross, J. (1971). Age, sex, race, and the perception of facial beauty. *Developmental Psychology, 5,* 433–439.

Cunningham, M.R. (1986). Measuring the physical in physical attractiveness: Quasiexperiments on the sociobiology of female facial beauty. *Journal of Social and Personality Psychology, 50,* 925–935.

Darwin, C. (1859). *On the origin of species by means of natural selection.* London: John Murray.

Dion, K.K. (1972). Physical attractiveness and evaluations of children's transgressions. *Journal of Personality and Social Psychology, 24,* 207–213.

Dion, K.K. (1973). Young children's stereotyping of facial attractiveness. *Developmental Psychology, 9,* 183–188.

Dion, K.K. (1974). Children's physical attractiveness and sex as determinants of adult punitiveness. *Developmental Psychology, 10,* 772–778.

Dion, K.K., & Berscheid, E. (1974). Physical attractiveness and peer perception among children. *Sociometry, 37,* 1–12.

Dion, K.K., Berscheid, E., & Walster, E. (1972). What is beautiful is good. *Journal of Personality and Social Psychology, 24,* 285–290.

Dion, K.L., & Dion, K.K. (1987). Belief in a just world and physical attractiveness stereotyping. *Journal of Personality and Social Psychology, 52,* 775–780.

Eibl-Eibesfeldt, I. (1975). *Ethology: The biology of behavior* (2nd Ed.). New York: Holt, Rinehart & Winston.

Ekman, P. (1976). *Pictures of facial affect.* Palo Alto, CA: Consulting Psychologists Press.

Enlow, D.H. (1968). *The human face: An account of the postnatal growth and development of the craniofacial skeleton.* New York: Harper & Row.

Enlow, D.H. (1982). *Handbook of facial growth.* Philadelphia: Saunders.

Fagan, J.F., & Singer, L.T. (1979). The role of simple feature differences in infants' recognition of faces. *Infant Behavior and Development, 2,* 39–45.

Fantz, R.L. (1965). Visual perception from birth as shown by pattern selectivity. In H.E. Whipple (Ed.), *New issues in infant development. Annals of New York Academy of Science, 118,* 793–814.

Fantz, R.L., & Fagan, J.F. (1975). Visual attention to size and number of pattern details by term and preterm infants during the first six months. *Child Development, 46,* 3–18.

Farkas, L.G. (1987). Age- and sex-related changes in facial proportions. In L.G. Farkas & I.R. Munro (1987). (Eds.), *Anthropometric facial proportions in medicine.* Springfield, IL: Charles C. Thomas.

Farkas, L.G., & Munro, I.R. (1987). *Anthropometric facial proportions in medicine.* Springfield, IL: Charles C. Thomas.

Farkas, L.G., Munro I.R., & Kolar, J. (1987). Linear proportions in above- and below-average women's faces. In L.G. Farkas & I.R. Munro (1987). (Eds.), *Anthropometric facial proportions in medicine.* Springfield, IL: Charles C. Thomas.

Field, T.M., & Vega-Lahr, N. (1984). Early interactions between infants with cranio-facial anomalies and their mothers. *Infant Behavior and Development, 7,* 527–530.

Gewirtz, J.L., & Hernandez, J.P. (1985, August). Gender can be determined from the baby's live face and from slide photographs of the baby's face. Paper presented at the meeting of the American Psychological Association, Los Angeles, CA.

Goldberg, R.T. (1974). Adjustment of children with invisible and visible handicaps: Congenital heart disease and facial burns. *Journal of Counseling Psychology, 21,* 428–432.

Guthrie, R.D. (1970). Evolution of human threat display organs. In T. Dobzhansky, M.K. Hecht, & W.C. Steere (Eds.), *Evolutionary biology* (Vol. 4, pp. 257–302). New York: Appleton-Century-Crofts.

Haaf, R.A. (1974). Complexity and facial resemblance as determinants of response to facelike stimuli to 5- to 10-week-old infants. *Journal of Experimental Child Psychology, 18,* 480–487.

Hildebrandt, K.A. (1983). Effect of facial expression variations on ratings of infants' physical attractiveness. *Developmental Psychology, 19,* 414–417.

Hildebrandt, K.A., & Fitzgerald, H.E. (1979). Adults' perceptions of infant sex and cuteness. *Sex Roles, 5,* 471–481.

Iliffe, A.H. (1960). A study of preferences in feminine beauty. *British Journal of Psychology, 51,* 267–273.

Izard, C.E. (1977). *Human emotions.* New York: Plenum.

Johnson, R.W., Dannenbring, G.L., Anderson, N.R., & Villa, R.E. (1983). How different cultural and geographic groups perceive the attractiveness of active and inactive feminists. *The Journal of Social Psychology, 119,* 111–117.

Karraker, K.H. (1986, August). *Information conveyed by the newborn's face.* Paper presented at the meeting of the American Psychological Association, Washington, D.C.

Keating, C.F. (1985). Gender and the physiognomy of dominance and attractiveness. *Social Psychology Quarterly, 48,* 61–70.

Keating, C.F., & Bai, D.L. (1986). Children's attributions of social dominance from facial cues. *Child Development, 57,* 1269–1276.

Keating, C.F., Mazur, A., & Segall, M.H. (1977). Facial gestures which influence the perception of status. *Sociometry, 40,* 374–378.

Keating, C.F., Mazur, A., Segall, M.H., Cysneiros, P.G., Divale, W.T., Kilbride, J.E., Komin, S., Leahy, P., Thurman, B., & Wirsing, R. (1981).

Culture and the perception of social dominance from facial expression. *Journal of Personality and Social Psychology, 40,* 615–626.

Kendrick, K.M., & Baldwin, B.A. (1987). Cells in temporal cortex of conscious sheep can respond preferentially to the sight of faces. *Science, 236,* 448–450.

Kleck, R.E., Richardson, S.A., & Ronald, C. (1974). Physical appearance cues and interpersonal attraction in children. *Child Development, 45,* 305–310.

Korthase, K.M., & Trenholme, I. (1982). Perceived age and perceived physical attractiveness. *Perceptual & Motor Skills, 54,* 1251–1258.

LaBarbera, J.D., Izard, C.E., Vietze, P., & Parisi, S.A. (1976). Four- and six-month-old infants' visual response to joy, anger, and neutral expressions. *Child Development, 47,* 535–562.

Langlois, J.H. (1986). From the eye of the beholder to behavioral reality: The development of social behaviors and social relations as a function of physical attractiveness. In C.P. Herman, M.P. Zanna, & E.T. Higgins (Eds.), *Physical appearance, stigma, and social behavior: The Ontario symposium* (Vol. 3, pp. 23–51). Hillsdale, NJ: Erlbaum.

Langlois, J.H., & Downs, A.C. (1979). Peer relations as a function of physical attractiveness: The eye of the beholder or behavioral reality? *Child Development, 50,* 409–418.

Langlois, J.H., & Prestholdt, P.H. (1977). Information: A control for observer bias. *Journal of Social Psychology, 102,* 133–141.

Langlois, J.H., Roggman, L., & Rieser-Danner, L.A. (1990). Infants' differential social responses to attractive and unattractive faces. *Developmental Psychology, 26,* 153–159.

Langlois, J.H., Roggman, L.A., Casey, R.J., Ritter, J.M., Rieser-Danner, L.A., & Jenkins, V.Y. (1987). Infant preferences for attractive faces: Rudiments of a stereotype? *Developmental Psychology, 23,* 363–369.

Langlois, J.H., & Stephan, C. (1977). The effects of physical attractiveness and ethnicity on children's behavioral attributions and peer preferences. *Child Development, 48,* 1694–1698.

Langlois, J.H., & Stephan, C. (1981). Beauty and the beast: The role of physical attractiveness in the development of peer relations and social behavior. In S.S. Brehm, S.M. Kassin, & F.X. Gibbons (Eds.), *Developmental social psychology: Theory and research* (pp. 152–168). New York: Oxford.

Langlois, J.H., & Roggman, L.R. (1990). Attractive faces are only average. *Psychological Science, 1,* 115–121.

Langlois, J.H., Ritter, J.M., Roggman, L.A., & Vaughn, L.S. (1991). Facial diversity and infant preferences for attractive faces. *Developmental Psychology, 27,* 79–84.

Lasky, R.E., Klein, R.E., & Martinez, S. (1974). Age and sex discriminations in five- and six-month-old infants. *The Journal of Psychology, 88,* 317–324.

LaVoie, J.C., & Andrews, R. (1976). Facial attractiveness, physique, and sex role identity in young children. *Developmental Psychology, 12,* 550–551.

Lemperle, G., & Radu, D. (1980). Facial plastic surgery in children with Down's Syndrome. *Plastic and Reconstructive Surgery, 3,* 337–342.

Liggett, J. (1974). *The human face.* New York: Stein & Day.

Lorenz, K. (1943). Die angeborenen formen moglicher arfahrung. *Zietschrift fur Tierpsychologie, 5,* 233–409.

Lucker, G.W. (1981). Esthetics and a quantitative analysis of facial appearance. In G.W. Lucker, K.A. Ribbens, & J.A. McNamara (Eds.), *Psychological aspects of facial form.* Ann Arbor: Center for Growth and Human Development, University of Michigan.

Maier, R.A., Holmes, D.L., Slaymaker, F.L., & Reich, J.N. (1984). The perceived attractiveness of preterm infants. *Infant Behavior and Development, 7,* 403–414.

Maret, S.M. (1983). Attractiveness ratings of photographs of Blacks by Cruzans and Americans. *The Journal of Psychology, 115,* 113–116.

Maret, S.M., & Harling, G.A. (1985). Cross cultural perceptions of physical attractiveness: Ratings of photos of whites by Cruzans and Americans. *Perceptual Motor Skills, 60,* 163–166.

Mark, L.S., Todd, J.T., & Shaw, R.E. (1981). Perception of growth: A geometric analysis of how different styles of change are distinguished. *Journal of Experimental Psychology: Human Perception and Performance, 7,* 855–868.

Maruyama, G., & Miller, N. (1981). Physical attractiveness and personality. In B.A. Maher (Ed.), *Progress in experimental personality research* (Vol. 10, pp. 203–280). New York: Academic Press.

McArthur, L.Z., & Apatow, K. (1983–1984). Impressions of baby-faced adults. *Social Cognition, 2,* 315–342.

McArthur, L.Z., & Baron, R.M. (1983). Toward an ecological theory of social perception. *Psychological Review, 90,* 215–238.

McArthur, L.Z., & Berry, D.S. (1987). Cross-cultural agreement in perceptions of babyfaced adults. *Journal of Cross-Cultural Psychology, 18,* 165–192.

McCabe, V. (1984). Abstract perceptual information for age level: A risk factor for maltreatment? *Child Development, 55,* 267–276.

Mearig, J.S. (1985). Facial surgery and an active modification approach for children with Down Syndrome: Some psychological and ethical issues. *Rehabilitation Literature, 46,* 72–77.

Mueser, K.T., Grau, B.W., Sussman, S., & Rosen, A.J. (1984). You're only as pretty as you fell: Facial expression as a determinant of physical attractiveness. *Journal of Personality and Social Psychology, 43,* 469–478.

Napoleon, T., Chassin, L., & Young, R.D. (1980). A replication and extension of "physical attractiveness and mental illness." *Journal of Abnormal Psychology, 89,* 250–253.

Nelson, C.A. (1987). The recognition of facial expressions in the first two years of life: Mechanisms of development. *Child Development, 58,* 889–909.

O'Grady, K.E. (1982). Sex, physical attractiveness, and perceived risk for mental illness. *Journal of Personality and Social Psychology, 43,* 1064–1071.

Ohman, A. (1986). Face the beast and fear the face: Animal and social fears as prototypes for evolutionary analyses of emotion. *Psychophysiology, 23,* 123–145.

Perrett, D.I., Rolls, E.T., & Caan, W. (1982). Visual neurones responsive to faces in the monkey temporal cortex. *Experimental Brain Research, 47,* 329–342.

Pittenger, J.B., & Shaw, R.E. (1975). Aging faces as viscal-elastic events: Implications for a theory of nonrigid shape perception. *Journal of Experimental Psychology: Human Perception and Performance, 4,* 374–382.

Power, T.G., Hildebrandt, K.A., & Fitzgerald, H.E. (1982). Adults' responses to infants varying in facial expression and perceived attractiveness. *Infant Behavior and Development, 5,* 33–44.

Pueschel, S.M., Monteiro, L.A., & Erickson, M. (1986). Parents' and physicians' perceptions of facial plastic surgery in children with Down's Syndrome. *Journal of Mental Deficiency Research, 30,* 71–79.

Richardson, S.A., Goodman, N., Hastorf, A.H., & Dornbusch, S.M. (1961). Cultural uniformity in reaction to physical disabilities. *American Sociological Review, 26,* 241–247.

Richardson, S.A., Koller, H., & Katz, M. (1985). Appearance and mental retardation: Some first steps in the development and application of a measure. *American Journal of Mental Deficiency, 89,* 475–484.

Rinn, W.E. (1984). The neuropsychology of facial expression: A review of the neurological and psychological mechanisms for producing facial expressions. *Psychological Bulletin, 95,* 52–77.

Ritter, J.M., Langlois, J.H., & Casey, R.J. (1988, April). Adults' responses to infants varying in appearance of age and attractiveness. Paper presented at the Sixth Biennial International Conference on Infant Studies, Washington, D.C.

Roberts, C.W., Green, R., Williams, K., & Goodman, M. (1987). Boyhood gender identity development: A statistical contrast of two family groups. *Developmental Psychology, 23,* 544–557.

Samuels, C.A., & Ewy, R. (1985). Aesthetic perception of faces during infancy. *British Journal of Developmental Psychology, 3,* 221–228.

Schwartz, G.M., Izard, C.E., & Ansul, S.E. (1985). The 5-month-old's ability to discriminate facial expressions of emotion. *Infant Behavior and Development, 8,* 65–77.

Shapiro, B.A., Eppler, M., Haith, M.M., & Reis, H. (1987, April). *An event analysis of facial attractiveness and expressiveness.* Paper presented at the meeting of the Society for Research in Child Development, Baltimore, MD.

Shears, L.M., & Jensema, C.J. (1969). Social acceptability of anomalous persons. *Exceptional Children, 36,* 91–96.

Sherrod, L.R. (1979). Social cognition in infants: Attention to the human face. *Infant Behavior and Development, 2,* 279–294.

Snyder, M., Berscheid, E., & Matwychuk, A. (1988). Orientations toward personnel selection: Differential reliance on appearance and personality. *Journal of Personality and Social Psychology, 54,* 972–979.

Sorell, G.T., & Nowak, C.A. (1981). The role of physical attractiveness as a contributor to individual development. In R.M. Lerner & N.A. Busch-Rossnagel (Eds.), *Individuals as producers of their development: A life-span perspective* (pp. 389–446). New York: Academic Press.

Stephan, C., & Langlois, J.H. (1984). Baby beautiful: Adult attributions of infant competence as a function of infant attractiveness. *Child Development, 55,* 576–585.

Sternglanz, S.H., Gray, J.L., & Murakami, M. (1977). Adult preferences for infantile facial features: An ethological approach. *Animal Behavior, 25,* 108–115.

Stoller, R. (1968). *Sex and gender: On the development of masculinity and femininity.* New York: Science House.

Styczynski, L.E., & Langlois, J.H. (1977). The effects of familiarity on behavioral stereotypes associated with physical attractiveness in young children. *Child Development, 48,* 1137–1141.

Sussman, S., & Mueser, K.T. (1983). Age, socioeconomic status, severity of mental disorder, and chronicity as predictors of physical attractiveness. *Journal of Abnormal Psychology, 92,* 255–258.

Symons, D. (1979). *The evolution of human sexuality*. New York: Oxford.

Thakerar, J.N., & Iwawaki, S. (1979). Cross-cultural comparisons in interpersonal attraction of females toward males. *Journal of Social Psychology, 108,* 121–122.

Thompson, P. (1980). Margaret Thatcher: A new illusion. *Perception, 9,* 483–484.

Todd, J.T., & Mark, L.S. (1981). Issues related to the prediction of craniofacial growth. *American Journal of Orthodontics, 79,* 63–80.

Walster, E., Aronson, V., Abrahams, D., & Rottmann, L. (1966). Importance of physical attractiveness in dating behavior. *Journal of Personality and Social Psychology, 4,* 508–516.

Webster's new collegiate dictionary. (1977). Springfield, MA: G. & C. Merriam Co.

Webster's new world dictionary. (1986). New York: Prentice Hall.

Weisfeld, G.E., Weisfeld, C.C., & Callaghan, J.W. (1984). Peer and self perceptions in Hopi and Afro-American third- and sixth-graders. *Ethos, 12,* 64–83.

Wernick, M., & Manaster, G.J. (1984). Age and the perception of age and attractiveness. *The Gerontologist, 24,* 408–414.

Yin, R.K. (1978). Face perception: A review of experiments with infants, normal adults, and brain-injured persons. In R. Held, H.W. Leibowitz, & H.L. Tenber (Eds.), *Handbook of sensory physiology* (Vol. VIII). New York: Springer-Verlag.

3
Beyond Beauty and After Affect: An Event Perception Approach to Perceiving Faces

Diane S. Berry

It has often been suggested that we make a life out of reading people's faces. In recent years, researchers have demonstrated a growing interest in just how we accomplish this feat. In fact, publications in the area of face perception have increased by more than 3,000% during the past 2 decades (Ellis, 1981). One line of this research has utilized our impressive capacity to recognize and recall faces as a domain in which to test ideas about human cognition (for a review, see Davies, Ellis, & Shepherd, 1981).

Two other areas of research on faces have also received extensive attention. First, work on the effects of facial attractiveness has contributed to our understanding of stereotyping and social interaction (see Langlois, 1986, this volume). Second, studies of emotional expression have increased our knowledge of social perception and coordination (for a review, see Ekman, 1982). Although these constitute important research questions, the combination of identity, attractiveness, and emotion seems unable to account fully for the richness and complexity of information derived from the face.

Why has research focused so exclusively on variables such as attractiveness and emotion? One factor may be that these characteristics are obvious and salient even to the layperson. However, the fact that these qualities are readily articulated by no means implies that they are the sole or the most important stimulus determinants of perceptions of faces. Consider, by analogy, the variables that contribute to depth perception. Based on intuition alone, most of us could probably articulate interposition as a cue for depth; that is, no theoretical framework may be needed to notice that close objects occlude more distant ones. However, it is less intuitively obvious that stimuli located at different distances from an observer move at different velocities across the retina. Nevertheless, this relationship, called motion parallax, also provides an important base for depth perception (e.g., Gibson, 1950). Perception is replete with such examples of nonintuitive bases for visual experience. Given this, attempts to articulate further the facial qualities that influence perceptions are diffficult in lieu of a theoretical framework from which relevant hypotheses can be generated.

With the exception of research on emotional expression, most approaches to face perception have incorporated the assumption that nondynamic structural characteristics provide most of the information available from the face (cf. Bruce & Green, 1985). Such perspectives view motion and change as noise that the perceptual system must disregard in order to analyze facial patterns. However, faces are animate and constantly changing. Moreover, many facial changes are the consequences of processes that are in themselves desirable to detect (e.g., emoting, aging). This presents a problem for a nondynamic approach: Why would a perceptual system evolve to dismiss prevalent and meaningful information as noise?

The intent of this chapter is to demonstrate the utility of an event perception approach (e.g., Johansson, von Hofsten, & Jansson, 1980) for the purpose of understanding face perception. A hallmark of the event perception model is that under normal conditions, dynamic ongoing styles of change are thought to constitute a primary basis for knowledge acquisition. In addition, a given event is defined by both what is transformed and what is preserved as it transpires. Both the changing and nonchanging characteristics of a stimulus undergoing an event can independently and simultaneously provide us with meaningful information. For example, when I see a friend smile, I detect something about his or her affective state from the particular pattern of facial deformation that I see. Moreover, I detect happiness from that pattern of change even when it appears on the face of a stranger. On the other hand, whether it is my friend or a stranger whom I see smile, some characteristics of their faces remain undisturbed through this event, allowing me to distinguish one face from the other.

Shaw and his associates have labeled these two potential sources of information transformational and structural invariants (cf. Shaw & Pittenger, 1977; Warren & Shaw, 1985). A transformational invariant may be defined as an abstract event, or style of change that makes available the same information across different underlying structures. For example, emotional expressions are recognizable across different faces. Structural invariants are those aspects of an underlying structure that remain constant through a particular change or event. For example, skin color does not change as a function of facial expression. From an event perception perspective, either of these classes of invariants can provide the basis for knowledge acquisition.[1]

[1] Not all sympathetic to this view are entirely comfortable with the terminology proffered by Shaw et al. However, most do agree that events can provide information apart from structure (cf. Cutting, 1986).

At least two assumptions regarding transformational invariants, or events, are unique to this view, and warrant emphasis. First, it is proposed that during normal, ongoing perceptual activity, people can and do extract meaning directly from the abstract style of change that characterizes a particular event. For example, the transformation that specifies a smile communicates affect independent of the appearance of the facial features at the apex of the smile (Bassili, 1978). A second characteristic of events is that they can vary in their temporal duration. For example, the transformation that gives rise to a smile may take place in only a few seconds. Such events, whose temporal dimension allows them to be identified as motion, are referred to as rapid or fast events. Other changes take place over a longer period of time. For example, the craniofacial changes produced by growth occur over a period of years. These are referred to as slow events. Despite the variations in duration which characterize these transformations, they are both defined as events because each incorporates a temporal dimension. The present chapter will consider the impact of both slow and rapid facial changes on perception.

What are the advantages of this theoretical position for the study of face perception? One is that the consideration of both structural and transformational invariants as conveyors of information can provide solutions to some of the logical problems encountered by a pattern perception approach to face perception. Consider, for example, the perception of facial identity: Despite evidence that different individuals may develop idiosyncratic styles of general facial behavior (Malatesta, Fiori, & Messina, 1987) and that identification accuracy in dynamic "mug" shots is superior to that found for still displays (Schiff, Banka, & de Bordes Galdi, 1986), researchers have virtually ignored the potential role of dynamic facial qualities in the recognition of personal identity (see Bruce & Valentine, 1988, for an exception). This phenomenon has instead generally been treated as a complex case of pattern recognition. However, if one conceptualizes facial changes as noise that disturbs facial patterns, difficulties arise in explaining how recognition of identity is relatively undisturbed by either the rapid deformations associated with expression changes or by the slower craniofacial changes that accompany growth. An event perception view can provide at least two potential solutions to this problem: First, variables such as personal identity may be revealed by some set of structural invariants that are not destroyed by these changes; and second, patterns of facial change may themselves provide some basis for facial recognition.

As this implies, an additional advantage of this perspective is that the consideration of facial events as potential sources of knowledge leads to some unique hypotheses regarding face perception. In particular, it is predicted that a facial event that shares a lawful relationship with a particular social variable may communicate that variable. It is further predicted that perceivers will be most sensitive to facial changes that convey adaptive information. Thus, it is predicted that facial events reveal a variety of person characteristics that have not been considered in previous research. Moreover, it is proposed that this social knowledge is specified in the visual information available in faces; thus, the use of stored representations or inferential processes to recognize these person qualities is deemed unnecessary. The research presented in this chapter assesses these hypotheses. First, analyses of the impact of the slow event of facial growth on social perception will be reviewed. Second, research examining the relationships among patterns of rapid facial motion and the detection of person qualities will be presented. Finally, the implications of this work for basic research in social cognition as well as the treatment of craniofacial populations will be considered.

Slow Facial Events

Change as Information

Craniofacial growth has been the most widely studied slow event. From birth through early adulthood, the maturation of the facial structure combined with the influence of external forces such as gravity produce a particular remodeling of the cranium. When viewed in profile, this change is characterized by a lessening of the predominance of the brain capsule. This transformation also influences the placement of facial features. More specifically, increasing age is accompanied by a higher placement of the eyes, nose, and mouth on the vertical plane of the face. This results in a smaller forehead and a larger chin in faces that are older than in those that are younger.

These changes share a lawful relationship with aging and growth. Moreover, the detection of maturational status serves a highly adaptive function (e.g., Alley, 1986). Therefore, it has been proposed that this slow facial event should provide the perceptual support for the identification of age (cf. Shaw & Pittenger, 1977). A particular transformation that preserves the structural invariants maintained during facial growth has since been mathematically defined (Todd, Mark, Shaw, & Pittenger, 1980). This geometric transformation, called cardioidal strain (see Figure 3.1), closely predicts the actual profile changes that occur in developing faces (Todd & Mark, 1981). What is the impact of this event on perceptions of faces?

Perceptions of Age

Several studies have investigated the impact of cardioidal strain on age perception. This work has revealed that perceivers spontaneously identify facial profiles to which this transformation is applied as growing, whereas

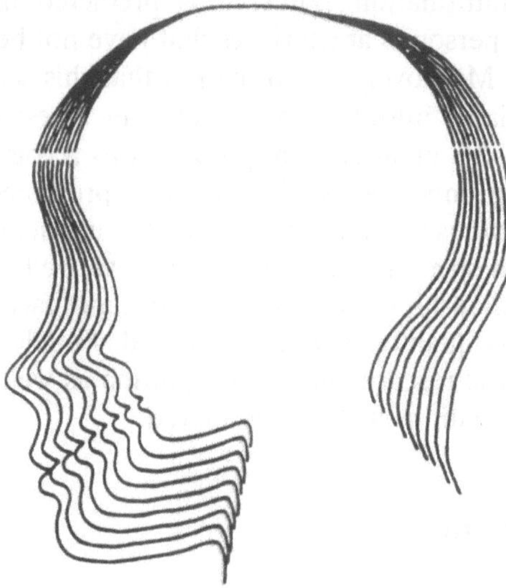

FIGURE 3.1. Consequences of the application of a growth-simulating cardioidal strain transformation to a standard profile. (From "The perception of human growth," by J.T. Todd, L.S. Mark, R.E. Shaw, and J.B. Pittenger, 1980, *Scientific American, 242,* p. 133. Reprinted by permission.)

growth is not perceived in profiles subjected to other geometric transformations. Moreover, judgments are influenced by these changes even when they only slightly exceed the threshold for visual sensitivity. Parallel results have been revealed when three-dimensional facial models are subjected to cardioidal strain (Mark & Todd, 1983, 1985; Mark, Todd, & Shaw, 1981; Pittenger & Shaw, 1975; Shaw & Pittenger, 1977). Sensitivity to this information has also been revealed at a very young age (Montepare & McArthur, 1986).

Thus, a particular, measurable facial event gives rise to the perception of growth or aging. Shaw and his colleagues further propose that information about age is specified by the abstract style of change simulated by cardioidal strain (e.g., Pittenger & Shaw, 1975). However, an alternative explanation of the data is that growth is recognized from a comparison of these stimuli with stored representations of what faces look like at different age levels. In order to assess this possibility, Pittenger, Shaw, and Mark (1979) presented subjects with stimuli produced by applying the strain transformation to drawings of Volkswagens. Pittenger et al. reasoned that if perceptions of aging were derived from experientially based stored representations, transformed inanimate objects would not be identified as growing; if we never see cars grow, on what could stored representations be based? However, if growth was instead specified by the *event* transforming a stimulus, nongrowing objects subjected to a growth transformation should also be perceived as aging. The results supported the event perception hypothesis: Volkswagens characterized by lower levels of strain were judged to be "younger" than were those featuring greater levels of strain. This effect has been replicated with other nongrowing objects (Shaw & Carello; 1979; see also Mark, Shapiro, & Shaw, 1986).

Perceptions of Age-Related Person Qualities

The configuration of the head and face undergoes a lawful set of changes as a function of age. Moreover, the work of Shaw and his associates suggests that knowledge about age is specified by the visual manifestations of that slow facial event. One reason for perceivers' keen sensitivity to this information is thought to be the adaptive significance of the recognition of maturational status. Extending this line of reasoning, it has been proposed that person qualities that are both correlated with maturational status and vital to detect may also be revealed by visible morphological consequences of growth. This idea finds its origins in the writings of the early ethologists. For example, Lorenz (1943) suggested that infants' facial characteristics, such as a large cranium and full cheeks, serve to elicit responses from adults that increase their chances of survival. More specifically, these characteristics were proposed to inhibit aggression and encourage caregiving toward an infant.

Some research has provided evidence that perceptions of age-related needs and abilities are influenced by growth-related craniofacial changes. For example, Alley (1983) showed subjects frontal versions of a schematic infant face to which a cardioidal strain transformation had been applied. Participants were asked to indicate which versions they would feel most obligated to defend from a beating. The "younger" profiles (in terms of strain level) were chosen as the most defense-provoking. Alley found parallel results when a similar judgment was made of profiles developed from cephalic x-rays of a child taken at 3, 57, 105, and 180 months: Younger profiles were thought to be more defense-provoking than were older profiles.

McArthur (1982, reported in Berry & McArthur, 1986) assessed the impact of craniofacial growth on a variety of additional perceptions. Subjects in this study were shown profiles representing seven different levels of cardioidal strain. These were viewed one at a time in different random orders. During each presentation, participants were asked to judge a profile on a different bipolar trait scale. Despite the subtle differences between adjacent levels of the profiles, increasing strain (age) exerted a powerful linear effect on perceptions. For example, more mature profiles were perceived to be stronger, more threatening, and sexier than were younger profiles.

The research just described reveals that perceivers are very adept at recognizing age-related person qualities on the basis of appearance characteristics. One interpretation of these data is that information about the needs and abilities of people of different ages is available in the facial consequences of growth. An alternative explanation, which warrants consideration, again relies on the use of preexisting knowledge structures: Perceivers may recognize that a stimulus person belongs to a particular age level and then use their relevant schema (or equivalent structure) to provide them with knowledge about the stimulus person's likely characteristics.

How can one test these competing hypotheses? They are not empirically distinguishable on the basis of the Alley and McArthur data just reported; cardioidal strain exerts a powerful impact on perceived age; thus, perceived age was confounded with age-related variations in facial appearance in these studies. However, if age level could be held constant and feature configuration varied, it would be possible to assess the impact of feature configuration on perception independent of age. In this situation, the age-mediation hypothesis predicts that variations in feature configuration will not influence perceptions of age-related behavioral propensities. Alternatively, if this information is specified in visible consequences of maturation, rather than dependent on stored knowledge about age, one would predict variations in these perceptions.

This provides a way to assess how perceivers acquire knowledge about age-related behavioral propensities. But if age and facial configuration indeed share a lawful relationship due to growth, how can configurations vary within a given age level? As discussed previously, growth exerts constraints on the style of *change* that accompanies age rather than on the underlying *structure* which grows. This transformation (and its accompanying facial consequences) is therefore invariant over different structures (faces): Everyone will have a smaller chin, larger forehead, and lower feature placement as a child than as an adult. However, due to individual differences in the facial structures transformed by growth, there will also be configural differences in faces at any particular age level: Some adults will have smaller chins, larger foreheads, and/or lower feature placements than will other adults. These naturally occurring differences in base structure allow an investigation of the impact of such stimulus variations on perceptions independent of age. Therefore, it was predicted that variations in characteristics such as the chin size and feature placement of adult faces would account for large proportions of the variance in perceptions of their power and approachability (Berry & McArthur, 1986).

Facial Babyishness

The issue of whether knowledge about age-related needs and abilities is specified in age-related facial qualities or dependent on a process of age-labeling gave rise to research on facial "babyishness." Berry and McArthur (1985) predicted that more childlike psychological qualities would be perceived in adult faces that exhibit relatively babyish feature configurations than in adult faces with more mature-appearing features. Moreover, it was predicted that these relationships would not be dependent on differences in the perceived ages of faces. In order to test these hypotheses, perceptions of 20 adult Caucasian male faces were obtained. Subjects rated the faces on trait dimensions, scales of attractive/unattractive, and mature-faced/baby-faced, and judged the age of each face. Measurements of the faces were also obtained.

Analyses revealed that, as expected, the judged babyishness of a face was positively correlated with its perceived warmth, honesty, kindness, and naiveté. Partial correlation analyses in which ratings of age and attractiveness were controlled further revealed that these variables did not account for the relationships observed between babyfacedness and impressions. Several facial measures were also found to correlate with perceived facial babyishness. In particular, a composite of two measures—chin width and eye size—together accounted for 57% of the variance in these ratings. These dimensions both reflect differences between infant and adult faces that result from growth and had been predicted to influence judgments of babyfacedness. Moreover, these two measures accounted for almost as much of the variation in trait ratings as had perceived babyishness. These results have since been replicated with a sample of Korean perceivers (McArthur & Berry, 1987; Experiment 2).

McArthur and Apatow (1983–1984) directly assessed the impact of variations in particular age-related facial characteristics on impressions by manipulating the babyishness of schematic adult faces. Facial configuration was manipulated along three dimensions that distinguish infant faces from those of adults: eye size, feature length, and the positioning of facial features on the vertical plane of the face. Results revealed that these manipulations were indeed successful in altering the perceived babyishness of the faces. In addition, variations in facial configuration exerted a strong impact on perceptions of the stimulus faces: those with babyish configurations (large eyes, short features, and low feature placement) were judged to be physically weaker and more submissive, naive, and honest than were those with more mature configurations (small eyes, long features, and high feature placement) (see Figure 3.2). As in earlier research, these effects were not attributable to differences in the perceived age or attractiveness of the faces. McArthur and Berry (1987, Experiment 1) replicated this work with native Korean subjects and again found impressive cross-cultural agreement in judgments of the stimulus faces.

The effects of facial babyishness on social perception have since been replicated with a number of samples of photographed and videotaped faces (e.g., Berry, 1990a, 1991a; Berry & Brownlow, 1989; Zebrowitz-McArthur & Montepare, 1989). In addition, several studies have provided evidence that facial babyishness exerts a predictable impact on more

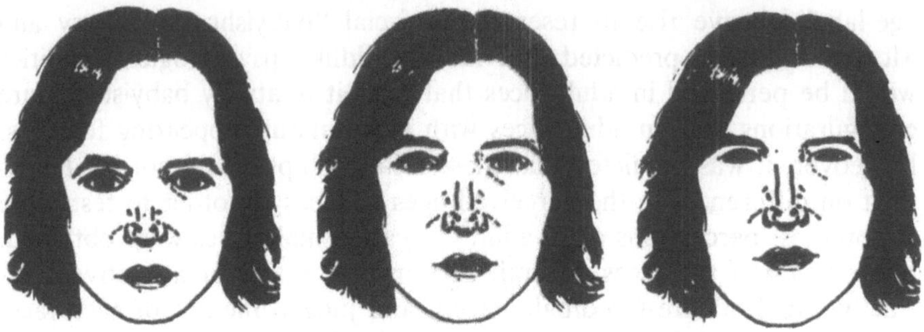

FIGURE 3.2. Sample schematic faces. Vertical feature placement, feature length, and eye size have manipulated to create high babyish (left); medium babyish (center); and low babyish (right) versions of the face. (From "Cross-cultural agreement in perceptions of babyfaced adults," by L.Z. McArthur and D.S. Berry, 1987, *Journal of Cross-Cultural Psychology, 18,* p. 171. Reprinted by permission.)

complex judgments of stimulus persons when information in addition to facial appearance is available. For example, Berry and McArthur (1988) reported that subjects were more likely to believe that a baby-faced male "defendant" had committed an offense resulting from negligence than from premeditated intent, whereas the opposite pattern was observed for maturefaced male "defendants." Zebrowitz, Tenenbaum, and Goldstein (1991) also found that subjects perceived baby-faced job applicants to be more appropriate than mature-faced applicants for a teaching position at a day-care center.

In a more naturalistic appraisal of the impact of facial babyishness on impressions, Brownlow and Zebrowitz (1990) asked subjects to judge the facial appearance of male and female actors who appeared in 146 television commercials. Different subjects also assessed the content of written transcripts of the commercials. Specifically, the transcripts were rated on the trustworthiness and expertise of the type of persuasive appeal featured in each. The results revealed that more mature-faced individuals appeared as spokespersons in commercials featuring appeals judged to be expert, whereas baby-faced persons were cast in those utilizing trustworthy appeals. Moreover, these effects could not be explained by differences in the perceived age or attractiveness of baby-faced and mature-faced spokespersons. Thus, casting directors appear to "know" that honest and trustworthy messages are most believable when communicated by baby-faced individuals, and messages characterized by knowledge and expertise are most convincing when provided by mature-faced individuals. Whether this knowledge is implicit or whether casting directors have explicit guidelines regarding the facial qualities of actors whom they select for different roles is an open question.

Accuracy of Perceptions Produced by Facial Babyishness

Investigations of first impressions of baby-faced adults have revealed that it is not necessary to identify individuals as varying in age in order to perceive them as differing in age-related person qualities. Rather, perceivers can extract information about physical and social power and approachability from the facial qualities that are correlated with maturational status. Moreover, when these facial qualities appear out of context, as in the case of a baby-faced adult, they continue to communicate this information. The expectations elicited by features such as large eyes, protruding foreheads, and narrow chins are clearly veridical in the case of infants. Is there any evidence of the validity of first impressions of adults with babyish facial configurations?

Berry (1990a) reported that impressions based on static facial appearance do persist over extended acquaintance. Specifically, subjects participating in a psychology course provided their impressions of one another during the first, fifth, and ninth weeks of the semester. Judgments of facial photographs of the subjects were also provided by a separate group of unacquainted raters. Impressions of the photographs were revealed to be significant predictors of classmates' impressions of one another at each point in the semester. For example, people judged to be dominant on the basis of a photograph were also thought to be dominant by classmates who had been acquainted with them for nine weeks.

Why might facially based impressions persist when additional information is made available to perceivers? One explanation of the data is the so-called kernel of truth hypothesis (Berry & Finch Wero, 1993; McArthur, 1982). This suggests that impressions based on facial appearance may be reliable because they are at least partially accurate. Berry (1990a) conducted a second study to evaluate the utility of the kernel of truth hypothesis for explaining the persistence of facially based perceptions. Stimulus persons completed several personality and self-report measures. In addition, a group of raters unacquainted with the stimulus persons made judgments of them on the basis of facial photographs. Analyses revealed substantial correspondence between facially based impressions and self-ratings. For example, people whose faces were judged to be dominant and powerful were also high scorers on the Rathus Assertiveness Scale (Rathus, 1973), high scorers on the Aggression subscale of the Multidimensional Personality Questionnaire (Tellegen, in press), and rated themselves as high on the trait scales of dominance and strength. Moreover, analyses revealed that facial babyishness mediates the relations between some of these self-ratings and the judged power of faces. In particular, aggression scores are negatively related to facial babyishness. At least two additional studies support this last point: Berry and Brownlow (1989) and Berry (1991b) also report negative correlations between self-reported aggression and facial babyishness in different samples of stimulus persons.

What mechanisms might produce the correspondence between facial configuration and these measures of disposition? One possible explanation is the self-fulfilling prophecy model (e.g., Langlois, 1986). Facial appearance may produce expectations that are repeatedly communicated to individuals and ultimately internalized. For example, a baby-faced person may be consistently treated as though he or she were submissive, and eventually consider him- or herself to be submissive. Such behavioral confirmation effects have indeed been found to occur as a function of facial attractiveness (Snyder, Tanke, & Berscheid, 1977). An alternative possibility that has received less attention is that a larger number of person qualities are perceptually specified than has been generally assumed. In fact, recent research has revealed that a variety of complex person characteristics are lawfully related to and revealed by dynamic, nonverbal information (Berry, 1988, 1990b). However, in the research just reported, impressions of *static* facial apearance predicted self-judgments and judgments after acquaintance. Why would personality share a lawful relationship with static facial appearance?

A study conducted by Malatesta, Fiore, and Messina (1987) provides one illustration of how such relationships might occur. Subjects were asked to rate neutral facial photographs of older adult women for emotion expression. In addition, the women depicted in the photographs completed Izard's (1972) Differential Emotions Scale (DES), which assesses the frequency with which individuals tend to experience particular emotions. Malatesta et al. found that neutral facial poses were often mistakenly identified as a particular facial expression. Moreover, individuals' scores on the DES predicted these errors. For example, people who reported experiencing much anger exhibited neutral expressions perceived as hostile. Malatesta et al. suggest that facial qualities such as wrinkle patterns may be influenced by the frequency with which particular facial expressions are expressed.

As the participants in the research described here were young adults, this particular determinant of personality–appearance relationships probably does not account for these effects. However, recent research has indicated that people can subtly alter their facial pose in a manner that influences the babyishness of their faces, and, in turn, people's perceptions of them (Berry & Finch Wero, 1993). This suggests that people may express their dispositional properties either consciously or unconsciously, through subtle facial manipulations. Although the correlational data described here cannot address the question of whether static facial appearance shapes one's disposition through behavioral confirmation, or whether dispositional attributes create perceptible differences in static facial appearance, this would seem an important focus for future research.

The craniofacial changes that accompany growth exert a strong impact on perceptions of faces. The research reviewed here reveals that the visible consequences of facial growth influence judgments of age.

Variations in these stimulus configurations also give rise to variations in perceptions of age-related person qualities, such as physical and social power. Moreover, these impressions persist when the stimulus configurations appear out of context, as in the case of baby-faced adults. This work provides support for the proposition that knowledge about qualities such as physical and social power is provided by age-related facial configurations. This research has also revealed a major source of consensus in perceptions of adult faces. Moreover, recent work has provided evidence for some validity in these impressions. Additional research is needed to understand fully how links between facial configuration and disposition may develop.

Rapid Facial Events

Change as Information

The work discussed thus far has considered the impact of *slow* facial events on social perception. In addition to slow changes, faces exhibit patterns of *rapid* deformation, many of which play a role in human communication. In the remainder of this chapter, we will consider perceivers' ability to extract person information from these facial events. An interest in rapid dynamic information mandates that moving facial displays, rather than photographs or drawings, should be used in this research. However, live and videotaped moving faces provide both dynamic and configural information to perceivers. The research reviewed thus far clearly reveals that configural characteristics that are produced by or mimic variations in facial growth exert a strong impact on perceptions. Thus, it is difficult to ascertain the independent contribution of facial movement to impressions from displays that confound both types of information.

One research methodology designed to circumvent this problem involves filming a moving object to which small light sources are attached. The films, or videotapes, are then presented on a black-and-white monitor, adjusted so that the display appears as a configuration of bright points moving against a black background. One advantage of this point-light technique is that it highlights dynamic information, or change, while concealing information about appearance and structure.

First introduced by Johansson (1973), point-light displays have been used most extensively in studies of human gait. These displays are created by attaching point-lights to the major joints of walking persons. Still versions of the displays look like random patterns of points. Facial point-lights, however, often feature as many as 50 or 100 points. This detail is necessary in order to pick up the rather fine-grained deformations that may influence perceptions. However, the level of detail available in these displays also raises the possibility that they may retain some configural information. Thus, the demonstration that some meaning is extracted from a dynamic display is not sufficient basis in itself for attributing the meaning to the patterns of motion; it also needs to be demonstrated that still versions of the displays do not exert the same impact on perceptions. If these criteria are met, we can conclude that the rapid facial deformations that are retained in moving displays indeed provide the informational basis for perceivers' judgments.

Research investigating perceivers' sensitivity to information about affect, age-related person qualities, and gender has been conducted with point-light facial displays. In each case, it was predicted that the transformations available in dynamic versions of the displays would be sufficient to reveal these person qualities.

Emotion Perception

Perceivers' ability to detect and convey emotional state has been one area of face perception that has received extensive attention (Buck, 1984; Ekman, 1982; Shepard and Malatesta, this volume). Although some individual differences in the ability to encode and decode affective displays have been revealed (e.g., Edwards & Eder, 1987; Halberstadt, 1986), the evidence for universality in the expression and perception of emotion is impressive (e.g., Ekman et al., 1987). In fact, the individual differences that do exist are often masked in standard recognition tasks, as nearly everyone attains the functional level of performance that these tasks assess. This high level of ability is also evident at an early age, making it difficult to examine developmental differences with standard tasks after age 4 or 5. In light of the adaptive significance of encoding and decoding abilities, such data have led many to posit a biological component to this system of social communication (e.g., Buck, 1984).

Evolution-based facial displays of emotion thus share invariant components across different persons. In fact, Ekman and Izard and their associates have provided detailed analyses of the sets of muscle contractions that are lawfully related to the basic emotions (e.g., Ekman & Friesen, 1978). Given this emphasis on muscular actions in the production of emotional expressions, it is somewhat surprising that many investigations of emotion perception do not feature dynamic displays. Studies using photographic stimuli do reveal that adults are proficient at identifying primary emotions from the appearance of the facial configuration at the apex of expression. Under natural conditions, however, is such configural information the sole or the primary basis for recognition? During an interaction, rapid and invariant patterns of deformation accompany a particular emotional display. Are these sufficient for the perception of emotion?

Bassili utilized facial point-light displays to examine this question. In one set of experiments (Bassili, 1978), 100 points were affixed to the faces of four stimulus persons, who were then videotaped while displaying expressions of happiness, sadness, disgust, fear, anger, and surprise. Standard full-face videotapes of these individuals exhibiting the same six expressions were also produced. Subjects viewed the displays, and chose one of the six emotion terms listed above to describe each. Bassili found that response accuracy to the point-light stimuli was 31%; this was significantly greater than the 16.7% that would be expected by chance. Full-face displays were recognized 64% of the time. This was significantly greater than either chance or the observed accuracy level for point-light faces.

Thus, the information provided by the patterns of change that characterize emoting faces was sufficient for the identification of their affective state, although the addition of configural information to full-face displays further contributed to accuracy. However, Bassili failed to include static control displays in this research. Therefore, an alternative explanation of the data is that feature-based information retained in the point-light faces was responsible for the greater-than-chance accuracy rates attained.

In order to evaluate this explanation, a second study was conducted (Bassili, 1979). Point-light displays of the facial expressions of six stimulus persons were filmed. In addition, still versions of the point-light expressions at their apex were prepared. Replicating the earlier study, dynamic displays received greater-than-chance recognition (53% versus 16.7%). Moreover, this level of accuracy exceeded that obtained for static displays (29.4%). Thus, feature-based information is not required for emotion recognition. Rather, the dynamic styles of change that characterize facial expressions of emotion are sufficient for their identification.

Research has further revealed that sensitivity to such patterns of motion may be present at an early age. McDaniel and Odom (1983) report that by age four months, infants prefer to look at point-light facial expressions than at either a standard photograph of the apex of an expression or a point-light display of a moving plastic mask. This may indicate that sensitivity to dynamic facial information actually appears prior to the ability to extract meaning from static facial characteristics (cf. Caron, Caron, & Myers, 1982, 1985; see also Soken, Smith, Bakec, & Pick, 1989). Additional research is needed in order to examine this issue.

Perception of Age-Related Person Qualities

Earlier in this chapter, research was described that revealed that the facial consequences of growth affected perceptions of age-related person qualities. Might rapid patterns of facial change also play a role in the communication of these characteristics? Although there has been little research devoted to uncovering the specific nature of age-related changes in patterns of facial motion, there is evidence that such differences do exist. For example, developmental differences have been documented in both the production of emotional expression (e.g., Field & Walden, 1982; Odom & Lemond, 1972) and the use of facial display rules (e.g., Cole, 1986; Malatesta & Haviland, 1982). Furthermore, Malatesta and Izard (1984) observed age-related differences in the facial behaviors of young, middle-aged, and older adults. Whereas these data reveal age-related changes in discrete facial behaviors, growth-determined differences in facial anatomy could affect the general style of motion characterizing faces of different ages.

In order to examine whether veridical differences in the physical and social power of children and adults are revealed by their facial movements, Berry (1990b) prepared point-light displays of stimulus persons drawn from different age levels. Displays of 8 children (*M* age = 5.5 yrs.), 8 middle-age adults (*M* age = 36.3 yrs.), and 8 older adults (*M* age = 70.8 yrs.) were created by randomly affixing 100 2 mm pieces of light-reflectant material to their faces. Half the faces at each level belonged to each gender. The height of the faces was also made equal prior to filming through the use of a zoom lens. The stimulus persons were then filmed while they recited the alphabet and while they were involved in an interaction with a research assistant; the stimulus persons were unaware that they were being filmed during the interation. Still versions of the facial displays were also prepared.

Subjects judged the facial displays on several dimensions designed to reflect physical and social power. As these judgments were highly correlated, a composite measure of perceived power was created by computing the mean rating received by a given face from a given subject on the original scales.

Analyses revealed a significant interaction of display type and age of stimulus face. Follow-up analyses revealed that although the judged power of still faces did not vary as a function of age of face, age did exert a reliable impact on the power perceived in moving faces. Consistent with predictions, moving point-light displays of children's faces were judged to be less powerful than were those of middle-age and older adults.

Analyses also revealed that the impact of age of face on judged power was greater for interacting than for reciting faces. However, follow-up analyses revealed that the impact of age of face on perceptions of power was reliable for reciting faces as well as for interacting faces. Moreover, the pattern of these effects paralleled that previously described: Children's faces were perceived to be less powerful than were either middle-age or older adult faces (see Figure 3.3).

Judgments of the perceived age of the faces were also obtained, and analyses revealed that stimulus persons at all three age levels were judged to be adults. Therefore, it seems unlikely that perceptions of power were based on a process of age-labeling. Moreover, covariance analyses paralleling those reported above in which age ratings were statistically controlled were performed. These revealed that the reliable effects of

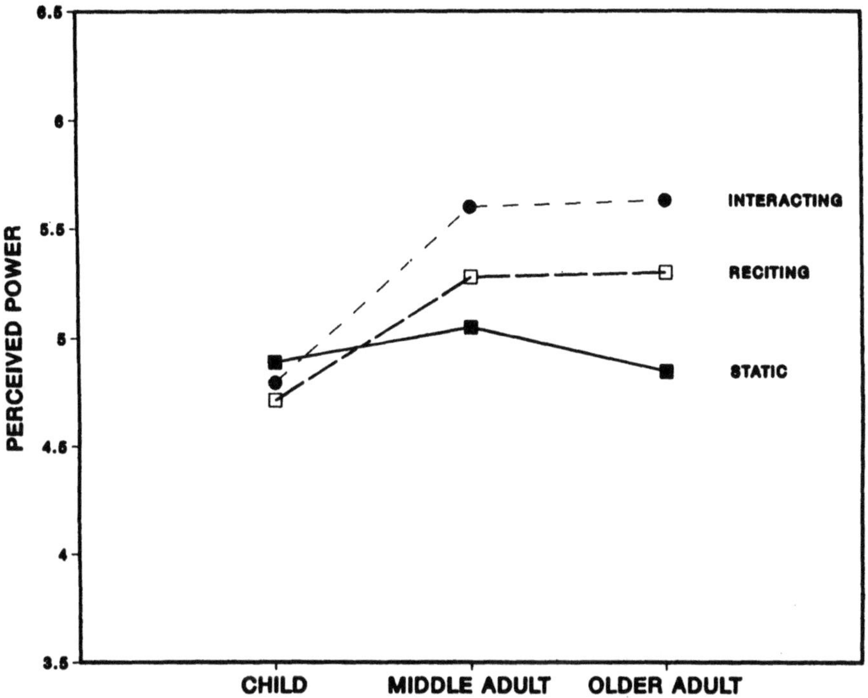

FIGURE 3.3. Judged power as a function of age of stimulus face for still, reciting, and interacting point-light faces. (From "What can a moving face tell us?," by D.S. Berry 1990, *Journal of Personality and Social Psychology, 58,* 1004–1014. Reprinted by permission.)

chronological age of face on the perceived power of the dynamic facial displays could not be explained by differences in the perceived age of the faces.

Thus, rapid facial events reveal veridical differences in the physical and social power of children and adults. The fact that parallel effects were not observed for still displays indicates that age-related variations in configural information retained in the displays were not responsible for these differences. Moreover, these effects do not require the recognition that one is viewing the face of a child or an adult. This indicates that perceptions of power were grounded in the patterns of motion that characterized the displays, rather than derived from an inferential process mediated by age-labeling. What might the specific basis of these perceptions be? The fact that the effect of age on perceived power was observed for reciting as well as interacting faces indicates that socially elicited patterns of expression are not necessary for this information to be communicated. This may suggest that some general invariant that influences all facial motion may be at least partially responsible for the effects. Additional research is needed before these questions can be satisfactorily answered.

Gender Perception

Our very presence attests to the fact that humans are skilled at differentiating others on the basis of sex, and it seems intuitive that facial qualities reveal gender. However, our understanding of the stimulus information on which such distinctions may be based is actually quite limited. For example, we know that even infants can differentiate people on the basis of gender (e.g., Lewis, 1981). Many of these studies have intentionally confounded potentially gender-revealing attributes such as facial appearance, facial movement, hairstyle, dress, and voice, in order to create prototypical male and female stimuli. As a result, they do not reveal the stimulus bases for these distinctions. There is also little known about the bases of adults' gender-identification abilities. Specifically, although it has been demonstrated that adults can identify the sex of a person from either vocal information or gait (e.g., Kozlowski & Cutting, 1977; Runeson & Frykholm, 1983), research has not assessed the impact of specific facial qualities on adults' perceptions of gender.

Both children and adults are adept at identifying the sex of a face. On what specific qualities are these discriminations based? There are several categories of facial information that could provide the basis for gender identification. First, it seems likely that gender is revealed by what Ekman (1978) calls "artificial signs": hairstyle and the presence or absence of facial hair and makeup. Second, gender identification may result from sex-related differences in facial structure or physiognomy (see Langlois, this volume). The fact that people can identify sex from standard photographs indicates that at least one of these factors does successfully convey information about gender.

A third possibility is that gender is revealed in sex-specific styles of facial motion. Although gender differences in facial movement have not been extensively studied, there is evidence that men and women exhibit different patterns of facial motion. Some of these differences appear to be socially elicited. For example, Berry (1987) found that moving female faces are judged to be more animated than are male faces, but only during an interaction. Hall has also reported that female faces are more socially expressive than are male faces (see Hall, 1985, for a review). In addition, some sex differences in facial motion may be anatomically based. For example, Alford (1983; Alford & Alford, 1981) provided evidence that males exhibit more asymmetrical facial expressions than do females and suggested that these differences may reflect gender differences in cerebral lateralization.

Using the still, reciting, and interacting point-light facial displays described previously, Berry (1991c) investigated whether patterns of facial motion are sufficient for greater-than-chance gender-identification accuracy. Adult subjects were shown 30-second clips of the point-light faces and then asked to identify whether each was male or female. As can be seen in Figure 3.4, gender was correctly identified 58% of the time for still displays. This rate was greater than what would be expected by chance, indicating that some gender information was available in the nondynamic characteristics retained in the displays. However, recognition accuracy was significantly greater for both the reciting (68%) and interacting (69%) faces than for the still displays. Thus, the patterns of facial motion available in the dynamic faces did provide gender information to adult perceivers. Interestingly, the kind of facial motion viewed did not influence accuracy; adults were as proficient at identifying the gender of faces that were reciting the alphabet as they were at recognizing the sex

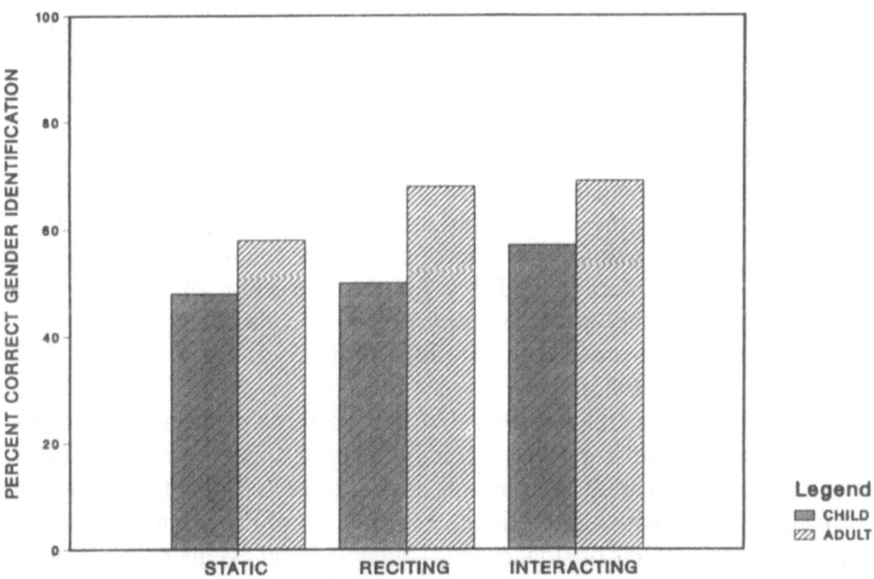

FIGURE 3.4. Proportion of accurate gender identifications as a function of subject age for still, reciting, and interacting point-light faces. (From "The perceiver as naive scientist or the scientist as naive perceiver? An ecological view of social knowledge acquisition," by D.S. Berry, 1990, *Contemporary Social Psychology*, p. 148. Reprinted by permission.)

of faces involved in a social interaction. This suggests that socially elicited facial behaviors did not constitute the informational basis for adults' judgments. Rather, some sex-related difference in the movement available in both types of displays appears to be sufficient for the perception of gender.

Berry (1991c) also measured 5-year-olds' sensitivity to gender information in point-light faces. Specifically, children viewed the facial displays that had been judged previously by adults and indicated whether they thought each was a "she" or a "he." Although their accuracy level was significantly lower than that observed for adults, children were also able to identify sex from patterns of facial movement (refer to Figure 3.4). Specifically, the proportion of correct responses for still displays (48%) and reciting faces (50%) did not differ from chance. However, the accuracy rate observed for interacting faces was greater than chance (58%). It is interesting to note the difference in the pattern of results observed for children and adults. First, unlike adults, children were not sensitive to whatever gender-revealing structural information was retained in the still displays. Second, although the addition of movement to the displays significantly increased the accuracy level for both age groups, each responded differently to the type of movement available. Specifically, the type of motion in the displays did not affect adults' gender-perception abilities: Adults were as good at extracting gender information from faces that were reciting the alphabet as they were at identifying the sex of faces involved in an interaction. However, children were only able to identify the gender of interacting faces. It seems unlikely that children, unlike adults, were sensitive to gender-linked differences in socially elicited patterns of expression. Rather, children may only detect gender-revealing invariants when they appear in the more complex, yet more natural, patterns of motion that characterize interacting faces. This may reflect a tendency for the extraction of meaning from higher-order stimulus configurations to precede the detection of information from lower-order configurations (e.g., J. J. Gibson, 1979; F. J. Gibson & Spelke, 1983).

In summary, research has revealed that patterns of facial deformation can exert a powerful impact on the identification of person characteristics. For example, both adults and infants appear to be sensitive to the patterns of facial motion that characterize the expression of the primary emotions. Paralleling the effects of slow growth–related facial events on perception, age-variant patterns of facial motion also influence the detection of age-related person qualities. Finally, 5-year-olds and adults are both able to identify the gender of a moving point-light face, although this ability improves significantly with age. These data indicate that rapid facial changes play an important role in human communication. Moreover, the kinds of person qualities revealed by these patterns of motion include, but are not limited to, affect-related states.

Summary and Implications

Recent years have witnessed a surge of interest in the topic of face perception. However, research directed toward uncovering the determinants and consequences of perceptions of faces has primarily dealt with attractiveness and emotional expression. One reason for this limited focus is the lack of a theoretical framework from which to make predictions regarding what other facial qualities give rise to what perceptions. It has been proposed here that the application of an event perception model to the study of faces can be useful for developing new hypotheses regarding relationships among facial qualities and impressions. Moreover, empirical tests of these predictions have revealed that both slow and rapid facial changes exert a powerful impact on judgments of faces. What are some of the implications of these data?

Theoretical Implications

There are at least two important implications of this work for basic research in psychology. First, it is clear that the abundance and complexity of information available in the human face is only beginning to be recognized. Moreover, the successful explication of additional stimulus–percept relationships is unlikely to be accomplished through atheoretical approaches to the problem. Facial dynamics are apparently one rich source of knowledge, and additional research on this topic seems warranted. However, the adoption of other theoretical perspectives to this domain may also prove valuable. The most crucial point may be that "breaking set" and adopting novel approaches to the problem of face perception can be a useful strategy.

A second implication of these data extends beyond the domain of face perception and takes issue with current conceptualizations of social-knowledge acquisition. A hallmark of these models is their strong emphasis on the inferential and indirect nature of social knowing. At the heart of this position is the assumption that person qualities, unlike object qualities, are "*nonobservable* attitudes . . . [For example,] both a person and a cup can be fragile, but that inferred characteristic is . . . more directly seen in the cup" (Fiske & Taylor, 1984, p. 16). However, the work described here adds to an emerging body of research on social-event perception that subjects this supposition to empirical test (cf. Baron, 1990; Berry, 1988, 1990c; McArthur & Baron, 1983). The results of these investigations challenge the claim that social qualities are not perceptually specified. For example, attributions regarding causation and intention are directed by both relational motions specifying interactions and the movement of individuals in isolation (e.g., Kassin & Baron, 1985; Runeson & Frykholm, 1983). Runeson and his associates (e.g., Runeson & Frykholm, 1983) have further demonstrated that information about deceptive intent is revealed in point-light representations of a person's actions. Berry's demonstrations that veridical differences in stimulus persons' characteristics and behavioral propensities are communicated by both static facial appearance and point-light displays of facial movement (Berry, 1990a, 1990b, 1991b) indicate that dispositional qualities can be perceptually specified. Finally, recent work has further provided evidence that the nature of the relationship between two people involved in an interaction can be recognized from point-light displays of their movements (Berry, 1990d; Good, 1987).

To the extent that perceptually based social-knowledge acquisition can be demonstrated, the assumed primacy of cognitive inference in social perception comes into question. These data do not imply that social knowledge *cannot* be attained in lieu of perceptual information. In fact, much social cognition research has repeatedly indicated that it can be. However, these investigations have been conducted in contexts void of stimulus information, thus leaving cognitive inference as the only available route by which to make a social judgment. In real life, instances of person perception almost never occur in such an environment. If it could be demonstrated that social information is not perceptually specified, this might not be particularly problematic. However, this is not the case. Person qualities do structure stimulus information, and perceivers can extract meaning from that structure. This gives rise to the rather worrisome possibility that social cognition research has provided us with a sophisticated account of the nature of social knowledge acquisition in unusual contexts which perceivers rarely encounter outside of the laboratory.[2] Clearly, an important goal of future research must be to consider the potential contribution of *both* perceptual and cognitive processes to social perception.

Implications for Craniofacial Populations

In addition to their implications for basic research, the data reported in this chapter have relevance to decisions that practitioners must make regarding the treatment of craniofacial populations. Perhaps the most fundamental implication of this research is that treatment programs that focus solely on increasing facial attractiveness are not adequate.[3] A variety

---

[2] It is also true that stimuli such as point-light displays are unusual and rarely encountered outside of the laboratoy. However, studies utilizing such displays do reveal that social knowledge acquisition *can* be perceptually based. Thus, this work emphasizes the need for a programmatic assessment of the roles of both perception and cognition in this process.

[3] Such interventions may also be questioned on the basis of two points which are beyond the scope of this discussion. First, one may question if the presence of facial anomalies is indeed equivalent to low facial attractiveness, either in terms of

of other facial qualities have also been found to exert a strong impact on person perception. Surgical procedures that impact on any of these variables may alter how individuals are perceived.

One such variable is facial babyishness. Interventions that affect the facial characteristics associated with babyishness may produce changes in how a person is perceived along dimensions such as power and approachability. Whereas a sudden shift in the nature of the expectations held about them by others could prove traumatic for adults, the alteration of features related to facial babyishness might be particularly risky for children. For example, McCabe (1984) reported that samples of abused children exhibit less babyish craniofacial proportions than nonabused samples matched on age, sex, and socioeconomic status. One explanation of these data can be drawn from Lorenz's (1943) proposition that babyish physical characteristics function to inhibit aggression in adults. Alternatively, children who exhibit mature facial features may produce expectations about their behavior that are not appropriate for their actual age level. When unable to meet those high expectations, these children may be placed at risk for abuse. Given the correlational nature of McCabe's study, additional research is needed before a causal relationship between facial configuration and abuse can be assumed. Such work would seem to have important implications for interventions that alter children's craniofacial characteristics.

The potential impact of surgical interventions on rapid patterns of facial motion also warrants consideration. For example, a procedure that improves facial attractiveness at the expense of the ability to produce a full range of facial movements may be of dubious value. An individual's social communication skills could be seriously impaired if his or her ability to produce recognizable emotional expressions, or to convey information about age- and gender-related characteristics, were limited. Thus, a full consideration of the stimulus characteristics that influence perceptions of faces is vital to making reasonable decisions about the treatment of craniofacial patients.

A second domain in which uninformed assumptions could lead to inappropriate intervention decisions involves the social and psychological

---

its impact on perception or interaction. Although most researchers and practitioners have apparently assumed this is the case, the point has not received much empirical attention (see Bull & Ramsey, 1988, for a review). Thus, research that applies principles derived from studies of attractiveness to craniofacial populations may suffer from problems with construct validity. Second, it is not clear that surgical interventions successfully improve the attractiveness of craniofacial populations. At least two lines of research give rise to this skepticism. First, researchers have had limited success in defining what the parameters of facial attractiveness indeed are. Second, pre- and postoperative judgments of the appearance of recipients of such surgeries do not provide strong support for postsurgical improvement in attractiveness (cf. Bull & Ramsey, 1988).

ramifications of exhibiting a particular appearance. When do the ultimate consequences of a change in facial appearance justify surgery? In certain cases, the objective of surgery seems clear and sound. For example, a surgical intervention that enables an individual to produce identifiable emotional expressions may be warranted. On the other hand, surgery strictly aimed at improving overall facial attractiveness may be less reasonable. Although it is certainly the case that attractiveness is accompanied by certain benefits, there are also exceptions (e.g., Dermer & Thiel, 1975; Heilman & Sarvwatari, 1979). Moreover, the relationship between attractiveness and social experience is neither straightforward nor well understood (Reis & Hodgins, this volume). Given this, surgical interventions that produce minor increases in attractiveness may not ultimately warrant either the medical risk or the financial burden they incur.

When other dimensions of facial appearance are considered, the question of what type of appearance will reap the most benefits becomes even less clear. For example, is it preferable to be baby-faced and perceived to be warm, weak, submissive, and naive; or to be mature-faced and impress others as cool, powerful, dominant, and shrewd? The answer to this question may depend upon a variety of factors, such as whether one is male or female; whether one is, in fact, submissive or dominant; and whether one's aspirations involve becoming a nursery school teacher or president of the United States.

Finally, it should be noted that the psychological impact of alterations in facial appearance will not be completely revealed by research on the social and psychological correlates of exhibiting a stable appearance. For example, the experiences of a person whose face is altered to be babyish cannot be assumed to be equivalent to those of a person who has always been baby-faced. Learning to adjust to a new set of appearance-based expectations may have unique consequences. Additional research is needed to address this issue.

Due to the highly compartmentalized nature of scientific investigation, several lines of research related to fact perception have developed in virtual isolation from one another. For example, perceptual psychologists have concentrated on identifying the stimulus determinants of perceptions of faces; social psychologists have studied the functions and consequences of those perceptions; and medical researchers have explored the anatomical bases of facial structure and motion and have developed surgical interventions by which they may be altered. One intent of this chapter is to emphasize the importance of integration among these lines of work. For example, perceptual psychologists could benefit from an understanding of the communicative and interpersonal functions of facial appearance and expression. Similarly, research in social cognition would be well served by a consideration of the perceptual bases of person perception, including those available in the face. And medical practitioners need to attain a working knowledge of both the stimulus information that gives rise to perceptions of faces and the psychological consequences of those impressions before informed decisions regarding intervention can be made. Based on intuition alone, most laypersons would probably agree that we make a life out of reading people's faces. However, only through the integration of theoretically guided research from a variety of areas will we develop a comprehensive understanding of *what* we read, and *why*.

Acknowledgments. Preparation of this chapter was supported by NIMH Grant #1-R03-MH43850-01.

References

Alford, R.D. (1983). Sex differences in lateral facial facility: The effects of habitual emotional concealment. *Neuropsychologia, 21,* 567–570.

Alford, R.D., & Alford, K.F. (1981). Sex differences in asymmetry in the facial expression of emotion. *Neuropsychologia, 19,* 605–608.

Alley, T.R. (1983). Growth produced changes in body shape and size as determinants of perceived age and caregiving. *Child Development, 54,* 241–248.

Alley, T.R. (1986). An ecological analysis of the protection of primate infants. In V. McCabe and G.J. Balzano (Eds.), *Event cognition: An ecological perspective* (pp. 239–258). Hillsdale, NJ: Erlbaum.

Baron, R.M. (1990). Towards an ecological specification of the nature of the effective stimulus for social knowing and action. *Contemporary Social Psychology, 14,* 136–144.

Bassili, J.N. (1978). Facial motion in the perception of faces and of emotional expression. *Journal of Experimental Psychology: Human Perception and Performance, 4,* 373–379.

Bassili, J.N. (1979). Emotion recognition: The role of facial movement and the relative importance of the upper and lower areas of the face. *Journal of Personality and Social Psychology, 37,* 249–258.

Berry, D.S. (1987). *Perceiving faces: Contributions of dynamic information.* Unpublished doctoral dissertation, Brandeis University, Waltham, MA.

Berry, D.S. (1988). The visual perception of people: A reply to Schmitt. *Journal for the Theory of Social Behavior, 18,* 345–354.

Berry, D.S. (1990a). Taking people at face value: Evidence for the kernel of truth hypothesis. *Social Cognition, 8,* 343–361.

Berry, D.S. (1990b). What can a moving face tell us? *Journal of Personality and Social Psychology, 58,* 1004–1014.

Berry, D.S. (1990c). The perceiver as naive scientist or the scientist as naive perceiver? An ecological view of social knowledge acquisition. *Contemporary Social Psychology, 14,* 145–153.

Berry, D.S. (1990d). *Social kinematics: An event perception view of social action and interaction.* Paper presented at the Nag's Head Conference on Interaction and Close Relationships, Nag's Head, NC.

Berry, D.S. (1991a). Attractive faces are not all created equal: Joint effects of facial babyishness and attractiveness on social perception. *Personality and Social Psychology Bulletin, 17,* 523–553.

Berry, D.S. (1991b). Accuracy in social perception: Contributions of facial and vocal information. *Journal of Personality and Social Psychology, 61,* 298–307.

Berry, D.S. (1991c) Child and adult sensitivity to gender information in patterns of facial motion. *Ecological Psychology, 3,* 349–366.

Berry, D.S., & Brownlow, S. (1989). Were the physiognomists right? Personality correlates of facial babyishness. *Personality and Social Psychology Bulletin, 15,* 266–27.

Berry, D.S., & Finch Wero, J.L. (1993). Accuracy in face perception: A view from ecological psychology. *Journal of Personality, 61,* 497–520.

Berry, D.S., & McArthur, L.Z. (1985). Some components and consequences of a babyface. *Journal of Personality and Social Psychology, 48,* 312–323.

Berry, D.S., & McArthur, L.Z. (1986). Perceiving character in faces: The impact of age-related craniofacial changes on social perception. *Psychological Bulletin, 100,* 3–18.

Berry, D.S., & McArthur, L.Z. (1988). What's in a face? Facial maturity and the attribution of legal responsibility. *Personality and Social Psychology Bulletin, 14,* 22–33.

Brownlow, S., & Zebrowitz, L.A. (1990). Facial appearance, gender, and credibility in television commercials. *Journal of Nonverbal Behavior, 14,* 51–60.

Bruce, V., & Green, P. (1985). *Visual perception*. Hillsdale, NJ: Erlbaum.

Bruce, V., & Valentine, T. (1988). When a nod's as good as a wink: The role of dynamic information in facial recognition. In M.M. Gruneberg, P.E. Morris, & R.N. Sykes (Eds.), *Practical aspects of memory,* Vol. 1 (pp. 169–174). New York: Wiley.

Buck, R. (1984). *The communication of emotion*. New York: Guilford Press.

Bull, R., & Ramsey, N. (1988). *The social psychology of facial appearance*. New York: Springer-Verlag.

Caron, R.F., Caron, A.J., & Myers, R.S. (1982). Abstraction of invariant face expressions in infancy. *Child Development, 53,* 1008–1015.

Caron, R.F., Caron, A.J., & Myers, R.S. (1985). Do infants see emotional expressions in static faces? *Child Development, 56,* 1552–1560.

Cole, P.M. (1986). Children's spontaneous control of facial expression. *Child Development, 57,* 1309–1321.

Cutting, J.E. (1986). *Perception with an eye for motion*. Cambridge, MA: MIT Press.

Davies, G., Ellis, H., & Shepherd, J. (1981). *Perceiving and remembering faces*. New York: Academic Press.

Dermer, M., & Thiel, D. (1975). When beauty may fail. *Journal of Personality and Social Psychology, 31,* 1168–1176.

Edwards, L.A., & Eder, R.A. (1987). *Individual differences in young children's sensitivity to social cues: The emergence of self-monitoring*. Paper presented at the Meeting of the Society for Research in Child Development, Baltimore, MD.

Ekman, P. (1978). Facial signs: Facts, fantasies and possibilities. In T.A. Sebeok (Ed.), *Sight, sound and sense*. Bloomington, IN: Indiana University Press.

Ekman, P. (1982). *Emotion in the human face.* Cambridge, England: Cambridge University Press.

Ekman, P., & Friesen, W.V. (1978). *The Facial Action Coding System: A technique for the measurement of facial movement.* Palo Alto, CA: Consulting Psychologists Press.

Ekman, P., Friesen, W.V., O'Sullivan, M., Chan, A., Diacoyanni-Tarlatzls, T., Heider, K., Krause, R., LeCompte, W.A., Pitcairn, T., Ricci-Bitti, P.E., Scherer, K., Tomita, M., & Tzavaras, A. (1987). Universals and cultural differences in in judgments of facial expressions of emotion. *Journal of Personality and Social Psychology, 53,* 712–717.

Ellis, H. (1981). Introduction. In G. Davies, H. Ellis, & J. Shepherd (Eds.), *Perceiving and remembering faces* (pp. 1–8). New York: Academic Press.

Field, T.M., & Walden, T.A. (1982). Production and discrimination of facial expressions by preschool children. *Child Development, 53,* 1299–1311.

Fiske, S.T., & Taylor, S.E. (1984). *Social cognition.* New York: Random House.

Gibson, E.J., & Spelke, E.S. (1983). The development of perception. In P.H. Mussen (Ed.), *Handbook of Child Psychology,* Vol. 3 (pp. 1–76). New York: Wiley.

Gibson, J.J. (1950). *The perception of the visual world.* New York: Houghton-Mifflin.

Gibson, J.J. (1979). *The ecological approach to visual perception.* Boston: Houghton Mifflin.

Good, J.M.M. (1987). *Perception, action, and inter-action: An ecological social psychology of social knowing.* Paper presented at the Fourth International Conference on Event Perception and Action, Trieste, Italy.

Halberstadt, A.G. (1986). Family socialization of emotional expression and nonverbal communication styles and skills. *Journal of Personality and Social Psychology, 51,* 827–836.

Hall, J.A. (1985). *Nonverbal sex differences.* Baltimore, MD: Johns Hopkins.

Heilman, M., & Sarvwatari, L. (1979). When beauty is beastly. *Organizational Behavior and Human Performance, 23,* 360–372.

Izard, C.E. (1972). *The Maximally Discriminative Facial Movement Coding System (Max.).* Newark, DE: University of Delaware.

Johansson, G. (1973). Visual perception of biological motion and a model for its analysis. *Perception and Psychophysics, 14,* 202–211.

Johansson, G., von Hofsten, C., & Jansson, G. (1980). Event perception. *Annual Review of Psychology, 31,* 27–63.

Kassin, S.M., & Baron, R.M. (1985). Basic determinants of attribution and social perception. In J. Harvey & G. Weary (Eds.), *Attribution: Basic issues and applications* (pp. 37–64). New York: Academic Press.

Kozlowski, L.T., & Cutting, J.E. (1977). Recognizing the sex of a walker from a dynamic point-light display. *Perception and Psychophysics, 22,* 575–580.

Langlois, J.H. (1986). From the eye of the beholder to behavioral reality: Development of social behaviors and social relations as a function of physical attractiveness. In C.P. Herman, M.P. Zanna, & E.T. Higgins (Eds.), *Physical appearance, stigma, and social behavior: The Ontario symposium,* Vol. 3 (pp. 23–52). Hillsdale, NJ: Erlbaum.

Lewis, M. (1981). Self-knowledge: A social cognitive perspective on gender identity and sex-role development. In M.E. Lamb & L.R. Sherrod (Eds.), *Infant social cognition* (pp. 395–414). Hillsdale, NJ: Erlbaum.

Lorenz, K. (1943). Die angeborenen Formen Moglicher Arfahrung. *Zietschrift für Tierpsychologie, 5,* 234–409.

Malatesta, C.Z., Fiore, M.J., & Messina, J.J. (1987). Affect, personality, and facial expressive characteristics of older people. *Psychology and Aging, 2,* 64–69.

Malatesta, C.Z., & Haviland, J.M. (1982). Learning display rules: The socialization of emotion expression in infancy. *Child Development, 53,* 991–1003.

Malatesta, C.Z., & Izard, C.E. (1984). The facial expression of emotion: Young, middle-aged and older adult expressions. In C.Z. Malatesta & C.E. Izard (Eds.), *Emotion in adult development.* Beverly Hills, CA: Sage.

Mark, L.S., Shapiro, B.A., & Shaw, R.E. (1986). Structural support for the perception of growth. *Journal of Experimental Psychology: Human Perception and Performance, 12,* 149–159.

Mark, L.S., & Todd, J.T. (1983). The perception of growth in three dimensions. *Perception and Psychophysics, 33,* 193–196.

Mark, L.S., & Todd, J.T. (1985). Describing geometric information about human growth in terms of geometric invariants. *Perception and Psychophysics, 37,* 249–256.

Mark, L.S., Todd, J.T., & Shaw, R.E. (1981). Perception of growth: A geometric analysis of how different styles of change are distinguished. *Journal of Experimental Psychology: Human Perception and Performance, 1,* 374–382.

McArthur, L.Z. (1982). Judging a book by its cover: A cognitive analysis of the relationship between physical appearance and stereotyping. In A. Hastorf & A. Isen (Eds.), *Cognitive Social Psychology.* New York: Elsevier/North-Holland.

McArthur, L.Z., & Apatow, K. (1983–1984). Impressions of baby-faced adults. *Social Cognition, 2,* 315–342.

McArthur, L.Z., & Baron, R.M. (1983). Toward an ecological theory of social perception. *Psychological Review, 90,* 215–238.

McArthur, L.Z., & Berry, D.S. (1987). Cross-cultural agreement in perceptions of babyfaced adults. *Journal of Cross-Cultural Psychology, 18,* 165–192.

McCabe, V. (1984). Abstract perceptual information for age level: A risk factor for maltreatment? *Child Development, 55,* 267–276.

McDaniel, C., & Odom, R.D. (1983). *Preferences for expressive patterns of movement in infancy.* Paper presented at the Meeting of the Society for Research in Child Development, Detroit, MI.

Montepare, J.M., & McArthur, L.Z. (1986). The influence of facial characteristics on children's age perceptions. *Journal of Experimental Child Psychology, 42,* 303–314.

Odom, R.D., & Lemond, C.M. (1972). Developmental differences in the perception and production of facial expressions. *Child Development, 43,* 359–369.

Pittenger, J.B., & Shaw, R.E. (1975). Aging faces as viscal-elastic events: Implications for a theory of nonrigid shape perception. *Journal of Experimental Psychology: Human Perception and Performance, 1,* 374–382.

Pittenger, J.B., Shaw, R.E., & Mark, L.S. (1979). Perceptual information for the age-level of faces as a higher order invariant of growth. *Journal of Experimental Psychology: Human Perception and Peformance, 5,* 478–493.

Rathus, S.A. (1973). A 30-item schedule for assessing assertive behavior. *Behavior Therapy, 4,* 398–406.

Runeson, S., & Frykholm, G. (1983). Kinematic specification of dynamics as an informational basis for person and action perception: Expectation, gender recognition, and deceptive intention. *Journal of Experimental Psychology: General, 112,* 580–610.

Schiff, W., Banka, L., & de Bordes Galdi, G. (1986). Recognizing people seen in events via dynamic mugshots. *American Journal of Psychology, 99,* 219–231.

Shaw, R.E., & Carello, C. (1979). *Are faces special?* Paper presented at the Meeting of the Psychonomics Society, Phoenix, AZ.

Shaw, R.E., & Pittenger, J.B. (1977). Perceiving the face of change in changing faces: Implications for a theory of object perception. In R. Shaw & J. Bransford (Eds.), *Perceiving, acting and knowing: Toward an ecological psychology.* Hillsdale, NJ: Erlbaum.

Snyder, M., Tanke, E.D., & Berscheid, E. (1977). Social perception and interpersonal behavior: On the self-fulfilling nature of social stereotypes. *Journal of Personality and Social Psychology, 35,* 656–664.

Soken, N., Smith, L., Bakec, C., & Pick, A.D. (1989). *Intermodal perception of fully illuminated and point-light displays of dynamic facial expressions by 7-month-old infants.* Paper presented at the Meeting of the Society for Research in Child Development, Kansas City, MO.

Tellegen, A. (in press). *The Multidimensional Personality Questionnaire.* Minneapolis, MN: National Computer Services.

Todd, J.T., & Mark, L.S. (1981). Issues related to prediction of craniofacial growth. *American Journal of Orthodontics, 79,* 63–80.

Todd, J.T., Mark, L.S., Shaw, R.E., & Pittenger, J.B. (1980). The perception of human growth. *Scientific American, 242,* 106–114.

Warren, W.H., & Shaw, R.E. (1985). Events and encounters as units of analysis for ecological psychology. In W.H. Warren, Jr. & R.E. Shaw (Eds.), *Persistence and change* (pp. 1–28). Hillsdale, NJ: Erlbaum.

Zebrowitz-McArthur, L., & Montepare, J.M. (1989). Contributions of a babyface and childlike voice to impressions of moving and talking faces. *Journal of Nonverbal Behavior, 13,* 189–203.

Zebrowitz, L.A., Tenenbaum, D., & Goldstein, L. (1991). The impact of job applicants' facial maturity, sex, and academic achievement on hiring decisions. *Journal of Applied Social Psychology, 21,* 525–548.

4
Socioemotional Development in Children with Craniofacial Anomalies

BETH SHEPARD AND CAROL MAGAI

Infants suffering from facial disfigurement would seem to be at risk in their socioemotional development. In adults, facial disfigurement tends to provoke discomfort and gaze aversion in others. There is no reason to assume that infants with facial disfigurement provoke less discomfort in observers. Moreover, it is conceivable that even caregivers may experience such feelings, perhaps compounded by a sense of guilt, and yet they must interact closely with their infants. This poses an emotional dilemma for the parents as well as a real risk for the infants.

The above assumptions seem intuitively reasonable but need to be examined more critically in light of current theoretical formulations about socioemotional development as well as research findings. This is the task we have undertaken in this chapter.

We begin with a brief historical overview of the study of emotions, followed by a more detailed presentation of what is meant by socioemotional development. We then consider the relative contributions of mother and infant to this process. In considering the impact of craniofacial anomalies on socioemotional development, we examine what limited data already exist and draw on other areas of research that might have a bearing on this topic. Finally, we present suggestions for future research in this area.

History of the Study of Emotions

Before discussing what is included under the rubric of "socioemotional development," a brief history of the study of emotions in psychology is warranted as a means of understanding how and why socioemotional development has become such a rich and timely area of study.

Historically, the study of emotions has captured both intense interest and heated debate (Cannon, 1927; James, 1884) and, at the other extreme, scornful indifference and even predictions of its demise (Duffy, 1934). The earliest work on emotion concerned itself with questions of causation, the importance of expression, and the ordering of physiological events (Cannon, 1927; Darwin, 1872 [1975]; James, 1884). Developmental aspects were rarely considered. During the 1920s and 1930s, as behaviorism became a dominant theoretical force, the study of facial expression, as directly observable behavior, became a natural focus of research, and infants became natural subjects for observation and study as a means of testing ideas concerning innate vs. learned behavior (see, for example, Pratt, 1954; Sherman, 1927a, 1927b; Watson & Raynor, 1920). One of the first developmentally oriented theories of emotion was also to emerge during this time. Encouraged by the new attention to emotion and by her own observational studies of infants and children, Bridges (1930, 1932) was led to propose an ontogenetic theory of early emotion. She was to argue that infants enter the world in an emotionally undifferentiated state and that only through maturation do more discrete emotions evolve.

Little further headway on the development of emotions was made during the decades of the 1940s and 1950s, due to the hegemony of activation theory, a view that discredited the notion of discrete emotions as meaningful constructs, behaviors, or experiences. During the 1960s, there were a few scattered studies involving emotional behaviors, including those of Kagan (1962), who explored social smiling; Walk and Gibson (1961), who examined the response of infants to placement on the visual cliff; and Schacter and Singer (1962), who examined the influence of context on emotion attribution. Upon closer inspection, however, these studies were primarily concerned with memory, depth perception, and cognitive processes, respectively, rather than with emotions as important independent variables in their own right (Campos, Barrett, Lamb, Stenberg, & Goldsmith, 1983).

Beginning in the 1970s, in part because of Spitz's pioneering work with institutionalized infants (Spitz, 1965), and in part because of Bowlby's and Ainsworth's seminal research on infant attachment (Ainsworth, Blehar, Waters, & Wall, 1978; Bowlby, 1969) a dramatic reevaluation of the importance of emotions in development began to replace the earlier neglect of emotions theory and research (Campos et al., 1983; Lamb, 1988; Malatesta, Culver, Tesman, & Shepard, 1989). An additional impetus for the study of emotions in general and their development in infancy more specifically came from advances in technology that facilitated measurement of emotional responses.

Socioemotional Development: The New Terrain

The term *socioemotional development* is used to denote an emerging field of inquiry that is concerned with intra- as well as interpersonal aspects of emotional development. Intrapersonal issues include feeling states and nonverbal behaviors, vocalization, gesture, and facial expressions of emotion and "personality" (Campos et al., 1983). Interpersonal concerns include "mechanisms underlying the formation of enduring emotional bonds or relationships to specific people. . . ." (Lamb, 1988, p. 360). As the field has matured, there has emerged a number of different theoretical perspectives on socioemotional development, including those of Campos et al. (1983), Izard (1977, 1979), Lewis and Michaelson (1983), and Sroufe (1979). Lewis and Michaelson (1983), for example, suggest that the infant enters the world in an emotionally undifferentiated state. In the course of cognitive maturation and in the context of socialization by caregivers, the infant learns how and what to feel. In this framework, facial expressions per se have little to do with emotional experiences. Sroufe (1979) has advanced a position that similarly emphasizes the role of cognition, arguing that "true" emotions do not emerge until emotional growth and differentiation begins and other cognitive milestones have been achieved. Facial activity is relatively unimportant, since affective experience is based on cognition, not facial expressions. Refer to Campos et al. (1983), Izard (1977), and Malatesta et al. (1989) for a more detailed treatment of these positions as well as those of other theorists.

Our perspective on socioemotional development coincides with that of Izard's discrete emotion theory. Proponents of discrete emotions theory (Ekman, 1973; Izard, 1971, 1977; Plutchik, 1980) typically accept Darwin's original premise that basic human emotions are essential for both biological and social adaptation of the species and, more specifically, that the facial expressions of emotion serve both as motivational signals to the self and communicative links with the social surround. Emotions are considered the primary motivators of behavior and contribute to the growth and differentiation of personality.

The theory itself derives its name from emphasis on a limited number of discrete, differentiated, fundamental emotions, which are characterized as having distinct phenomenological, motivational, and signal properties. Each of the primary emotions is said to affect broad domains of behavior in distinctive and characteristic ways. Because discrete emotions have individual signal properties (i.e., differential facial, vocal, and gestural features), they provide important communicative links between individuals. In early development, facial and vocal expressions of emotion figure prominently in the child's ability to communicate his or her needs and establish affective bonds with the caregiver. The eight basic emotions are joy, interest/excitement, surprise/startle, distress/anguish, shame/shyness, sadness, fear, and anger; while certain of these are functionally present at birth, others emerge as a result of maturation and adaptational demands. Each of the basic emotions includes motor-expressive, neurochemical, and mental components. Cognition plays in increasingly important role as the system matures and the child learns to label his or her emotions. However, since emotions are grounded on neurophysiological behaviors, much of early emotional behavior is innate and stereotyped. Discrete emotion theory is considerably more complex than can be described here. For a more complete discussion of the theory, refer to Izard (1977), Izard and Malatesta (1987), and Malatesta et al. (1989).

The ability to identify discrete emotions was greatly enhanced during the late 1970s, with the development of microanalytic facial coding systems. One such system, specifically designed for application with infant facial expressions, is called the Maximally Discriminative Facial Movement Coding System, or MAX (Izard, 1979). In this system, three regions of the face are individually assigned numerical codes based on a second-by-second analysis of changes in the facial musculature. The codes are then used in conjunction with formulas that are provided in a manual that accompanies the training videotape. The formulas distinguish the eight fundamental emotions enumerated above. We should note, however, prior to proceeding to the literature on children with craniofacial anomalies, that the MAX system may be difficult to apply to such children. Malformations of bone structure and muscular deviations may preclude the use of such a microanalytic system as MAX with these infants, although this has yet to be established.

Microanalytic facial coding systems such as MAX have allowed us to discern the subtleties of a primary avenue of affective communication. The MAX system becomes particularly significant when it is considered that, despite the fact that the human face makes up only 3% of total body surface (Epsteen, 1958), it is one of the most important vehicles for interpersonal communication and is the basis for the expression and communication of emotion (Ekman, 1978). In the infant, prior to the development of language, facial expressions and other signs of emotion, such as gestures and vocalizations, constitute the only medium of communication. This early form of expressivity is also essential for the establishment of the attachment relationship between caregiver and child.

The study of the facial expression of emotion during infancy has helped to illuminate the process of emotions ontogenesis and the development of attachment as well as aid in the clarification of the contributions of both infant and mother to this process. Studies of face-to-face interaction have been popular paradigms for the study of early emotional development; recently, this methodology has been extended to include special groups, such as blind infants (Fraiberg, 1979), abused and neglected infants (Gaensbauer & Mrazek, 1981; Schneider-Rosen, Braunwald, Carlson, & Cicchetti, 1985), and handicapped infants (Wasserman & Allen, 1985). Obviously, this method of investigation can be of use with mothers and infants with craniofacial anomalies as well.

Turning now to the group of focus in this chapter, it is believed that children with craniofacial anomalies are at risk for disturbances in socioemotional development as well as in their attachments to their caregivers. Since children with facial disfigurement have, by definition, deformities in the facial area, the sensory feedback that they receive from their own expressions may alter the nature of their affective experiences. Correspondingly, caregivers may find their expressions difficult to interpret or to empathize with. The caregiver's ability to relate to such a child may also be impaired because of the parents' sense of dealing with a "damaged" child; despite their best intentions, parents may be repelled by the defective child, which may cause avoidance or, conversely, overcompensatory nurturance. It should also be considered that many infants suffering from craniofacial anomalies and, indeed, many other high-risk children, such as preterm infants, often have extended hospital stays immediately following birth. If this is not enough to impede the establishment of the affectional tie between mother and infant, the process of corrective surgery for many facial disfigurements is often a long, drawn-out process, which may further impede normal bonding and socioemotional growth and development (Field & Vega-Lahr, 1984). In any case, it is clear that both partners will be affected by the nature of the disfigurement, although the extent to which they are affected and the relative impact on parent and child has yet to be determined. Still, some initial research would seem to shed some light on the topic.

In the next section of this chapter, we discuss both infants' and mothers' contributions to the process of socioemotional development.

Maternal Contributions to Socioemotional Development

Caregivers play an important role in the socialization of emotional expression and in the affective, experiential development of their children. Mothers "read" and respond to behavioral signs of emotional expression and, in so doing, influence the subsequent expression of emotion (Haviland, Malatesta, & Lelwica, 1984). Bowlby (1969) has argued that early face-to-face interaction between mother and infant is of paramount importance for the development of the attachment bond. A substantial body of literature now exists detailing the manner in which affectional ties develop; this literature highlights the special importance of infant affective signals (their clarity, reliability, and signal value) as well as the nature of maternal responsivity (its appropriateness, contingency, and sensitivity). These factors would seem to be no less important for mothers and infants with craniofacial anomalies. However, the developmental profile of such dyads may differ considerably from that of their nonaffected counterparts. Indeed, there is mounting evidence that differences in affective communication exist between this group and nonafflicted mother–infant pairs.

These differences may begin as early as birth. Several researchers interested in maternal reactions to the birth of facially disfigured infants have conducted retrospective interviews with mothers. Tisza and

Gumpertz (1962) reported that mothers of infants born with cleft palates experience acute grief reactions and often express feelings of sadness, hurt, shame, resentment, self-blame, and isolation. In a study that contrasted the experience of normal and cleft palate mother–infant pairs, Brantley and Clifford (1980) found that mothers of cleft palate infants experienced more anxiety concerning their infants' futures and less positive feelings about themselves than did mothers of normal infants. Clifford and Crocker (1971), using similar populations, found that all mothers expressed positive changes in themselves as a result of giving birth; however, mothers of normal infants expressed a greater degree of positive change, while mothers of cleft palate infants additionally reported experiencing "shock" when told that their infants suffered from facial disfigurement. Aamot (1978) argues that the initial reaction of fear to infants with anomalies is automatic. Easson contends that parents of facially disfigured infants must cope with anger, disappointment, and bitterness (Easson, 1966).

While all these studies concur that there are a number of negative emotions evoked upon giving birth to a facially disfigured infant, it is important to point out that all studies were retrospective; children ranged in age from approximately 6 months to 18 years of age when mothers completed the study questionnaires. As such, there had perhaps been ample time for mothers to adjust to their infants' anomalies as well as to distance themselves from their initial emotional reactions. Thus, original emotional reactions may be even more profound than those described above. There is debate within the literature as to the duration of the negative emotional response. While some studies report that initial negative emotional reactions are replaced fairly quickly with more positive responses (Tisza & Gumpertz, 1962), other studies imply that negative feelings continue unabated for an extended period of time (Clifford & Crocker, 1971; Norval, Larson, & Parshall, 1964).

In what is perhaps the most comprehensive attempt to date to specify parental reactions to infants with facial disfigurement, Wasserman and Allen (1985) videotaped normal, preterm, and a mixed group of physically handicapped infants at 9, 12, 18 and 24 months of age in a "free play" paradigm with their mothers. At 12 months, the Bayley Mental Development Scale was administered to all infants; and at 24 months, all verbal children were administered the Stanford-Binet. Videotapes were scored for maternal ignoring behavior. Results reveal that maternal ignoring was uncommon for any group under the age of 18 months; however, at 24 months, mothers of physically handicapped infants showed significantly more ignoring than either of the other two groups. When this handicapped group was broken down more discretely, it was determined that mothers of children suffering from facial anomalies accounted for all ignoring behavior. When cognitive capacities were taken into account, it was revealed that maternal ignoring was specific to the combination of congenital facial disfigurement and poor cognitive performance. Wasserman and Allen acknowledge that while the immediate postpartum period may be particularly tumultuous for mothers of facially disfigured infants, they argue that their results indicate continuing disturbance of mother–infant interaction.

Mothers of children suffering from craniofacial anomalies may also be at risk for conveying "mixed emotional messages" to their infants, albeit quite unwittingly. Mixed messages occur when emotional expression from different channels (for example, the face and the voice) present conflicting and incongruent information to the infant. Mothers struggling with feelings of guilt and depression while simultaneously attempting to interact normally with their infants may present a confusing affective picture. In a study with normal infants, Barrett (1984) had an experimenter present an angry voice/happy face (or vice versa) to infants in a novel situation. Infants responded with ambivalence, as indexed by the increased expression of a concerned smile, an atypical expression combining a smile with a knit brow. They also spent greater amounts of time looking at the face of the experimenter, the thinking being that the infant was attempting to disambiguate the conflicting message. While there have been no studies to date that have examined the long-term consequences of such confusing messages, Barrett's study revealed that even brief exposure to mixed messages had a significant effect on infants' emotional behavior. We would hypothesize similar findings for infants suffering from craniofacial anomalies.

While maternal reactions to their infants' disfigurement are clearly implicated in the children's socioemotional development, the reactions of others may be similarly contributory, as the literature on perceived infant attractiveness would seem to indicate. Very little research has explored adults' reactions to facially disfigured infants, though studies exploring adults' reactions to facially disfigured adults reveal that adults express disgust and revulsion, immediately followed by pity, that they avoid eye contact with the facially disfigured (Epsteen 1958), and that physically normal persons feel "uncomfortable" when interacting with a physically handicapped person (Davis, 1961; Kleck, 1966). When considering infants, experimental and observational studies have shown that more physically attractive infants are perceived and evaluated in a more positive light (Adams, 1977; Berschied & Walster, 1974). Ethological studies reveal that infantile facial features rated most attractive include large eyes in the middle of the face, fat cheeks, a small nose and mouth, and a high forehead (Gardner & Wallach, 1965; Hess, 1970). Features associated with attractiveness are also perceived in terms of "babyishness" (Berry & McArthur, 1985). Studies have shown that perceived attractiveness is related to the similarity of features that the infants share with the parents and that this results in enhancing mothers' feelings of closeness to their infants (Robson & Moss, 1970). Another study showed that judges gazed longer at infant faces that they perceived as "cuter" (Hildebrandt & Fitzgerald, 1979), and yet another (Power, Hildebrandt, & Fitzgerald, 1982) revealed that judges were influenced by the expression on the infant's face. In a study designed to understand the Power et al. finding more fully, Hildebrandt (1983) utilized photos of infants in various emotional states and asked one set of judges to rate the infants on "cuteness" and another set of judges to rate the same photos on a continuum of positive to negative expression. This study attempted to determine how perceived cuteness can be influenced by changes in facial expression. While infants were rated as cuter when they exhibited more positive facial expressions than when rated as displaying negative expressions, the most important determinant was the overall cuteness rating; those infants judged more cute overall were rated more highly for both positive and negative facial expressions, leading the author to conclude that the general perception of cuteness is more important than changes in facial expression in determining overall attractiveness.

Collectively, the research of the two literatures just cited help to interpret a study by Field and Vega-Lahr (1984). This study is one of the few investigations that has compared infants with craniofacial anomalies to normal counterparts. The two groups of infants were videotaped in face-to-face interaction with their mothers at three months of age; researchers then examined the tapes for differences in patterns of gazing, smiling, and vocalization. Results indicated that mothers of infants with craniofacial anomalies spent similar amounts of time looking at their infants as mothers of normal infants; however, they smiled and vocalized less with their infants than did the other mothers. The craniofacial anomaly infants themselves also smiled and vocalized less than did their nondisfigured counterparts. Field and Vega-Lahr find their results puzzling when compared to other studies of high-risk mother–infant interactions. Studies with other such groups find that mothers of these infants are often more active in their attempts to engage their infants (Beckwith & Cohen, 1980; Field, 1977; Goldberg, Brachfeld, & DiVitto, 1980). However, over time, mothers may become disengaged when their babies remain unresponsive, gaze avert, or cry in order to escape the excessive stimulation, as indicated in a study by Malatesta et al. (1989). Another reason for disengagement may stem from the difficulty that caregivers have in accurately reading the expressions of craniofacial anomaly infants; such difficulty would impair their ability to sustain continued responsive contact with their infants. Finally, it is also possible that maternal depression and sadness over the children's deformities continues beyond the postpartum period, and this may account for the mothers' decreased rates of smiling and vocalizing to their infants. In light of the above, it is clear that both mothers and children may be affected by the children's disfigurement and that their interactive competence will conceivably be compromised. It is apparent that interactive patterns between mothers and their facially disfigured children are already different from those of nonaffected dyads at an early age and that such patterns may lead to continuing interactive difficulties.

The importance of maternal facial affective communication is also underscored in studies of social referencing (Sorce, Emde, Campos, & Klinnert, 1981). One-year-old infants, placed on a visual cliff, looked toward their mothers before crossing the "deep side." When mothers were instructed to pose fear faces, infants did not cross the cliff. If, however, mothers were asked to pose happy faces, infants did, in fact, cross to the "deep side." Similar results were obtained for posed expressions of anger and interest. Thus, infants actively used facial information in helping them negotiate ambiguous stimulus situations (Feinman, 1992). One assumes that infants rely on this information because they have come to understand its communicative significance. It is conceivable that the previously mentioned possibility of reduced facial expressivity from mothers of facially disfigured infants may make them less favored reference objects in later development. If, for example, mothers smile less to their infants (Field & Vega-Lahr, 1984), or, as results showed in the Malatesta et al. study with preterm infants (1989), mothers tend to disengage when their infants are unresponsive to attempts to engage them, the infants themselves will, over time, become less involved with their mothers in face-to-face interaction—the process ceases to be pleasurable.

Even very young infants are clearly sensitive to the facial signals of their mothers. Cohn and Tronick (1983) show that alteration in mothers' normal facial activity maternally affects 3-month-old infants' own emotional behavior. Mothers were instructed to appear "depressed" by using monotonous voices, slow speech, minimal movement, and an absence of touching. Infants reacted with increased crying, gaze aversion, and protest behavior as compared to a control condition in which mothers interacted as they normally would. The authors conclude that their findings are evidence of the sensitivity of young infants to their mothers' emotional states. There is no reason to assume that infants suffering from facial disfigurement are less sensitive; thus, there is every possibility that they may detect their mothers' feelings of guilt, sadness, and depression, and be affected by these feelings.

As we have attempted to indicate, maternal sensitivity to infant facial expressivity is critically important, as is a mother's own expressivity toward her infant. Several studies have investigated individual differences in maternal responsivity to infant expressions (e.g., Denham, 1986; Kochanska, Kuczynski, Radke-Yarrow, & Welsh, 1987; Zahn-Waxler, Cummings, McKnew, & Radke-Yarrow, 1984). Kochanska et al. (1987) found that depressed mothers become less tolerant and less affectionate and concerned when faced with their children's anger. In addition, mothers react in idiosyncratic ways to their infants' expressions of emotion (Frodi, Lamb, Leavitt, & Donovan, 1978; Haviland & Malatesta, 1981). A study by Malatesta, Grigoriev, Lamb, Albin, & Culver (1986) revealed that high rates of maternal modeling of infants' interest and joy were associated with increases in infants' expressions of these affects between 2½ and 7½ months of age. Thompson and Lamb (1983) have argued that insensitive and/or unresponsive mothers appear immune to their infants' attempts to engage them. They further postulate that such infants will later develop a flattened affect, with neutral or subdued expressivity.

Although it would be erroneous to assume that mothers of infants suffering from craniofacial anomalies are generally insensitive or unresponsive to their infants' attempts to interact, these mothers are most certainly at risk and are also at a distinct disadvantage when considering the area of maternal contingent responding. Depending on the severity of the disfigurement, the infants will have difficulty facially expressing their emotions. Mothers may be unable to discern their expressions reliably and respond to them appropriately, thus setting up a vicious and frustrating interactive style for both mothers and infants.

Alternatively, let us consider the possibility that, as these mothers become increasingly attuned to their infants in terms of their temperament, sleep–wake cycles, eating patterns, and so on, they may also become more adept at reading their infants' facial expressions. Once again, depending on the nature of the disfigurement, facial musculature will be more or less intact, thus allowing mothers to interpret more accurately their infants' expressions. The crucial variable we believe to be considered, however, is time. Face-to-face mother–infant interaction begins soon after birth; and rather than enjoying normal facial interaction from the onset of their relationship, these mothers must learn, over time, the precise meanings of their infants' expressions. An additional obstacle to consider that compounds this situation is that should an infant require surgery to correct facial disfigurement, it is quite plausible that, to some extent, the mother will have to relearn her infant's expressions postsurgically. This relearning process could continue well into the infant's development.

In this section, we have attempted to explore some of the maternal variables that contribute to socioemotional development. While it may be argued that it is the mothers who hold the balance of power in terms of the amount and quality of the interaction, infants also posess certain means by which they may still affect the directionality of affective exchange. We will explore some of these sources of infant influence in the next section.

Infant Contributions to Socioemotional Development

For many years it was assumed that very young infants did not express emotions. Indeed, as Haviland (1976) notes, smiles were attributed to "gas" "until linked to eye contact and the mother's smile" (p. 375). Early smiles, frowns, and grimaces were considered to be the result of rapid eye movement (REM) states (Emde, Gaensbauer, & Harmon, 1976). While many of these behaviors have a reflexlike quality, they appear to be more complex than simple infant reflexes. Malatesta (1985) argues that these early behaviors are more akin to transition behaviors, midway between random, spontaneous responses and more complex, instrumental behavior. From a slightly different perspective, when mothers are asked about their infants' affective expressivity, they attribute a variety of emotions to their infants as early as 2 months of age—affects including interest, distress, enjoyment, shame, disgust, anger, surprise, fear, sleepy, and passive-bored (Emde et al., 1976). It has been demonstrated by Oster (1978) that both premature and full-term infants can utilize the facial musculature necessary for adult facial expressions.

How early in development might we expect to observe distinct facial expressions in normal infants? Joy, interest, disgust, and physical distress can be observed in neonates (Izard, 1977). Field and Walden (1982) also report observing sadness and surprise expressions in neonates undergoing a Brazelton exam. Malatesta and Haviland (1982) have observed and coded anger expressions in 3-month-olds who were not immediately picked up by their mothers following a separation, and mild limb restraint has resulted in anger expressions in 4-month-olds (Stenberg, 1982).

Earlier we discussed the importance of face-to-face interaction as it applies to maternal contributions to infants' socioemotional development. This early form of communication serves an important function for infants as well as parents. For the infant, there is the opportunity to learn the roles of reciprocal social interaction. These early social interchanges are evident as early as the first trimester of life (Stern, 1985; Thompson & Lamb, 1983). While admittedly the infant's repertoire of interactive behaviors is rather limited, even in the early months following birth the infant can smile in an attempt to maintain interaction and cry to cease interaction altogether. Gaze is an additional influence on maternal responsiveness. While gazing at the mother tends to promote interaction, gaze averting effectively terminates an interaction, at least temporarily (Fogel, 1982; Stern, 1974).

There are further indications of infants' abilities to communicate affectively very early in their lives. We stated previously that the human face is the locus of emotional communication. Infants seem to find the face a fascinating source of stimulation, although they show preferences for types of expression. When presented with slides of facial expressions, for example, infants as young as 6 months spent more time gazing at smiles than at negative or neutral expressions (LaBarbara, Izard, Vietze, & Parisi, 1976). Charlesworth and Kreutzer (1973) showed infants between 4 and 10 months of age happy, sad, angry, and neutral facial expressions accompanied by appropriate vocalizations. While the 4-month-olds did not discriminate, infants of all other ages responded differentially to the expressions.

Earlier in this chapter, we discussed infants' reactions to simulated depressive affect in their mothers (Cohn & Tronick, 1983). In an attempt to determine whether infants at 10 weeks of age would respond in similar ways when other affective states were posed by mothers, Lelwica and Haviland (1983) trained mothers to pose expressions of happiness, sadness, and anger to their 10-week-old infants. Both mothers' and infants' faces were coded using MAX (Izard, 1979). The results are complicated but include the findings that infants were able to discriminate the three maternal affects of happiness, sadness, and anger. They were also able to match joy and sometimes anger, and all changes in facial expression by the mothers produced changes in the infants. The authors argue that not only is their study evidence of a very young infant's ability to discriminate the emotional state of his or her mother, but it also points to the importance of the quality of interaction during the first year of life. The implications of this study for infants with craniofacial anomalies is clear: Mothers of infants with a craniofacial anomaly who appear to suffer from depression and/or guilt may unwittingly transmit some of their depressed affect to their children, which may ultimately result in a less responsive infant.

On a more general level, it is obvious that infants suffering from facial disfigurement will experience a different interactive environment than normal children. The ability of the mothers to discern facial expression will depend on the severity of disfigurement: lack of appropriate responding will add to the frustration of both infants and mothers in their attempts to communicate affectively, as mentioned earlier.

Let us consider the implications of this with an example from the domain of discrete emotions theory. The specific facial displays of emotion affected in the infant will depend on the part of the face involved. Consider that the mouth will be the affected area in an infant with cleft palate. Facial displays of emotion that involve the mouth include joy, interest/excitement, surprise/startle, sadness, anger, and fear—in short, nearly all the basic emotions. While it is true that the brow area is also involved in the display of these emotions, conceivably it is more difficult to decipher a particular emotion when one of the areas necessary for its expression is compromised. As discussed previously, the mothers may learn to understand their infants' idiosyncratic facial displays, but a considerable amount of trial and error may be involved that may, in turn, affect the quality of their early interactions.

An additional issue to consider is that, because these infants are unable to exhibit the prototypic facial displays of emotion that unaffected infants display, there is the possibility that they may not experience the same kinds of internal states that normal infants experience. Admittedly, this is merely speculation, but it is speculation that is grounded in the facial feedback postulate of discrete emotions theory. That is, emotional experience is said to be derived from patterned feedback from contraction of facial musculature, and further, "there are distinct neurophysiological processes subserving each of the fundamental emotions and that these processes and their corresponding neuromuscular efferents are activated by biologically and psychologically meaningful stimuli" (Malatesta et al., 1989, p. 6). There is an additional theoretical assumption that, in young infants, there is a distinct correspondence between this patterned feedback and subjective feeling state, such that joyful expression is accompanied by joyful feelings. If, however, that musculature is deformed in some way, the patterning cannot be the same, thus impairing the innate concordance between expression and feeling. Suffice it to say that we believe that this issue will continue to be unresolved until we move beyond our current state of empirical knowledge.

Summary

The literature reviewed above indicates that even very young infants are capable of facially expressing a wide range of emotions. That same literature, though limited in nature, suggests that infants suffering from craniofacial disfigurement will have difficulty in facially expressing their emotions. From a discrete emotions perspective, it is predicted that they may also experience different internal states. However, these infants' disfigurements would not necessarily impair their ability to discriminate accurately their mothers' facial displays of affect, whose own dampened affectivity has been implied in the research literature. If this is indeed the case, such reactions could explain the apparently lowered responsivity in infants with craniofacial anomalies.

Implications for Research

The purpose of this chapter is to discuss the likely socioemotional development of infants with craniofacial anomalies. The above summary indicates that only a rough outline is available. It is clear that this is an area that is ripe for further exploration. What is needed is more longitudinal study of these infants from early on to determine the extent to which they are able to communicate facially their affective states as well as the quality that is involved. Additional studies of face-to-face interaction of infants with craniofacial anomaly and their mothers may not only clarify the quality of the interaction but may also enhance our understanding of the emotions that these mothers display to their infants. Only through the unique lens provided by microanalytic analyses of mothers of infants suffering from craniofacial anomalies and the infants themselves will we come close to a more detailed and accurate understanding.

A second point to consider is that of later development. What happens to these infants in terms of their emotional expressivity as they mature?

According to discrete emotions theory, the early concordance between expression and feeling state gives way to more mature forms of emotion expression and regulation. Children learn to modulate their emotions in terms of frequency, variability, and miniaturization (Izard & Malatesta, 1987). How might this be different in maturing children suffering from craniofacial anomalies, given that their developmentally earlier expressions of emotions differed from those of their nonfacially disfigured counterparts?

These are two questions we consider important in terms of gaining a better understanding of the socioemotional development in infants with craniofacial anomalies from our theoretical perspective.

Implications for Treatment

Infants with facial disfigurement almost inevitably undergo surgical procedure to correct their deformities. Surgeons might consider videotaping their young patients in face-to-face interactions with their mothers or in a free-play situation, in order to obtain a more dynamic perspective on their facial movements. Having a more "active" view of the faces they surgically correct (as opposed to still photographs) may provide a unique perspective in terms of the decisions that they make for surgical corrections.

When considering how the quality of interaction between the mother–infant dyad might be improved, we suggest programs such as those offered to mothers of preterm infants. These programs help mothers understand the special circumstances involved in having a preterm child as well as how to cope with many of the difficulties that they may face. Support groups might provide the mother with a sense of belonging—there are others who are familiar with the issues that she must cope with on a daily basis. We also suggest an intervention focused on helping these mothers interact with their infants, perhaps filming early interactions and viewing the tapes with the mothers to help them learn to identify their infants' facial expressions and to serve as guides to assist them in learning what an optimal interaction consists of for both mothers and their children.

Recent Findings

Since the completion of this chapter, several empirical studies utilizing mother–infant dyads in which the infants suffer craniofacial anomalies have been completed. The results of these studies are important to discuss when considering the socioemotional development of these young children.

Barden, Ford, Jensen, Rogers-Salyer, and Salyer (1989) hypothesized that facial deformity impacts on the mother–infant relationship, and that early corrective surgery would have a positive influence on the quality of the relationship. It was further proposed that the mothers of facially disfigured infants defended against negative feelings they may experience toward their infants through the utilization of denial (as measured via paper and pencil measures). Ten dyads (5 with infants with a variety of craniofacial anomalies) with a mean age of 15 weeks were videotaped for observation in three episodes: 10 minutes of free play, a 5-minute vocal elicitation, and 3 minutes of imitation (mothers asked to imitate their babies facial displays). Measures assessing social support, general life satisfaction, and life experiences were collected from the mothers. Results demonstrated that mothers of the facially disfigured infants "manifested a consistent pattern of less nurturant behavior" (p. 821). Further, the facially disfigured infants were less responsive toward their mothers in their vocalizing, touching, and smiling behaviors. Finally, on self-report measures, mothers of the infants with craniofacial anomalies reported being more satisfied with parenting than did mothers of nondisfigured infants. The authors interpreted this finding as the mothers' use of denial.

Speltz, Armsden, and Clarren (1990) examined the relationship between toddlers with facial disfigurement and their mothers, with a goal of identifying early precursors to psychosocial deficits observed during the early school years in this group. Thirty-three children (ages 12 to 36 months) with facial disfigurement (cleft palate, cleft lip and palate, and sagittal synostosis) and their mothers were matched with 22 nonfacially disfigured children and their mothers. Pairs were videotaped in a 5-minute free play episode and a 5-minute teaching task. Mothers completed paper and pencil measures of stress, general well-being, marital adjustment, and social health. In contrast to differences found by previous studies, Speltz et al. did not find any significant differences between the two groups during either the play or teaching task. However, mothers of the children with facial disfigurement reported higher stress levels, a reduced sense of general well-being, and lower marital adjustment scores.

A third study relevant to this discussion was completed by Wasserman, Lennon, Allen, and Shilansky (1987). They explored attachment classifications in physically handicapped (cleft lip and palate or limb reduction) children. Children participated at 9 and 12 months of age; all had had surgical intervention prior to their taking part in the study. The Ainsworth Strange Situation procedure (Ainsworth et al., 1978) was completed at the 12-month visit. No differences in attachment classification between the physically handicapped group and a group of matched controls were found. Results did demonstrate, however, significant differences in maternal styles of interaction between the two groups. The authors argued that these differences are ameliorated as the disfigured children are more "normalized" by surgical intervention, and that attachment classification is not ultimately affected.

Collectively, these more recent studies begin to shed light on the complexities involved in the early relationship and interactions between infants with craniofacial anomalies and their mothers. Longitudinal investigations exploring quality of interaction, attachment classification and coping strategies in these dyads will assist both researchers and clinicians with more effective interventions for this special group of children.

References

Aamot, S. (1978). Reactions to facial deformities: Automatic and social psychological. *European Journal of Social Psychology, 8,* 315.

Adams, G.R. (1977). Physical attractiveness research: Toward a developmental psychology of beauty. *Human Development, 20,* 217–239.

Ainsworth, M.D.S., Blehar, M.C., Waters, E., & Wall, S. (1978). *Patterns of attachment.* Hillsdale, NJ: Erlbaum.

Barden, R.C., Ford, M.E., Jensen, A.G., Rogers-Salyer, M., & Salyer, K.E. (1989). Effects of craniofacial deformity in infancy on the quality of mother–infant interaction. *Child Development, 60,* 819–824.

Barrett, K.C. (1984). *Infants' use of conflicting emotional signals.* Unpublished doctoral dissertation, University of Denver, Denver, CO.

Beckwith, L., & Cohen, S.E. (1980). Interactions of preterm infants with their caregivers and test performance at age two. In T. Field, S. Goldberg, D. Stern, & A. Sostek (Eds.), *High risk infants and children: Adult and peer interactions.* New York: Academic Press.

Berry, D.S., & McArthur, L.Z. (1985). Some components and consequences of a babyface. *Journal of Personality and Social Psychology, 48, 2,* 312–323.

Berschied, E., & Walster, E. (1974). Physical attractiveness. In L. Berkowitz (Ed.), *Advances in experimental social psychology,* Vol. 7. New York: Academic Press.

Bowlby, J. (1969). *Attachment and Loss: Vol. I Attachment.* New York: Basic Books.

Brantley, H.T., & Clifford, E. (1980). When my child was born: Maternal reactions to the birth of a child. *Journal of Personality Assessment, 44, 6,* 620–623.

Bridges, K.M. (1930). A genetic theory of the emotions. *Journal of Genetic Psychology, 37,* 514–527.

Bridges, K.M. (1932). Emotional development in early infancy. *Child Development, 3,* 324–341.

Campos, J.J., Barrett, K.G., Lamb, M.E., Stenberg, C., & Goldsmith, H.H. (1983). Socioemotional development. In M.M. Haith & J.J. Campos (Eds.), *Infancy and developmental psychobiology* (Vol. 2). In P.H. Mussen (Gen. Ed.), *Handbook of child psychology.* New York: Wiley.

Cannon, W.B. (1927). The James-Lange theory of emotion: A critical examination and an alternative theory. *American Journal of Psychology, 39,* 106–124.

Charlesworth, W., & Kreutzer, M. (1973). Facial expressions of infants and children. In P. Ekman (Ed.), *Darwin and facial expression.* New York: Academic Press.

Clifford, E., & Crocker, E.C. (1971). Maternal responses: The birth of a normal child as compared to the birth of a child with a cleft. *Cleft Palate Journal, 8,* 298–306.

Cohn, J.F., & Tronick, E.Z. (1983). Three-month-old infants' reaction to stimulated mother depression. *Child Development, 54,* 185–193.

Darwin, C. (1872/1975). *The expression of emotion in man and animals.* Chicago: University of Chicago Press.

Davis, F. (1961). Deviance disavowal: The management of strained interaction by the visibly handicapped. *Social Problems, 9,* 120–32.

Denham, S.A. (1986). Social cognition, prosocial behavior and emotion in preschoolers. *Child Development, 57, 1,* 194–201.

Duffy, E. (1934). Emotion: An example of the need for reorientation in psychology. *Psychological Review, 41,* 184–198.

Easson, W.M. (1966). Psychopathological environmental reaction to congenital defect. *Journal of Nervous and Mental Disease, 142, 5,* 453–459.

Ekman, P. (1973). Cross cultural studies of facial expression. In P. Ekman (Ed.), *Darwin and facial expression: A century of research in review.* New York: Academic Press.

Ekman, P. (1978). Facial signs: Facts, fantasies and possibilities. In T.A. Sebeok (Ed.), *Sight, sound and sense,* Bloomington, IN: Indiana University Press.

Emde, R., Gaensbauer, T., & Harmon, R. (1976). Emotional expression in infancy: A biobehavioral study. *Psychological Issues* (Vol. 10). New York: International Universities Press.

Epsteen, C.M. (1958). Psychological impact of facial deformities. *American Journal of Surgery, 96,* 745–748.

Feinman, S. (1992). *Social referencing and the social construction of reality in infancy*. New York: Plenum.

Field, T. (1977). Effects of early separation, interactive deficits and experimental manipulations on face-to-face interaction. *Child Development, 48,* 767–771.

Field, T., & Walden T. (1982). Perception and production of facial expression in infancy and early childhood. In H. Reese & L. Lipsett (Eds.), *Advances in child development and research* (Vol. 16). New York: Academic Press.

Field, T.M., & Vega-Lahr, N. (1984). Early interactions between infants with craniofacial anomalies and their mothers. *Infant Behavior and Development, 7,* 527–530.

Fogel, A. (1982). Affect dynamics in early infancy: Affective tolerance. In T. Field & A. Fogel (Eds.), *Emotion and early interaction.* Hillsdale, NJ: Erlbaum.

Fraiberg, S. (1979). Blind infants and their mothers: An examination of the sign system. In M. Bullowa (Ed.), *Before speech.* New York: Cambridge University Press.

Frodi, A.M., Lamb, M.E., Leavitt, L.A., & Donovan, W.L. (1978). Fathers and mothers' responses to infant smiles and cries. *Infant Behavior and Development, 1,* 187–198.

Gaensbauer, T.J., & Mrazek, D. (1981). Differences in the patterning of affective expression in infants. *Child Development, 20,* 673–691.

Gardner, B.T., & Wallach, L. (1965). Shapes of figures identified as a baby's head. *Perceptual and Motor Skills, 20,* 135–142.

Goldberg, S., Brachfeld, S., & DiVitto, B. (1980). Feeding, fussing and playing: Parent-infant interaction in the first year as a function of prematurity and perinatal problems. In T. Field, S. Goldberg, D. Stern, & A. Stosek (Eds.), *High-risk infants and children: Adult and peer interactions.* New York: Academic Press.

Haviland, J. (1976). Looking smart: The relationship between affect and intelligence. In M. Lewis (Ed.), *Origins of intelligence: Infancy and childhood.* New York: Plenum.

Haviland, J., & Malatesta, C.Z. (1981). A description of the development of sex differences in nonverbal signals: Fallacies, facts, and fantasies. In C. Mayo & N. Henley (Eds.), *Gender and nonverbal behavior.* New York: Springer-Verlag.

Haviland, J., Malatesta, C.Z., & Lelwica, M.L. (1984). Emotional communication in early infancy. *Infant Mental Health Journal, 5, 3,* 135–147.

Hess, E.H. (1970). Ethology and developmental psychology. In P. Mussen (Ed.), *Carmichael's manual of child psychology,* Vol. I. New York: Wiley.

Hildebrandt, K.A. (1983). Effect of facial expression variations on ratings of infant attractiveness. *Developmental Psychology, 19, 3,* 414–417.

Hildebrandt, K.A., & Fitzgerald, H.E. (1979). Facial feature determinants of perceived infant attractiveness. *Infant Behavior and Development, 2,* 329–339.

Izard, C.E. (1971). *The face of emotion.* New York: Appleton-Century-Crofts.

Izard, C.E. (1977). *Human emotions.* New York: Plenum.

Izard, C.E. (1979). *The maximally discriminative facial movement scoring system.* Unpublished manuscript, University of Delaware, Newark, DE.

Izard, C.E., & Malatesta, C.Z. (1987). Perspectives on emotional development I: Differential emotions theory of early emotional development. In J. Osofsky (Ed.), *Handbook of infant development.* New York: Wiley.

James, W. (1884). What is emotion? *Mind, 19,* 188–205.

Kagan, J. (1962). A study in psychological development. *Birth to maturity.* New York: Wiley.

Kleck, R. (1966). Emotional arousal in interactions with stigmatized persons. *Psychological Reports, 19,* 1226.

Kochanska, G., Kuczynski, L., Radke-Yarrow, M., & Welsh, J. (1987). Resolutions of control episodes between well and affectively ill mothers and their young children. *Journal of Abnormal Child Psychology, 15, 3,* 441–456.

LaBarbara, V.D., Izard, C.E., Vietze, P., & Parisi, S.A. (1976). Four and six month old infants' visual responses to joy, anger and neutral expressions. *Child Development, 47,* 535–538.

Lamb, M.E. (1988). Social and emotional development in infancy. In M.H. Bornstein & M.E. Lamb (Eds.), *Developmental psychology: An advanced textbook.* Hillsdale, NJ: Erlbaum.

Lelwica, M., & Haviland, J.M. (1983). Infant's reactions to mother's affect expressions. Paper presented at Society for Research on Child Development, Detroit, MI.

Lewis, M., & Michaelson, L. (1983). *Children's emotions and moods: Developmental theory and measurement.* New York: Plenum.

Malatesta, C.Z. (1985). Developmental course of emotion expression in the human infant. In G. Zivin (Ed.) *The development of expressive behavior: Biology-environment interactions*. New York: Academic Press.

Malatesta, C.Z., Culver, C., Tesman, J., & Shepard, B. (1989). The development of emotion expression during the first two years of life. Monographs of the *Society for Research in Child Development, Serial No. 219, Vol. 54, Nos. 1–2,* pp. 1–104.

Malatesta, C.Z., Grigoriev, P., Lamb, C., Albin, M., & Culver, C. (1986). Emotion socialization and expressive development in pre-term and full-term infants, *Child Development, 57,* 316–330.

Malatesta, C.Z., & Haviland, J.M. (1982). Learning display rules: The socialization of emotion expression in infancy. *Child Development, 53,* 991–1003.

Norval, M., Larson, T., & Parshall, P. (1964). The impact of the cleft lip and palate child on the family: A preliminary survey. Minnesota: Crippled Children Services, Mimeographed Report. Minneapolis, MN. Unpublished manuscript.

Oster, H. (1978). Facial expression and affective development. In M. Lewis, & L. Rosenbloom (Eds.), *The development of affect.* New York: Plenum.

Plutchik, R. (1980). *Emotion: A psychoevolutionary synthesis.* New York: Harper & Row.

Power, T.G., Hidebrandt, K.A., & Fitzgerald, H.E. (1982). Adults' responses to smiling and crying infants. *Infant Behavior and Development, 5,* 33–44.

Pratt, K. (1954). The neonate. In P. Musson (Ed.), *Carmichael's manual of child psychology*. New York: Wiley.

Robson, K.S., & Moss, H.A. (1970). Patterns and determinants of maternal attachment. *Pediatrics, 77,* 976–985.

Schacter, S., & Singer J.E. (1962). Cognitive, social and physiological determinants of emotional state. *Psychological Review, 69,* 379–399.

Schneider-Rosen, K., Braunwald, K.G., Carlson, V., & Cicchetti, D. (1985). Current perspectives in attachment theory: Illustrations from the study of maltreated infants. In I. Bretherton & E. Waters (Eds.), *Growing points of attachment theory and research. Monograph for the Society of Research in Child Development, 50 (1–2, Serial No. 209).* Chicago: University of Chicago Press.

Sherman, M. (1927a). The differentiation of emotional responses in infants: I. Judgments of emotional responses from motion picture views and from actual observations. *Journal of Comparative Psychology, 7,* 265–284.

Sherman, M. (1927b). The differentiation of emotional responses in infants: II. The ability of observers to judge the emotional characteristics of the crying of infants and of the voice of an adult. *Journal of Comparative Psychology, 7,* 335–351.

Sorce, J., Emde, R.N., Campos, J.J., & Klinnert, M. (1981, April). Maternal emotional signaling: Its effect on the visual cliff behavior of one year olds. Paper presented at the meeting of the Society for Research in Child Development, Boston, MA.

Speltz, M.L., Armsden, G.C., & Clarren, S.S. (1990). Effects of craniofacial birth defects on maternal functioning postinfancy. *Journal of Pediatric Psychology, 15,* 117–196.

Spitz, R. (1965). *The first year of life.* New York: International Universities Press.

Sroufe, L.A. (1979). Socioemotional development. In J. Osofsky (Ed.), *Handbook of infant development.* New York: Wiley.

Stenberg, C. (1982). The development of anger facial expressions in infancy. Unpublished doctoral dissertation, University of Colorado, Boulder, CO.

Stern, D. (1985). *The interpersonal world of the infant.* New York: Basic Books.

Stern, D. (1974). Mother and infant at play: The dyadic interaction involving facial, vocal and gaze behavior. In M. Lewis & L. Rosenbloom (Eds.), *The effect of the infant on its caregiver.* New York: Wiley.

Thompson, R.A., & Lamb, M.E. (1983). Individual differences in dimensions of socioemotionsl development in infancy. In R. Plutchik & H. Kellerman (Eds.), *Emotion: Theory and research.* New York: Academic Press.

Tisza, V.B., & Gumpertz, M.S.W. (1962). The parents' reaction to the birth and early care of children with cleft palate. *Pediatrics, 30,* 86–90.

Walk, R.D., & Gibson, E.J. (1961). A comparative and analytical study of visual depth perception. *Psychological Monographs, 75, (15, whole No. 519).*

Wasserman, D.A., Lennon, M.C., Allen, R., & Shilansky, M. (1987). Contributors to attachment in normal and physically handicapped infants. *American Academy of Child and Adolescent Psychiatry, 26,* 9–15.

Wasserman, G.A., & Allen, R. (1985). Maternal withdrawl from handicapped toddlers. *Journal of Child Psychology and Psychiatry, 26, 3,* 381–387.

Watson, J.B., & Raynor, R. (1920). Conditioned emotional reactions. *Journal of Experimental Psychology, 3,* 1–14.

Zahn-Waxler, C., Cummings, E.M., McKnew, D.H., & Radke-Yarrow, M. (1984). Young offspring of depressed parents: A population at risk for affective problems. In D. Cicchetti & K. Schneider-Rosen (Eds.), *Childhood Depression.* San Francisco: Jossey-Bass.

Part 2
Attachment and Parenting

5
Early Interaction of Infants with Craniofacial Anomalies

TIFFANY FIELD

Physical attractiveness appears to affect interpersonal attraction and social interaction. The development of these social processes begins in very early infancy. Infants who are less attractive, such as infants with craniofacial anomalies, may be at risk for a number of later psychosocial problems. Infants with craniofacial anomalies may be more difficult to interact with because their facial deformity makes them less physically appealing to look at and their facial expressions may be dampened, making them appear to look less responsive and more "difficult to read" than normal infants. The purpose of this chapter is to review literature on the risks associated with physical unattractiveness and data specifically suggesting that infants with craniofacial anomalies experience less optimal interactions during early infancy.

Effects of Physical Attractiveness on Social Behavior

Several investigators studying the effects of physical attractiveness on social development have postulated a similar model (Adams, 1978a; Langlois & Stephan, 1977; Tobiasen, 1984). They have suggested that people have different expectations about the behavior of infants and children with differing levels of attractiveness. These expectations, they maintain, may lead to the differential treatment of attractive and unattractive infants and children by their peers and by adults. Differential treatment may, in turn, lead to differences in how attractive and unattractive infants and children behave and develop.

Differential expectations may derive from the stereotype that relates physical beauty to personality characteristics that are highly valued. The preference for physically attractive faces appears to occur as early as infancy, with very young infants preferring photographs of attractive faces (Langlois, Roggman, Casey, Riffer, Rieser-Danner, & Jenkins, 1987).

This preference is also characteristic of young children (Adams, 1978a) and has consistently been noted in adult samples (Berscheid & Walster, 1974). That physically attractive infants and children are expected to show more optimal development has been reflected in a number of studies. Teachers believe that attractive children are more popular with their peers and are more likely to succeed academically (Adams, 1978b; Clifford, 1975; Rich, 1975). Even attractive newborns have been given a better prognosis for later development by nurses (Corter et al., 1978). Not only adults but also peers hold greater expectations for their attractive colleagues. For example, grade school–age children have been noted to rate more attractive children as smarter, more likeable, and more socially skilled in at least two samples of young children (Langlois & Stephan, 1977; Lerner & Lerner, 1977).

Very different expectations are held for infants and children who are physically unattractive. For example, in studies by Richardson, Goodman, Hastorf, and Dornbusch (1961), children ranked other children who had a cleft lip as being less liked than normal children or children with various other physical handicaps. Similarly, children who are asked to rank drawings of children with a normal face, "bat ears," eye squint, protruding teeth, cleft lip, and misshapen nose consistently ranked the children with the cleft lip or misshapen nose as the least liked (Landsdown & Polak, 1975). These data suggest, then, that infants and children with craniofacial anomalies are less preferred than normal children and that different expectations are held for the children by both adults and peers.

Since differential expectations typically lead to differential treatment, it is not surprising that attractive and unattractive infants and children receive differential treatment. As early as infancy, individuals are treated differentially based on their attractiveness. Attractive infants, for example, are looked at significantly longer than infants rated as less attractive when photographs of infants are presented to child and adult judges (Hildebrandt & Fitzgerald, 1978). Mothers also engage in more eye contact and more holding and kissing of attractive babies as compared to mothers of less attractive babies (Parke & Sawin, 1975). These same authors noted that the fathers also stimulate their attractive neonates more frequently than less attractive neonates, by touching, kissing, and holding them. The attractiveness ratings of the infants were significantly related to the fathers' actual participation and caregiving of their infants three months later. Similar data have been reported by Langlois and Stephan (1981), who showed that physically attractive neonates were held closer and given more physical contact. The interactions between these physically attractive infants and their mothers were also rated as more positive than the interactions of mothers with physically unattractive infants.

Although there are very limited data on the differential treatment of craniofacial anomaly infants and children by their parents, parents have reported that they have more difficulty accepting a child with facial anomalies than a normal child (Clifford, 1969; Richman & Harper, 1978). And, in turn, children with oral facial clefts have described their birth and infancy as more difficult for their parents than children who were born either normal or born with cerebral palsy (Richman & Harper, 1978).

Finally, that differential expectations and differential treatment might lead to differential *behavior* on the part of infants and children is not at all surprising. Observational studies of attractive and unattractive preschool children suggest that more attractive children spend significantly more time engaging in interactions with their peers than do less attractive children, who more often play alone (Trnavsky & Bakeman, 1976). Despite their more frequent playing alone, unattractive preschoolers reportedly are more aggressive toward their playmates than are their more attractive peers (Langlois & Downs, 1979). In contrast, children with craniofacial anomalies such as cleft palate and cleft lip are rated by parents and teachers as being more shy and socially inhibited than are normal children (Richman, 1978; Simonds & Heimburger, 1978; Spriesterbach, 1973). This is disconcerting, inasmuch as social acceptance and being liked by others in young children is highly related to later social confidence and positive mental health (Roff, Sells, & Golden, 1972). Thus, it would appear that there are differential expectations for attractive infants and children vs. unattractive infants and children such as those with craniofacial anomalies; and that the more attractive children, in turn, receive differential treatment by adults as well as their peers. It is not, then, surprising that the unattractive children show less competence in social development.

Most of the previously reviewed research has been conducted with infants and children within the normal range of physical attractiveness rather than the extremes of unattractiveness such as is experienced by infants and children with craniofacial anomalies. Deformity may be an extreme version of unattractiveness. However, some research suggests that a normal configuration vs. a deformed configuration may exist on a different continuum than attractiveness vs. unattractiveness. For example, Kleck and Strenta (1980) reported that people respond differently to deformed individuals as compared to unattractive normal people. Being normal and unattractive and being deformed and unattractive may have different consequences. For example, whereas unattractive children were noted to be more aggressive toward their peers than were attractive ones (Langlois & Downs, 1979), children with craniofacial anomalies such as cleft lip and cleft palate are more shy and socially inhibited than noncleft children (Richman, 1978; Simonds & Heimburger, 1978; Spriesterbach, 1973). The behavior of these 2 groups of children may serve different functions; the behavior of unattractive children may elicit more attention, whereas the behavior of deformed children may serve to make them less noticeable. Both unattractive and deformed children may show less social competence. However, their actual behaviors (and perhaps the reasons for their behavior) may differ.

Nonetheless, the importance of investigating the early behavior of infants with craniofacial anomalies is highlighted by the likelihood that infants with facial deformities of this kind are at high risk for problems of social and emotional development and by the relatively high prevalence of this problem, with as many as 15,000 infants born each year, or 1 in every 600 live births with such anomalies (U.S. Census). Despite the significance of this problem, to date there appear to be only two studies in the literature on the behavior of young infants with craniofacial anomalies (Barden, Ford, Jensen, Rogers-Salyer, & Salyer, in press; Field & Vega-Lahr, 1984).

Early Interactions Between Infants with Craniofacial Anomalies and Their Mothers

In the first study on early interactions of infants with craniofacial anomalies, Field and Vega-Lahr (1984) speculated that infants with craniofacial anomalies may be more difficult to interact with because their facial deformity makes them physically unappealing to look at. Alternatively, their facial expressions may be dampened, making them appear to be less responsive and more "difficult to read" than normal infants (Field, 1978; Goldberg, 1979). The purpose of the Field and Vega-Lahr study was to compare the early face-to-face interactions of craniofacial anomaly infants and their mothers with those of normal infant–mother dyads to determine the degree to which early interactions appear to be impaired by the infants' facial deformity. The sample was comprised of 24 3-month-old infants, 12 of whom had craniofacial anomalies (cleft lip and palate). None of the infants had received surgical repairs for their anomalies. The craniofacial anomaly infants and their mothers were recruited from a craniofacial anomaly clinic during their first visit, and the normal sample was recruited from a normal control group sample attending a clinic in the same institution. Only infants with normal perinatal histories and primiparous, middle socioeconomic–status adult mothers were recruited. These criteria were used, inasmuch as early interactions are noted to vary as a function of these factors (Field, 1980). In addition, because bottle feeding of the craniofacial anomaly infants might confound the data, only bottle-fed infants were recruited.

For the study of face-to-face interaction, the infants were placed in an infant seat on a table with the mothers seated approximately 1½ feet from the infants in a face-to-face position. The mothers were informed that we were studying face-to-face play behaviors of infants and were simply asked to play with their infants as they would play with them at home. Their play was videotaped for a 10-minute period, and the videotapes were coded for time spent by the infants and mothers looking and smiling at each other and vocalizing to each other. The mothers' looking-at-the-infant behavior was coded to test the hypothesis that the mothers of craniofacial anomaly infants may look at their infants less frequently because they are unattractive. The infants' smiling and vocalizing behaviors were coded to test the hypothesis that these infants' facial and vocal expressions may be dampened, making them appear to be less responsive and "more difficult to read" than normal infants. In addition, the tapes were rated on the interaction rating scale (Field, 1980). this is a 3-point Likert-type scale on the following behaviors: 1) infant's state, physical activity, head orientation, gaze behavior, facial expressions, vocalizations, and fussiness; and 2) mother's state, physical activity, head orientation, gaze behavior, silencing during infant gaze aversion, facial expressions, vocalizations, imitative behaviors, contingent responsivity, and game playing.

The data analyses revealed that, although the mothers of craniofacial anomaly infants looked at their infants as much of the time as mothers looked at their normal infants, the craniofacial anomaly infants vs. normal infants looked at their mothers for a lesser amount of the interaction time (see Figure 5.1). In addition, the craniofacial infants engaged in less

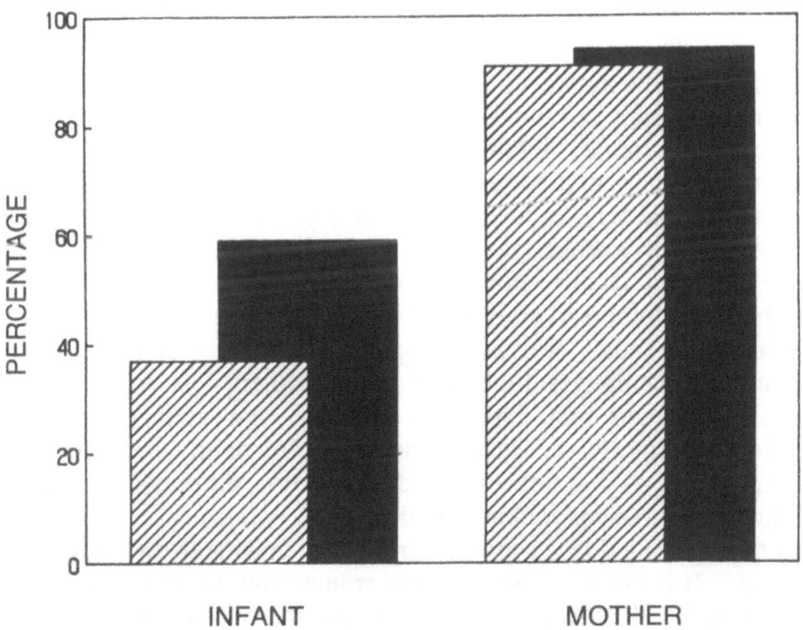

FIGURE 5.1. The percentage of time that infants looked at mothers and mothers looked at infants (□-craniofacial anomaly, ■-normal).

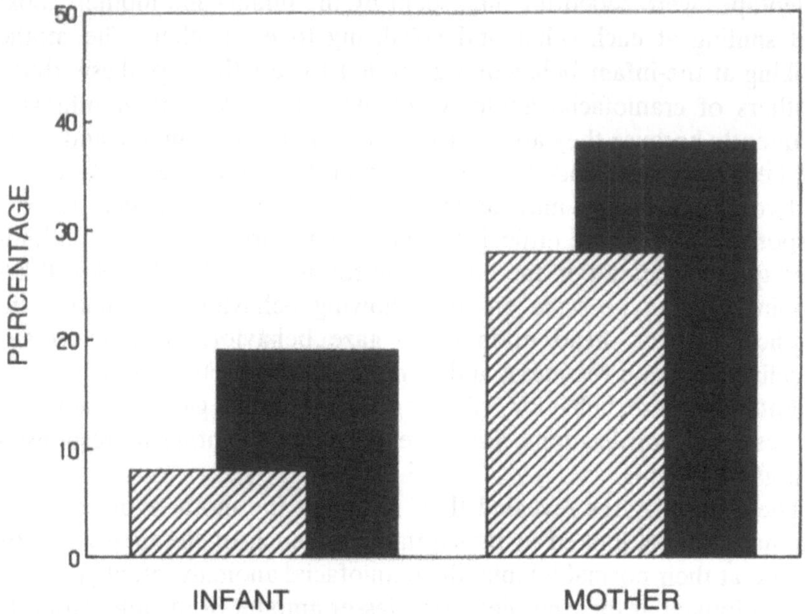

FIGURE 5.2. The percentage of time that infants and mothers smiled at each other.

frequent smiling and vocalizing than did the normal infants (see Figures 5.2 and 5.3). The mothers of the craniofacial anomaly infants also showed less frequent smiling, and vocalizing (Figures 5.2 and 5.3). Finally, the craniofacial anomaly infants received lower interaction rating-scale scores on head orientation, gaze behavior, facial expressions, and vocalizations (see Table 5.1). In turn, the mothers of craniofacial anomaly infants received lower ratings on facial expressions, vocalizations, imitative behaviors, contingent responsivity, and game playing.

While the mothers of craniofacial anomaly infants did not differ in their looking-at-the-infant behavior, despite their infants' facial deformities, the infants themselves looked at their mothers less frequently. This suggests that our first hypothesis—that is, that mothers would look at their craniofacial anomaly infants less frequently because of their unattractiveness—was not confirmed. In contrast, the craniofacial anomaly infants' less frequent looking, smiling, and vocalizing to their mothers may have provided fewer interaction signals, making them "more difficult to read." It is not clear whether the craniofacial anomaly infants' lesser eye contact and/or less smiling and vocalizing may have contributed to the mothers' less frequent smiling, vocalizing, and use of imitation and game playing. Without the eye contact, turn taking, and signals from the infant, the mothers are less likely to initiate social behaviors (Beebe,

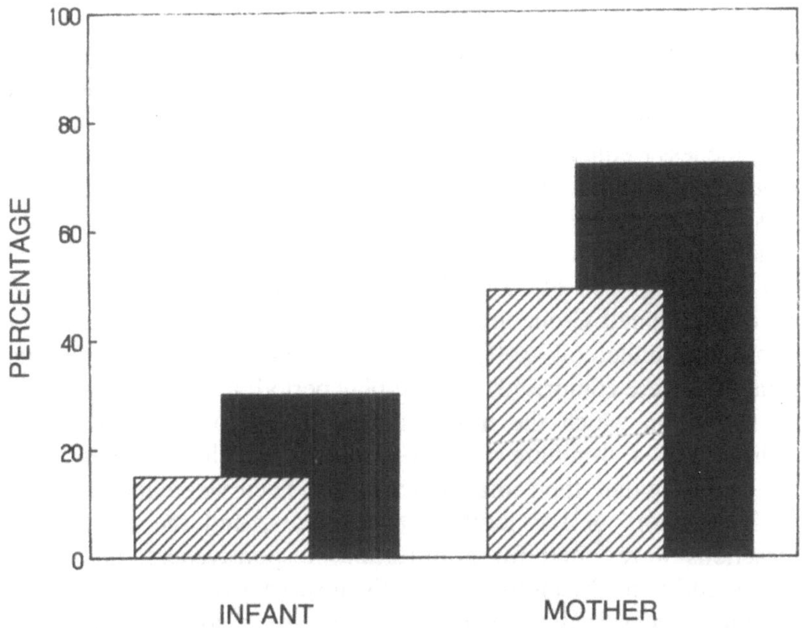

FIGURE 5.3. The percentage of time that infants and mothers vocalized to each other.

Table 5.1. Interaction behaviors of craniofacial anomaly and normal infants and their mothers.

	M for groups		
	Craniofacial anomaly	Normal	*p* values
Behavior ratings[1]			
Infant-state	1.8	2.2	N.S.
Physical activity	1.8	2.1	N.S.
Head orientation	1.5	2.4	.01
Gaze behavior	1.4	2.5	.005
Facial expressions	1.6	2.7	.005
Fussiness	1.8	2.3	N.S.
Vocalizations	1.2	2.8	.001
Mother-state	2.2	2.4	N.S.
Physical activity	1.8	2.1	N.S.
Head orientation	2.9	3.0	N.S.
Gaze behavior	2.9	2.9	N.S.
Silence during infant gaze aversion	1.4	1.9	N.S.
Facial expressions	1.7	2.8	.01
Vocalizations	1.7	2.9	.01
Imitative behaviors	1.1	2.7	.001
Contingent responsivity	1.3	2.4	.005
Game playing	1.2	2.5	.005

[1] Higher rating is optimal.

Jaffe, Feldstein, Mays, & Alson, 1985; Mayer & Tronick, 1985). Alternatively, or at the same time, because so many of the mothers' face-to-face behaviors are imitations of the infants' behaviors (Field, 1977; Pawlby, 1977), the less frequent social behavior of the craniofacial anomaly infants provides fewer stimulus opportunities for the mothers' imitative behaviors.

A similar study was conducted on the early interactions of craniofacial anomaly infants by Barden and his colleagues (Barden et al., 1987). Their study was comprised of 10 infants, 5 with craniofacial anomalies. Their diagnoses included Crouzon's Syndrome, Apert's Syndrome, microfacial microsomia, unilateral cleft, and bilateral cleft. Their mother–infant interactions were comprised of a free-play period; a 5-minute vocal elicitation period, in which the mothers were asked to get their infants to vocalize; and a 3-minute imitation, during which the mothers were instructed to imitate their infants' behaviors. Their videotapes were coded on 12 behaviors of the mothers and infants, and the mother–infant interactions were rated for gratification, responsiveness, and affective tone. In addition, the mothers were given surveys to provide background information and self-assessments of their life stress, social support, general life satisfaction, and parental satisfaction. Their data analyses revealed that the mothers of craniofacial anomaly infants engaged in less tactile / kinesthetic stimulation, less affectionate touching, and less responsivity to their infants' behavioral cues. The infants, in turn, touched their mothers less frequently, averted their heads more often, engaged in less smiling and laughing, and were less responsive to their mothers' behavior. In contrast to these behavioral data, the mothers of craniofacial anomaly infants expressed more satisfaction with parenting and more positive life experiences following their pregnancy than did the mothers of normal infants. The authors interpreted these more optimal reports of background stress as denial of stress by mothers of craniofacial anomaly infants.

Summary

Implications for Research

These two studies combined suggest that craniofacial anomaly infants are less active and less responsive and, in turn, that their mothers are less active and less responsive. This lesser activity of the mothers of craniofacial anomaly infants is inconsistent with several studies that have reported greater activity in mothers of high-risk infants (Beckwith & Cohen, 1980; Field, 1977; Goldberg, Brachfeld, & DeVito, 1980). Mothers of typically less responsive high-risk infants have been described as being more active in their attempts to model social behaviors and elicit more social behavior from their less responsive infants. It is not clear, then, why the mothers of these less responsive, craniofacial anomaly infants were less active. Field and Vega-Lahr (1984) suggest that one possibility is that, unlike the mothers of high-risk premature infants, these mothers view their infants' condition as long term and are somewhat "depressed" by this reality. The "depression" that they feel regarding their deformed infant may also contribute to the denial of experienced stress noted by Barden et al. (1987). Thus, interaction problems may not be the same for different samples of high-risk infants. Infants from different samples (e.g., preterm vs. craniofacial anomaly infants) may experience different early interactions and different later social competence. A characterization of these differences in early interaction and later social competence might lead to a better understanding of the functions and implications of particular aspects of early interactions for later social development.

In a future study, it would be important to tap the mothers' perceptions of their infants' condition and behavior. It is of considerable concern that these less than optimal interactions may contribute to the later social interaction problems that have been noted in studies on the relationships between early interactions and later social development (Bakeman & Brown, 1980; Field, Dempsey, & Shuman, 1983; Sigman, Cohen, & Forsythe, 1981).

Implications for Treatment

The data from these two studies provide empirical support for performing infant craniofacial surgery as soon as possible on these infants. Unfortunately, corrective surgery is often not performed on infants with craniofacial anomalies until later in infancy or later in childhood, when facial anatomy and musculature are more developed (Kapp-Simon, 1980). By that time, infants with craniofacial anomalies may have already experienced irreversible effects of unresponsive early interactions. Longitudinal studies will be required to address the question of whether craniofacial anomaly infants continue to be less attentive and responsive during face-to-face interactions or whether corrective surgery facilitates a reversal of this process and an increase in the infants' social responsivity. In addition, other studies will be required to address what other important developmental processes are affected by the less than optimal early interactions of craniofacial anomaly infants and their mothers.

The literature on physical attractiveness suggests that differential expectations are held for physically attractive and unattractive infants and children, which contributes to differential treatment by adults as well as peers. These differential expectations and treatment may contribute to differential behavior in less attractive children. This process appears to start very early in infancy, as manifested by the less than optimal interaction behavior of craniofacial anomaly infants and their mothers, as has been reported in at least two studies. It is not clear to what degree the infants' physical unattractiveness or the infants' lesser responsivity and the mothers' receiving fewer behavioral cues or less reinforcement from the infants contributes to these less optimal interactions. However, because less than optimal interactions contribute to later social–emotional problems and because it is unclear how these might be attenuated by corrective surgery in early infancy, further research is needed on these important problems.

Acknowledgments. The author would like to thank the children, mothers, and nursing staff who participated in this study. This research was supported by an NIMH Research Scientist Development Award #MH00331. Reprint requests can be sent to Tiffany Field, University of Miami Medical School, Touch Research Institute, P. O. Box 016820, Miami, FL 33101.

References

Adams, G.R. (1978a). Physical attractiveness research: Toward a developmental social psychology of beauty. *Human Development, 20,* 217–323.

Adams, G.R. (1978b). Racial membership and physical attractiveness effects on preschool teachers' expectations. *Child Study Journal, 8,* 29–41.

Bakeman, R., & Brown, J. (1980). Early interaction: Consequences for social and mental development at three years. *Child Development, 51,* 437–447.

Barden, R.C., Ford, M.E., Jensen, A.G., Rogers-Salyer, M., & Salyer, K.E. (1987). *Effects of physical unattractiveness/craniofacial deformity in infancy on the quality of mother-infant interactions.* Unpublished manuscript, University of Utah, Salt Lake City, UT.

Beckwith, L., & Cohen, S.E. (1980). Interaction of preterm infants with their caregivers and their performance at age two. In T. Field, S. Goldberg, D. Stern, & A. Sostek (Eds.), *High-risk infants and children: Adult and peer interactions* (pp. 155–178). New York: Academic Press.

Beebe, B., Jaffe, J., Feldstein, S., Mays, K., & Alson, D. (1985). Matching of timing: The application of an adult dialogue model to mother-infant vocal and kinesic interactions. In T. Field & N. Fox (Eds.), *Social perception in infancy* (pp. 217–248). Norwood, NJ: Ablex.

Berscheid, E., & Walster E. (1974). Physical attractiveness. In L. Berkowitz (Ed.), *Advances in experimental social psychology* (Vol. 7). New York: Academic Press.

Clifford, E. (1969). Parental ratings of cleft palate infants. *Cleft Palate Journal, 6,* 235–244.

Clifford, M.M. (1975). Physical attractiveness and academic performance. *Child Study Journal, 5,* 201–209.

Corter, C., Trehub, S., Bonkydis, C., Ford, L., Celhoffer, L., & Minde, K. (1978). *Nurses' judgements of the attractiveness of premature infants.* Unpublished manuscript, University of Toronto, Toronto, Ontario, Canada.

Field, T. (1977). Effects of early separation, interactive deficits, and experimental manipulations on infant-mother face-to-face interaction. *Child Development, 48,* 767–771.

Field, T. (1978). The three R's of infant-adult interactions: Rhythms, repertoires and responsivity. *Journal of Pediatric Psychology, 3,* 131–136.

Field, T. (1980). Interactions of preterm and term infants with their lower and middle-class teenage and adult mothers. In T. Field, S. Goldberg, D. Stern, & A. Sostek (Eds.), *High risk infants and children: Adult and peer interactions* (pp. 113–132). New York: Academic Press.

Field, T., Dempsey, J., & Shuman, H.H. (1983). Five-year follow-up of preterm respiratory distress syndrome and post-term postmaturity syndrome infants. In T. Field & A. Sostek (Eds.), *Infants born at risk: Physiological, perceptual and cognitive processes* (pp. 317–336). New York: Grune & Stratton.

Field, T., & Vega-Lahr, N. (1984). Early interactions between infants with craniofacial anomalies and their mothers. *Infant Behavior and Development, 7,* 527–530.

Goldberg, S. (1979). Premature birth: Consequences for the parent-infant relationship. *American Scientist, 67,* 214–220.

Goldberg, S., Brachfeld, S., & DeVito, B. (1980). Feeding, fussing, and playing: Parent-infant interaction in the first year as a function of prematurity and perinatal problems. In T. Field, S. Goldberg, D. Stern, & A. Sostek (Eds.), *High-risk infants and children: Adult and peer interactions* (pp. 133–154). New York: Academic Press.

Hilebrandt, K.A., & Fitzgerald, H.F. (1978). Adults' responses to infants varying in perceived cuteness. *Behavioral Processes, 3,* 267–273.

Kapp-Simon, K. (1980). Psychological adaptations of patients with craniofacial malformations. In G.W. Lucker, K.A. Ribbens, & J. McNamara (Eds.), *Psychological aspects of facial form.* Ann Arbor, MI: Center for Human Growth and Development.

Kleck, R.E., & Strenta, A. (1980). Perceptions of the impact of negatively valued physical characteristies on social interaction. *Journal of Personality and Social Psychology, 39,* 861–873.

Landsdown, R., & Polak, L. (1975). A study of the psychological effects of facial deformity in children. *Child Care, Health, & Development, 4,* 85–91.

Langlois, H.J., & Downs, A.C. (1979). Peer relations as a function of physical attractiveness: The eye of the beholder or behavioral reality? *Child Development, 50,* 409–418.

Langlois, J.H., Roggman, L.A., Casey, R.J., Ritter, J.M., Rieser-Danner, L.A., & Jenkins, V.Y. (1987). Infant preferences for attractive faces: Rudiments of a stereotype. *Developmental Psychology, 23,* 363–369.

Langlois, J.H., & Stephan, C.F. (1977). The effects of physical attractiveness and ethnicity on children's behavioral attributions and peer preferences. *Child Development, 48,* 1694–1698.

Langlois, J.H., & Stephan, C.F. (1981). Beauty and the beast: The role of physical attractiveness in the development of peer relations and social behavior. In S.S. Brehm, S.M. Kassin, & F.X. Gibbons (Eds.), *Developmental social psychology: Theory and research.* New York: Oxford University Press.

Lerner, R.M., & Lerner, J.V. (1977). Effects of age, sex, and physical attractiveness on child-peer relations, academic performance, and elementary school adjustment. *Developmental Psychology, 3,* 585–590.

Mayer, N.K., & Tronick, E.Z. (1985). Mothers' turn-giving signals and infant turn-taking in mother–infant interaction. In T. Field & N. Fox (Eds.), *Social perception in infancy* (pp. 199–216). Norwood, NJ: Ablex.

Parke, R.D., & Sawin, D.B. (1975, April). *Infant characteristics and behavior as elicitors of maternal and paternal responsivity in the newborn period.* Paper presented at the meeting of the Society for Research in Child Development, Denver, CO.

Pawlby, S. (1977). Imitative interaction. In H.R. Schaffer (Ed.), *Studies in mother-infant interaction* (pp. 203–26). London: Academic Press.

Rich, V. (1975). Effects of children's physical attractiveness on teachers' evaluations. *Journal of Educational Psychology, 67,* 599–609.

Richardson, S.A., Goodman, N., Hastorf, A, & Dornbusch, S.M. (1961). Cultural uniformity in reaction to physical disabilities. *American Sociological Review, 26,* 241–247.

Richman, L.C. (1978). The effects of facial disfigurement on teachers' perception of ability in cleft palate children. *Cleft Palate Journal, 15,* 155–160.

Richman, L.C., & Harper, D.C. (1978). Observable stigmata and perceived maternal behaviors. *Cleft Palate Journal, 19,* 251–257.

Roff, M., Sells, S.B., & Golden, M.M. (1972). *Social adjustment and personality development in children.* Minneapolis, MN: University of Minnesota Press.

Sigman, M., Cohen, S.E., & Forsythe, A.B. (1981). The relations of early infant measures to later development. In S.L. Friedman & M. Sigman (Eds.), *Preterm birth and psychological development* (pp. 313–328). New York: Acdemic Press.

Simonds, J.F., & Heimburger, R.E. (1978). Psychiatric evaluation of youth with cleft lip-palate matched with a control group. *Cleft Palate Journal, 15,* 193–201.

Spriesterbach, D.C. (1973). *Psychological aspects of the cleft palate problem,* Vols. 1 and 2. Iowa City, IA: University of Iowa Press.

Tobiasen, J.M. (1984). Psychosocial correlates of congenital facial clefts: A conceptualization and model. *Cleft Palate Journal, 21,* 131–139.

Trnavsky, P.A., & Bakeman, R. (1976, August). *Physical attractiveness: Stereotype and social behavior in preschool children.* Paper presented at the meeting of the American Psychological Association, Washington, D.C.

6
The Experience of Attachment in Infants with Disabilities

SANDRA H. PETERSEN, JEREE H. PAWL, AND ALICIA F. LIEBERMAN

Imagine a baby crying. Her lip quivering. Her cheeks red. Her little fingers clenched in fists, arms drawn up to her chest. Her mother comes to her murmuring, "It's OK. It's all right, little one. You're OK." The baby stops crying as her mother lifts her to her shoulder, nuzzles her cheek, suffuses her with a glow of loving looks and words and touch. It would be hard to imagine this picture and not to know first the distress and then the comfort felt by the infant. We know by both our instincts and the study of infancy how rich a subjective experience infants enjoy. The literature on infant development is filled with descriptions that speak to us of the child's experience of interaction with the parent, of the child's development of trust, of the child's joy in learning about the workings of the world. We are keenly aware of the depth and range of feelings of infants and their parents as they learn their unique, synchronous dance of relationship.

Imagine again the crying baby. This time, though, the baby is noteworthy not only for her distress but also for a flaccid muscle tone, a slant to her eyes, a small nose. This crying baby has Cerebral Palsy. She is not so readily comforted by her mother. She cries on and on. As imaginary observers, we feel sympathy for this mother, who has a difficult baby to care for, a baby who does not easily stop crying. Each time we look at this baby, we are reminded that she has extra challenges in her future; and as we look at this mother and child, our feeling response, our empathic response, shifts from the child to the mother. "How hard it must be," we think to ourselves, "to raise a child with disabilities."

This empathic shift from the baby's feelings to the mother's is not unique to individual observers. It is a phenomenon as well of the research literature, to look at "atypical" dyads and then to consider the experience only of the mothers. The literature is replete with studies of how mothers behave differently with their disabled infants (Blacher, 1984; Hanson, 1984), how stressed these mothers are by their babies' special needs

(Gallagher, Beckman, & Cross, 1983; Breslau, Staruch, & Mortimer, 1982) and their own grief as their children do not achieve the developmental milestones in the time and manner of typically developing infants (Blacher, 1984). Research analyzes the resources that mothers draw upon to cope with the extraordinary demands of an infant with disabilities—but the literature does not tell us how babies with disabilities find ways to touch and engage their parents' hearts. Even the traditional concept of attachment, which focuses on the child's experience of the relationship, has been reversed in the special needs literature to describe the mother's feelings rather than the child's.

Hard as it was in the study of typically developing infant–parent relationships for us to come to appreciate the impact of the infant on the parent or other caregiver, it would seem as if it has been all too easy to dwell exclusively on the impact of the infant with disabilities on his or her parents. In reviewing the literature, it is striking how differently we think about interaction and attachment when the child has a disability. In a physically intact baby–mother dyad, we think about how the mother's personality and experiences with relationships affect her style of caring for the baby and what effect that style has on the baby's development. We consider the other stresses and supports acting upon the woman's life—for example, her family history and current marital situation. We wonder about the many meanings that the baby might hold for the mother: Is the baby a symbol of love and fulfillment, for example, or a disturbing reminder of an abusive spouse? We evaluate both the mother's and the baby's abilities to send and receive cues. We watch for whether they look at each other and touch each other (Brazelton, Koslowski, & Main, 1973).

When babies have disabilities, however, the studies concentrate on grief, mourning, stress, and depression. While these are significant and important factors in the lives of families who have infants with challenges they should be elements to consider in addition to all the things we look at in intact dyads. Instead, they have come to define how we see the dyad, robbing our perception of the relationship between a baby with disabilities and his or her parents of its essential human qualities.

In the following discussion of attachment and the parent–infant relationship of children with disabilities, we have chosen to include infants with craniofacial abnormalities. This inclusion seems appropriate under the Individuals with Disabilities Education Act of 1986, Public Law 99-457, which defines infants or toddlers as being disabled if they:

> have a diagnosed physical or mental condition which has a high probability of resulting in developmental delay in one of the following areas: cognitive development, physical development, language and speech development, psychosocial development, or self help skills.

Children with craniofacial abnormalities are documented as being at risk for language and speech delays, hearing loss, and secondary effects from poor nutrition (Batshaw & Perret, 1986). Craniofacial abnormality may be present as one aspect of multiple malformations due to lack of room or fluid in the womb (Batshaw & Perret, 1986), with varying related disabling effects. And, for our purposes, it is most pertinent that the presence of craniofacial abnormalities in infants may affect the infants' ability to communicate with their parents and may affect the parents' perceptions of and feelings about the infants (Daly & Wilson, 1981).

As the discussion of the parent–infant relationship proceeds, it is the transactional nature of the parent–infant relationship that we wish to emphasize. Thomas and Chess (1980) propose that the child and the parent each brings unique characteristics to the relationship, and the quality of development in the child will depend somewhat on how well those two sets of characteristics work together. Thomas and Chess refer to this as "goodness of fit," suggesting that there is no one right way to parent a child and that parents and children must, in many ways, match each other. A hovering father may be acting appropriately to his newborn, but his 2-year-old daughter needs some opportunities for independence; that is, the parent must respond to both particular and changing needs in the child. The child needs a parent who can help him or her in making relationships, feeling safe, and learning about the world.

In this way, we see all children on a continuum of specific abilities and challenges and all parents on a continuum of capacities with which to meet the needs of their children. In a sense, we see disability as one important factor in placing a child on that continuum, rather than the overriding characteristic of the child or the relationship.

In this chapter, we would like to disallow the assumption that a baby, a parent, or their relationship can or should be fully defined or described exclusively by the existence of a disability. While making full acknowledgment of the impact of a disabling condition on individuals and families, we would like to look at the many facets of the parent–infant with disabilities relationships, as we do all parent–infant relationships. We will particularly consider what it is that any baby (including a baby whose limbs, or sensors, or brain work differently) needs to experience in relationship to his or her parents.

Attachment Theory

Current research on the interactions of parents and babies tends to be organized around the theory of attachment. This presents both opportunities and difficulties for studying this population. It is confusing, for example, when the term *attachment* is broadly and incorrectly used, as though it fully describes all aspects of the parent–child relationship. The concept of attachment as introduced by Bowlby (1969) was a narrower one. Bowlby described attachment as a behavioral system that allows an infant to seek one discriminated adult (the attachment figure) for comfort and protection when the infant's sense of security is threatened. This move toward a protector on the part of the frightened infant, and the feelings inspired in the adult partner to protect the infant, serve a biological purpose in providing safety for the young, vulnerable member of the species from predators.

Ainsworth, Blehar, Waters, & Wall (1978) expanded the concept by suggesting that the quality of the patterns of an infant's approach to the mother reflect the quality of the child's experience of being with the mother. Although Ainsworth found a bond between almost all infants and mothers whom she studied, she found that "securely attached" infants were able freely to seek proximity to their mothers when frightened, and the mothers were willing and able to comfort their babies. These mothers were generally more sensitive and responsive to their babies than mothers of "insecurely attached" infants. Insecure infants had found their mothers to be inconsistently available for caregiving, or even hostile or rejecting of them. Securely attached babies also:

> have a more harmonious mother-infant relationship; the infants are more cooperative, cry less, spend more time in exploratory play, are more outgoing toward and cooperative with a moderately familiar adult, and subsequently show higher scores on a variety of problem-solving and socio-affective measures than "insecure" dyads. (Hinde, 1982, p. 68)

Children develop their ideas about who they are, at least in part, by how they are treated by the important people in their lives. If a mother and father protect and comfort their babies when the babies feel fearful or alarmed, the children grow up with a sense that they are worthy of someone's efforts to protect them and that they will have a measure of safety provided by their parents as they move out to explore the world. When parents are alert and responsive to their children's needs, the children develop a particular set of ideas—mental representations—of how it feels for them to be with other people, how they can expect to be treated by other people, and about how effective they are in letting people know their needs. Bowlby (1969) calls this set of ideas an "internal working model," a template, or filter, that affects what the children will expect of later relationships. These early experiences are influential, though not the sole determining force in all later relationships. The dynamic nature of these internal models also allows them to be affected by experiences that disconfirm the expectations, perhaps through relationships with siblings, peers, teachers, and other relatives.

Although parents and babies have many aspects to their relationship, it is the complementary aspects of intimacy and exploration that concern attachment theory. The safety provided by intimacy allows children's natural curiosity to propel them into the world. This poses particular challenges for the parents of children with disabilities. These parents may be drawn toward overprotection of children who seem vulnerable or they may feel an urgency for their children to explore and learn from the world. These parents may also have conflicting feelings about their perceptions of the children as "defective" while experiencing the children as being "products" of themselves and belonging to them (Decarie, 1969, p. 168). We need to consider what effect the presence of disabilities might have on parents' desire and ability to provide a safe base from which children can explore the world.

It is difficult to approach this topic with direct comparisons of typical and atypical dyads because contrary to the classic definition of attachment, in the literature on infants with special needs, attachment is often described as an internal experience of the mothers. Blacher and Meyers, in an excellent review of the literature (1983), "propose that the nature of the mother's attachment is a critical variable in the development of family–severely impaired child dynamics" (p. 360). It is only in this population that we even have a concept of the "mother's attachment." In the traditional literature on attachment, it is the effect of the mother's behaviors and attitudes on the child that is discussed. In an article on babies without disabilities, Hinde (1982) writes:

> . . . the emphasis in the concept of attachment is clearly on the infant. Reference is made to the tie that the infant forms and to a stable propensity on behalf of the infant. It thus refers not to the mother-infant relationship as a whole but to the child's side of that relationship. (pp. 65–66)

The Expression and Evaluation of Attachment

Attachment is usually evaluated using an assessment paradigm called the "Strange Situation" (Ainsworth et al., 1978). This involves observations of a child's attempts, when feeling distressed by repeated separations from the parent, to seek proximity to his or her parent upon reunion. The experience of attachment refers to an internal sense of danger and a desire to feel protected, presumed to be demonstrated by proximity seeking behaviors to signal or reach an adult partner. This experience and these behaviors belong to the infant, although the quality of the attachment reflects the patterns of earlier transactions and therefore the nature of the adult partner's participation. Attachment studies usually observe the behaviors of both people in an attempt to understand the experience of attachment for the child. The determination of secure or insecure attachment catagories is then made from observations of the child's behaviors in the relationship, with the assumption that those behaviors reflect a corresponding internal experience for the child. While it is obvious that children with disabilities may not have the usual repertoire of signaling or approach behaviors available to them to demonstrate attachment, the contributions of particular impairments on a child's experience of attachment (desire for protection provided by a particular person) has not been thoroughly studied.

The impediments to doing this kind of research have included confusion over how to "read" the signals of a baby with challenges and how to determine the meaning of behaviors that may be more an effect of the disability than reflective of the quality of attachment. For example, in an early study, Stone and Chesney (1978) compared mothers' reports with observations of infant responses to being handled, smiling, crying, vocalizing, activity level, and visual search and eye contact in 15 infants with disabilities. These authors began by looking for typical attachment behaviors, such as proximity seeking, smiling, eye contact, and clinging. When, instead, the children with Down Syndrome were limp when held, the authors described the behavior as a "disturbance" in attachment behavior—disregarding the expectable hypotonicity of a child with Down Syndrome. Infants with brain-damage demonstrated "attachment disturbances," such as being tense when handled, unresponsive, and seldom smiling. In this early study, the authors took what are essentially physiological responses indicative of central nervous system disorders and attributed attachment meanings to them.

Serafica and Cicchetti (1976) made one of the earlier attempts to see if the Strange Situation was a useful tool for studying attachment and exploratory behaviors of children with Down Syndrome. The children with Down Syndrome were matched with normally developing peers for chronological but not mental age. Children with Down Syndrome were less likely to cry or vocalize than their peers, but there was no difference in smiling or locomotion to achieve closeness to the mothers. The authors saw more attachment behaviors in the normally developing peers than in the children with Down Syndrome. In their discussion, they suggest that the novel situation may not have been as threatening to the children with Down Syndrome as a result of an overall "generalized lower reactivity to stimuli" or because of a lower mental age. Perhaps another reason why there was little distress for the children with Down Syndrome was that the 3-minute segments of the Strange Situation did not allow them enough time to process and react.

Rather than beginning to look at attachment in this population by searching for behaviors that are found in normally developing children, qualitative studies are needed to determine what behaviors might signify attachment or proximity seeking for children with various disabilities. Surely the first attachment theorists began by assuming the existence of something that was internal to the child and then trying to determine what behaviors might signify or express its existence. We must now assume that infants with disabilities also form meaningful bonds with their parents; and, as careful observers, we will be able to determine which behaviors demonstrate the quality of those relationships.

In keeping with this perspective of studying attachment, we consider studies that evaluate an infant's experience of attachment and his or her ability to express attachment. Decarie (1969), in a study of the interrelationships of mothers and their infants with thalidomide-induced birth defects, considered how limited physical abilities might affect emotional development and the expression of attachment:

If, besides sucking, crying, and smiling, . . . clinging and following are instinctual behavior patterns that normally constitute basic elements of the tie of the human infant to his mother, what kind of attachment behavior will be observed in children for whom clinging (because of lack of arms) or following (because of lack of legs) is impossible? Will there be compensatory mechanisms? If so, from which partner will they originate? The mother? The child? Or through reciprocal adaptation? (p. 171)

Decarie reports that they found no relationship between severity of malformations and children's ability to form a relationship with their "love object." "[A] child suffering from severe malformations can show remarkable socialization, while a subject less handicapped may reveal a distressing lack of attachment to human persons" (p. 184). Decarie clearly differentiates the capacity for emotional experience in the infant from the experiences and limitations associated with the physical disability.

Stahlecker and Cohen (1985) studied the effect of severe physical impairment on attachment. They wanted to see if the Strange Situation and its classifications could be used with children with severe physical and mental impairments. The degree of impairment was measured by the mental and motor indices of the Bayley (Bayley, 1969), and social responsiveness and rhythmic habit patterns (stereotypic behaviors) were considered as correlates with measures from the Carolina Record of Individual Behavior (Simeonsson, Huntington, & Parse, 1980). Attachment was measured with a fairly straightforward use of the Strange Situation, with small adaptations for nonlocomotive children.

The subjects were infants with neurological impairments and developmental delays. Some of the infants could crawl, scoot, or walk; others were nonambulatory, but there were behaviors available to them with which they demonstrated approach, avoidance, or resistance. They were able to reach, grasp, make eye contact, or move their heads or some part of their bodies in ways that were meaningful to the mother.

The inclusion of a wider variety of behaviors as serving the mother–child relationship was an important adjustment in being able to use the Strange Situation paradigm in research with this population. Adaptive devices were also used as needed, and toys were placed within easy reach of children when mobility aids were used. With these small accommodations and the use of a clarifying category of NL (nonlocomotive), 80% of the infants were classifiable in the secure or insecure categories, with 14 of the 19 infants classified as secure. Measures of general development (Bayley MDI and PDI) did not differentiate secure and insecure attachment groups. Only the scale of social responsiveness (Carolina Record of Individual Behavior) correlated with the attachment classification.

The authors suggest that the more "responsive child may elicit greater responsiveness and involvement . . . and may better provide a sense of efficacy for the caregiver's efforts" (p. 505). Unfortunately, in their discussion, the burden of successfully achieving a secure attachment rests on the baby's ability to engage the mother. There is no discussion of how the experience of successfully "hooking" the mother or not might feel to the child.

Hanson (1988) also found that disabilities affected different developmental domains to different degrees, in a longitudinal study of the social–emotional development of young children with disabilities. The three groups of subjects were children with Down Syndrome, hearing impairments, and neurological impairments. This study evaluated the "quality of attachment, child developmental achievement, child social responsiveness, parent stress/adaptedness, and parent-child interaction when the children were in infancy" (p. 2). The groups of children differed significantly on cognitive development, but there were no differences "on the measures of attachment, maternal "adaptedness," or mother-infant interaction" (p. 35). This was true even though mothers of the children with neurological impairments rated themselves as "more restrained by parenting, more isolated, and as having less social support than other groups," and they rated their children as more problematic in terms of matching parental expectations, demandingness, and mood. Despite Hanson's expectation that maternal adaptedness and stress and children's social–emotional development would be related to attachment classification or interaction measures, this was not the case. The ratio of securely attached to insecurely attached children resembled that found in children without disabilities. Although there were proportionately more neurologically impaired children in the insecure group, Hanson suggest that this may in part reflect "difficulties in 'reading' their signals and evaluating their relationships" (p. 38). In her summary, she states:

> Perhaps the major implications of this research is the fact that observations . . . revealed relatively few differences from those found or expected with mother-child dyads where the children were nondisabled. . . . Though mothers revealed stresses associated with their children and their parenting situations, profiles did not emerge of families who were extremely dissatisfied or unable to cope with parenting a child with a particular disability. It is likely that other factors, such as socio-economic status, spousal relationships, and problems (e.g. alcohol abuse) played a greater role in determining family difficulties than did the presence of a child with disabilities . . . the presence of a disability may present a sressful situation, but it does not necessarily result in damaged parent-child relationships. (p. 38)

In naturalistic observations of blind children's interactional patterns, Fraiberg (1975) describes blind infants' developing attachment behaviors such as preferential smiling and postural comfort when being held. For blind children, this demonstration of preferential attachment follows the demonstration of object permanence developed through tactile and aural experiences. Without the ability to check visually on parents, children's assurance that the attachment figures are present at any time in the first year of life can only be made through touch or sound contact. In these babies, the demonstration of attachment coincided with the ability to coordinate reach and sound (the knowledge that there is an object producing the heard sound) and independent mobility.

The question of whether there is a relationship between mobility and attachment is often raised in studies of children with disabilities. The question is usually phrased like this: When the organization of the attachment system seems so closely linked to exploration and locomotion, what inspires the development of attachment in children who have not developed independent mobility? Mobility has a role in the expression of attachment, but it is not a necessary condition for attachment to develop. Babies move toward their attachment figures when they feel frightened or anticipate separation from their caregivers. Mobility offers the infants an avenue to gain access to the attachment figures, enhancing the strength of the relationships and, in turn, intensifying the expression of protest over separation. It is the experience of protection, however, that is relevant to attachment rather than mobility. We need to learn how infants with disabilities express their expectations about protection, within whatever physical constraints are present.

The Experience of Attachment in Infants with Disabilities

In the literature on parents and their infants with disabilities, there is a tendency to look at the broad range of parental reactions to their children's disabilities; to discuss internal factors in the parents, such as moral or religious beliefs, and external factors such as social support, economics, and the severity of the disabilities; and to call it all "attachment." It is reasonable to consider all of these factors as potentially influencing the parent–child relationship, from a parent's point of view. However, a parent's behavior in regard to these issues may or may not be reflected in a child's attachment. In normally developing children, it is the parents' mental representation of their relationship history that seems most pertinent. How these other issues play out in a reworking of that mental representation is unclear at this time. Attempts to draw at least theoretical associations between these factors and attachment are usually built on the following reasoning: Attachment may be threatened when parents fear for their children's medical survival, so they may "minimize . . . contact with and attachment to infants with medical complications in order to maintain lower distress and anxiety" (Blacher, 1984, p. 23). Here again we address the mothers' attachment, but the idea that the mothers' fears about their babies might affect their behavior toward the babies is relevant to attachment theory. Exemplifying the perspective that attachment in this population is a maternal experience, Blacher theorizes that reduced eye contact in infants may lead to "negative feelings in the mother[s] and subsequent attentuated maternal attachment." Many perceived differences in the babies may cause a considerable reworking of the parents' mental representation of relationships. Appearance, functional communication, and normal modes of eliciting contact, such as gaze, reciprocity, or smiling, may all be reduced in infants with severe disabilities. These child characteristics may affect parental attitudes, acceptance, and attachment. Parents may be inhibited from acting naturally with their children if the "disability dominates their attention" or even causes them to feel "repulsed," promoting "feelings of withdrawal, rejection, or minimal interaction" (Fraser, 1986, p. 143).

Yando and Zigler (1984) support changing the traditional view of attachment, saying it is impossible to look at families of infants with disabilities as though the family system were as closed as it is for nondisabled infants. The presence of many professionals and services changes the character of the infancy experience and the entire transactional process. Yet despite the insistence of those who would change the attachment paradigm when children have disabilities, the studies that have measured attachment from the children's point of view show clearly differentiated relationships. This is a finding with which most parents and early interventionists would readily agree.

In the traditional attachment literature, authors have tried to correlate the quality of the mother–infant relationship with later outcomes in the child. When authors in the special needs literature change the meaning of "attachment" to describe only mothers' experiences, they consider family-related outcomes as correlates of the mothers' attachment rather than considering the child outcomes of their attachment. For physically intact children, the reasoning is that if children can grow up feeling protected and confident to explore the world, they will have better self-esteem ("I am worthy of protection"). This self-esteem has been related to outcomes such as increased personal motivation, longer attention spans, and persistence in tasks (Bretherton, 1985). For infants with disabilities, however, Blacher and Meyers (1983) suggest the need to correlate attachment (mothers') with factors such as "family integrity, marital harmony, and consideration of institutionalization" (p. 361). The failure to consider child outcomes may be, in part, due to assumptions like those made by Yando and Zigler (1984), that the importance of infant attachment has to do only with later adult functioning and so is not relevant in its classical form for this group of children:

> The quality of infant attachment and the development of the attachment system is related to expectations of mature adult functioning. Positive infant attachment

results in a mentally and emotionally mature adult. Given that most severely handicapped children will not achieve either cognitive or affective maturity, as defined for the nonhandicapped population, investigators interested in pursuing the attachment model need to specify the significance of attachment for severely handicapped children and their parents. What, for example, are the behavioral indices, for both child and parent, that positive attachment has been achieved? (p. 407)

In babies with disabilities, the significance of attachment and the behaviors that reflect attachment come from the infants' current experience of feeling loved, valued, and protected. Attachment cannot be considered significant only in terms of adult functioning. Attachment is only one aspect of anyone's life experiences and only one of the influences on the achievement of fully realized maturity. Even if we could assume that there is a direct relationship between attachment and maturity, we cannot currently predict which children will achieve this cognitive or affective maturity. As an example, consider that children whose bodies are profoundly incapacitated by cerebral palsy once were thought to be severely cognitively delayed; sheer determination, in some cases, and the technology of computers, in others, freed productive, creative minds from the limits of their bodies—minds that 50 years ago we did not imagine could exist in those constrained bodies (Nolan, 1987). We need to be equally wary of assuming the nonexistence of a relevant emotional life in even the most severely disabled. It is important, however, that investigators "specify the significance of attachment" for infants with disabilities, as suggested by Yando and Zigler (1984, p. 407). Although the current emotional health of infants with disabilities is of greatest significance, there are additional issues to be understood from studies of children without disabilities. Bretherton (1985) associates positive attachment not only with feelings of security but also with increased "persistence, attention-span, and motivation" (pp. 20–21). These outcomes seem singularly relevant to children with disabilities, who must strive harder than nondisabled children to learn about their world. This suggests that an essential daily experience of infants with severe impairments must include attention to their need and ability to "feel secure." Quite possibly infants with Down Syndrome experience the same feelings of security or insecurity when they are with their mothers or suddenly away from their mothers as any other children. What do babies who cannot see or hear feel when their mothers are close by and when they are not?

We may need to learn whether there is, in fact, some point of severity of disability that is a cut-off line; below this level of brain functioning, babies can no longer feel with utter clarity that being held, touched, or talked to by mother or father is different and preferred than the same events with other people. Until we know this, we must assume the difference and work very hard to discover its expression.

Parental Contributions to Attachment

Infants, with or without disabilities, live in families. The experience of the family and the society in which they live affect the emotional experiences of the baby. Along with the sociological factors that Hanson (1988) identifies as affecting the functioning of families and relationships, we must consider the unique personal history of each parent in their relationships. Bretherton (1985) points out that the parent–child relationship is a product of two attachment systems: the child's and that of the parent's as a child. According to attachment theory, the parent also has an internal model of relationships that begins in his or her own infancy relationship with his or her parents. Main and Goldwyn (1984), using an adult attachment classification system, found that adults tend to repeat or reenact the attachment patterns that they had as children when they become parents. As attachment theory is extended into the life cycle, it is believed that the mental model (Bowlby's internal working model) will both be applied to and altered by other relationships, including the current one with this particular child. Therefore, the parent's history and mental representations of relationships should be expected to play a significant role in the shaping of any parent–child relationship.

A recent study by Crowell and Feldman (1988) considers some questions around these issues. Using an adult attachment classification measure (Main and Goldwin, 1984), the authors interviewed mothers of preschool children in 1 of 3 experimental groups: children with developmental delays and behavioral problems, children with behavioral problems and typical development, and a control group of typically developing preschoolers with no identified concerns. The adult attachment measure attempted to provide classifications of the mothers' mental representations of relationships as related to their own early attachment experiences. Classifications included "secure," "preoccupied," and "detached" attachments. The mothers were also observed in interaction with their children. Mothers classified as having mental representations of secure relationships were warm, supportive, and helpful to their children. Mothers classified as detached were "cool and remote" and "had a controlling, task-focused style" (p. 1283). The preoccupied mothers were inconsistent with their children, sometimes warm, sometimes angry, and presented the study task to the children in a "confusing or dyssynchronous manner," leaving the children "overwhelmed" (p. 1283). All of this suggests that mothers' responsiveness and sensitivity to their children are "selectively and qualitatively" affected by their own early experiences.

Acknowledging the transactional nature of relationships, the authors also question whether difficulties of the current relationships with their children with developmental delays had affected the mothers' mental construction of relationships. All the mothers of the children with developmental delays and behavioral problems were classified in the detached or preoccupied groups; not one was classified as having a secure mental construct of relationships. It would be interesting to pursue this inquiry with prospective studies of adult classification with a large sample, so that women could be interviewed during pregnancy and then followed for several years. Given a large sample size, at least a small percentage of the mothers could be expected to produce children with some level of delay or disability. Then we could learn if a woman's attachment classification would change as she coped with the unique challenges of living with a child with a disability.

Along with relationship histories, studies of parent–infant relationships with babies without disabilities evaluate the overall affective tone of the interaction–whether the partners seem to be enjoying each other and whether there is a sense of warmth and mutuality between them, and we note individual components of the interaction—the gazes, the touches, the cooing, babbling, or words (Stern, 1977). In evaluating interactions, we look to parents to be keen observers of their infants' subtle cues, little ways the babies have to say, "I want to play now" or, "Let's stop for a moment, while I rest." We look at how parents react to those cues and how responsive babies are to their parents' ministrations (Goldberg, 1978).

We are interested in these interactions both out of respect for the children's immediate experience of life and because we believe that the quality of these early experiences has long-term effects on the children's development (Rosenberg, Robinson, & Beckman, 1986). Parents' warmth, sensitivity, contingency of response, and encouragement of babies' achievements have all been related to positive outcomes in children. Punitive, restrictive parent behavior has been correlated with more negative child outcomes. The idea is that parents can, through sensitive interaction, help children to understand their own feelings; help children to express those feelings and needs more clearly; and, through interest and encouragement, help children develop internal motivation to learn about the world. Parents who restrict their babies' expression of feeling or need may also be preventing the babies from really knowing and responding to their own feelings. From this theoretical literature we have a picture of directive, demanding parents as people who do not help babies to understand their own experience and perhaps even make the world a more random and confusing place for the babies.

Research studies of parent–infant interaction involving babies with disabilities tend to suggest that the presence of a disability disrupts the normal pattern of parent–infant interaction. Parents of infants with developmental delays seem too directive (Jones, 1977), and parents of infants with visual impairments seem alarmingly physically stimulating (Fraiberg, 1975). Similarly, people who study medically fragile infants sometimes described parents as seeming to be emotionally removed (Field, 1977). These are often referred to as disturbances in the parent–

infant relationship rather than differences, and they are attributed to parents' negative response to the presence of the disabilities. We propose that these may be accommodations that parents make to their babies' special needs, adjusting their natural tendancies to improve the "goodness of fit" (Thomas & Chess, 1980) with their children. The directive parents may be trying to simplify and slow down the flow of information, in order to give the babies time to process it. The parents of medically fragile babies may be avoiding overstimulating and overwhelming the infants. We will review some studies of parent behaviors from the perspective that parents may be making *positive* adaptations to their special babies.

Fraiberg (1975) describes parents as using what initially seemed to observers to be a worrisome amount of gross tactile stimulation with their babies with visual impairment: they bounced, jiggled, tickled, and nuzzled the infants to a degree that the observers felt was "excessive by any standards" (p. 223). Subsequently, the researchers discovered that this kind of stimulation was the only stimulus that would almost guarantee a smile. The parents later articulated their need (just like that of any parent) for the affirmation of a positive response and how they had found this way to inspire their babies to smile. The babies also made accommodations. Instead of turning their heads to make visual contact with their parents, they froze, holding absolutely still, locating their parents by sound. This was not the typical engagement of a sighted baby, but it was a perfectly adequate signal when both partners recognized the meaning of the cues. Babies with visual impairment also used an eloquent hand language, manifesting their interest, their search for toys, and their anticipation with their fingers while maintaining the vacant look of their eyes. Parents, some spontaneously, some with guidance, were able to read these signals and give sensitive, appropriate responses to their infants. Other studies report parents whose infants can neither hear nor see trying hard to elicit a response, repeating their actions far more times than parents of sighted and hearing children (Rosenberg et al., 1986).

Other parents take very different routes to interact with their babies. Some highly irritable children with multiple disabilities are helped to remain engaged with the parents through slow, soothing tones and a program of "relaxation techniques such as rocking and warm water baths [and] progressive desensitization of sensitive body parts" (Rothbart, 1984). In a comparison between mothers of infants with cerebral palsy and mothers of infants with developmental delays, the mothers of infants with cerebral palsy stayed physically closer to their infants and made more efforts to arouse their children's interest and express themselves affectively (Brooks-Gunn & Lewis, 1984), presumably in response to their infants' more limited capacity to interact with toys and objects independently. Kogan and Tyler (1973) compared young children without disabilities to children with physical or mental disabilities. They found that mothers of children with physical disabilities showed both more assertive behaviors and more warmth to their children.

The most thoroughly studied group of infants with disabilities is children with Down Syndrome, one of the few disabilities recognizable at birth. Mothers of babies with Down Syndrome are often described as more directive and controlling than are mothers of normally developing infants (Jones, 1977). Mothers talk more simply and there are more verbal "clashes," with mother and baby speaking at the same time, making a truly reciprocal interchange more difficult. Hanson (1984) found mothers of children with Down Syndrome smiling more and giving more praise to their infants, while mothers of normally developing infants were more explanatory in their comments.

Children with general developmental delays have been described as responding less contingently to their mothers (Vietze, Abernathy, Ashe, & Faulstich, 1978) and as giving mixed cues such as having such rapid state changes that make it difficult for mothers to know if their child is awake or asleep (Thoman, Becker, & Freese, 1978). Mothers of these children with developmental delays do far more purely caregiving activities and have fewer social interactions with their babies.

These studies of parents and babies with developmental delays try to classify and describe the deviations from typical interaction behaviors such as smiling, turn taking, initiations, and responses. We believe that we need to consider the function of these elements in the relationship and the function of any compensatory behaviors that may emerge in adaptation to the disability. In a study that respects the adaptive functions of behaviors and the transactional nature of relationships, Crawley and Spiker (1983) address whether "controlling and directive" behavior on the part of a parent might be appropriate and effective for a child with Down Syndrome. They suggest that a directive mother who is helping a passive child become interested in his or her environment by presenting stimulating material in a warm, sensitive manner may be helping that child achieve more adequate development. They point out that directiveness "is not synonymous with intrusiveness; conversely directiveness and sensitivity are not neccessarily incompatible qualities" (p. 1320). Their research also highlights the questions raised by the transactional quality of mother–infant interaction. In their study, they found that mothers who "combine sensitivity and directiveness in ways that provide stimulation value may have more competent children" (p. 1320). But they acknowledge the possibility that the stimulation value apparent in the mothers' behavior may be a reflection of the more competent children's effect on the mothers. Mothers in their study seemed to alter their behavioral styles according to their children's level of responsiveness.

Yoder (1986) expands our abilities to struggle with the complexities of this topic in a study in which he discusses some measurement problems inherent in studies of babies with disabilities. He hypothesizes that mothers of children with severe disabilities may make fewer responses to their babies than do mothers of babies without such disabilities, but it may be because they have fewer opportunities to respond contingently. When he controls for these differences in opportunity, he finds no association between parent responsiveness and the degree of disability in the child. In fact, studies that report increased responsivity in mothers as their disabled infants grow older may simply reflect a greater number and growing clarity of cues given by the children. Secondly, researchers and mothers may differ significantly in evaluating when children with severe disabilities are making a communicative bid. In his study, Yoder asked mothers to code those behaviors that they felt to be attempts at communication on the part of their infants. He compared the mothers' lists to those of his trained coders. The mothers "identified a greater proportion of subtle cues than did the coders." The coders were tied to conventional and clearly defined cues. The mothers were able to code subtle, idiosyncratic cues that they understood to have meaning for their infants.

Yoder's is an attempt to match the research view of infants with a more experiential view. It would not surprise the parents of babies with disabilities to be told that their infants have feelings and can express their likes and dislikes. Parents know many things about babies that have not yet been formally verified by research studies. It is not unusual in the area of infancy research for that research to lag behind everyday experience. For example, parents knew for years that babies could see at birth and that they seemed to recognize the mother's voice. Until we developed the tools to study the questions, however, we could not "prove" these facts with research. The fact that we have not asked many questions about how it feels to be a baby whose body is malformed or whose brain confuses its information only means that we don't know much about what such babies experience. It does not take away any of the experience—for the baby.

It is difficult sometimes for us, as adults, to allow ourselves to think about and fully know the helplessness of young babies. That awareness can evoke uncomfortable and frightening feelings of dependency in us. So instead of imagining the baby's experience, we generally respond to infants with a desire to protect and nurture, feelings that reassure us of our internal strength and power. If the typical helplessness of a newborn evokes discomfort in us, how much harder would it be for us to imagine the emotional life of babies with severe challenges? Do we dare stop and wonder what these babies feel when they try to call their mothers? Maybe they even believe they are calling their mothers or letting the world know that they are wet and hungry and want comfort—yet all the while unable to create any intelligible signal? When mothers are unable to respond to their infants because of their own severe depression, babies become hopeless and stop trying to signal. Do infants with challenges have a similar emotional experience—an overriding sense of their own lack of effect and agency, or does a passive trust develop toward the world? We do not know. We have not asked. It is as though our vision has been too narrow when we focus on infants with disabilites. The disability blinds us to the whole, rich picture of the children with their parents.

What should children experience in relationship to their parents? They should develop the expectation that they will be able to let their parents know when they have needs and that the parents will respond. They should be comforted when distressed and helped to feel safe and protected. If they are lucky, they will also feel a glow from their parents that allows them to feel that they are the most wonderful thing in the universe. We need to learn more about how the impairment of child's ability to move, to communicate, to return a gaze or look in the direction of the mother's voice, how a body that will arch or hang limp when held or a face that is shaped differently may affect the expectations of the baby as well as the feelings of the parent. We need to find ways to study the meaning of each partner's behavior in interaction and the effects of those behaviors on the other partner. Most important, we need to respect the richness an complexity of each person's experience as we try to understand the development of the parent–infant relationship.

References

Ainsworth, M.D.S., Blehar, M., Waters, E., & Wall, S. (1978). *Patterns of attachment: A psychological study of the Strange Situation*. Hillsdale, NJ: Erlbaum.

Batshaw, M.L., & Perret, Y.M. (1986). Children with handicaps: A medical primer. Baltimore, MD: Brookes.

Bayley, N. (1969). Bayley scales of infant development. New York: Psychological Corporation.

Blacher, J. (1984). A dynamic perspective on the impact of a severely handicapped child on the family. In J. Blacher (Ed.), *Severely handicapped young children and their families: Research in review*. Orlando, FL: Academic Press.

Blacher, J., & Meyers, C.E. (1983). A review of attachment formation and disorder of handicapped children. *American Journal of Mental Deficiency, 87,* 359–371.

Bowlby, J. (1969). *Attachment and loss. Vol. 1: Attachment*. New York: Basic Books.

Brazelton, T.B., Koslowski, B., & Main, M. (1974). The origins of reciprocity: The early mother-infant interaction. In M. Lewis & L.A. Rosenplum (Eds.), *The effect of the infant on its caregiver*. New York: Wiley.

Breslau, N., Staruch, K.S., & Mortimer, E.A. (1982). Psychological distress in mothers of disabled child. *American Journal of Disorders of Childhood, 136,* 682–686.

Bretherton, I. (1985). Attachment theory: Retrospect and prospect. In I. Bretherton and E. Waters (Eds.), *Growing points of attachment theory and research. Monographs of the Society of Research in Child Development, 50 (1–2, Serial No. 209),* 3–35.

Brooks-Gunn, J., & Lewis, M. (1984). Maternal responsivity in interactions with handicapped infants. *Child Development, 55,* 782–793.

Crawley, S.B., & Spiker, D. (1983). Mother-child interactions involving two-year-olds with Down syndrome: A look at individual differences. *Child Development, 54,* 1312–1323.

Crowell, J.A., & Feldman, S.S. (1988). Mother's internal models of relationships and children's behavioral and developmental status: A study of mother-child interaction. *Child Development, 59,* 1273–1285.

Daly, M., & Wilson, M. (1981). Abuse and neglect of children in evolutionary perspective. In D. Tinkle & R. Alexander (Eds.), *Natural selection and social behavior: Recent research and new theory*. Concord, MA: Chiron Press.

Decarie, T.G. (1969). A study of the mental and emotional development of the thalidomide child. In B.M. Foss (Ed.), *Determinants of infant behavior* (Vol. 4). London: Methuen.

Field, T. (1977). Effects of early separation, interactive deficits, and experimental manipulation on mother-infant interaction. *Child Development, 48,* 763–771.

Fraiberg, S. (1975). The development of human attachments in children blind from birth. *Merrill-Palmer Quarterly, 21,* 315–334.

Fraser, B.C. (1986). Child impairment and parent/infant communication. *Child Care Health, and Development, 12/(3),* 141–150.

Gallagher, J., Beckman, P., & Cross, A. (1983). Families of handicapped children: Sources of stress and its amelioration. *Exceptional Children, 50 (1),* 10–19.

Goldberg, S. (1978). Prematurity: Effects on parent-infant interaction. *Journal of Pediatric Psychology, 3,* 137–144.

Hanson, M.J. (1984). Parent-infant interaction. In M.J. Hanson (Ed.), *Atypical infant development* (pp. 179–206). Austin, TX: PRO-ED.

Hanson, M.J. (1988). *Social-emotional development of preschoolers*. Final grant report.

Hinde, R.A. (1982). Attachment: Some conceptual and biological issues. In C.M. Parks and J. Stevenson-Hinde (Eds.), *The place of attachment in human behavior*. New York: Basic Books.

Individuals with Disabilities Education Act of 1986, Public Law 99-457 [S. 2294].

Jones, O.H.M. (1977). Mother-child communication with pre-linguistic Down's syndrome and normal infants. In H.R. Schaffer (Ed.), *Studies in mother-infant interaction* (pp. 379–401). New York: Academic Press.

Kogan, K.L., & Tyler, N. (1973). Mother-child interaction in young, physically handicapped children. *American Journal of Mental Deficiency, 77,* 492–497.

Main, M., & Goldwyn, R. (1984). Predicting rejection of her infant from mother's representation of her own experience: Implications for the abused-abusing intergenerational cycle. *Child Abuse and Neglect, 8,* 203–217.

Nolan, C. (1987). *Under the eye of the clock: The life story of Christopher Nolan*. New York: St. Martin's Press.

Rosenberg, S.A., Robinson, C.C., & Beckman, P.J. (1986). Measures of parent-infant interaction: An overview. *Topics in Early Childhood Special Education, 6 (2),* 32–43.

Rothbart, M.K. (1984). Social development. In M.J. Hanson (Ed.), *Atypical infant development* (pp. 207–230). Austin, TX: PRO-ED.

Serafica, F., & Cicchetti, D. (1976). Down's syndrome children in a strange situation. *Merrill-Palmer Quarterly, 22,* 137–150.

Simeonsson, R., Huntington, G., & Parse, S. (1980). Developmental assessment of young children with severe handicaps. *New Directions for Exceptional Children, 3,* 51–74.

Stahlecker, J., & Cohen, M. (1985). Application of the strange situation attachment paradigm to a neurologically impaired population. *Child Development, 56,* 502–507.

Stone, N., & Chesney, B. (1978). Attachment behaviors in handicapped infants. *Mental Retardation, 16,* 8–12.

Stern, D.N. (1977) The first relationship: Infant and mother. Cambridge, MA: Harvard University Press.

Thoman, E.B., Becker, P.T., & Freese, M.P. (1978). Individual patterns in mother–infant interactions. In G.P. Sackett (Ed.), *Observing Behavior.* Volume 1: *Theory and Applications in mental Retardation*. Baltimore: University Park Press.

Thomas, A., & Chess, S. (1980). *Dynamics of psychological development.* New York: Brunner-Mazel.

Vietze, P.M., Abernathy, S.R., Ashe, M.L., & Faulstich, G. (1978). Contingent interaction between mothers and their developmentally delayed infants. In G.P. Sackett (Ed.), *Observing Behavior.* Volume 1: *Theory and Applications in Mental Retardation.* Baltimore: University Park Press.

Yando, R., & Zigler, E. (1984). Severely handicapped children and their families: A synthesis. In J. Blacher (Ed.), *Severely handicapped young children and their families: Research in review* (pp. 401–416). Orlando, FL: Academic Press.

Yoder, P. (1986). Clarifying the relationship between degree of infant handicap and maternal responsivity to infant communicative cues: Measurement issues. *Infant Mental Health Journal, 7,* 281–293.

7
Implications of Attachment Theory for Infants and Preschoolers Who Require Hospitalization

JUDITH A. CROWELL, EVERETT WATERS, AND NATHAN SZAJNBERG

The concept of attachment and aspects of attachment theory are highly relevant when infants or very young children require hospitalization or surgery. In particular, these issues are important for children who require repeated hospitalizations or surgeries, such as children with birth defects or chronic illness. Attachment-related issues affect children and their families, and therefore the medical team, in predominantly three ways.

First, children's attachment to their parents is a resource on which medical, surgical, and pediatric psychosocial teams can draw to help the children manage the specific stresses of hospitalization, illness and/or surgery, and recovery. Second, aside from serving as a resource in the children's medical care, attachment relationships are a valuable asset to children in general. They are a source of comfort and confidence. They aid children in the development of peer relationships and relationships with adults other than the parents. The relationships are sustained beyond infancy and early childhood and are a continuing resource in meeting the challenges of later development (Waters, Kondo-Ikemura, Posada, & Richters, 1990). Disrupted attachment relationships should not and need not be among the sequelae of hospitalization or surgical intervention. Finally, attachment theory also bears on the fact that not only are children attached to their parents, but also parents are attached to their children. This has significant implications for the medical team's ability to connect with the parents in consultations prior to hospitalizations, to enlist their cooperation, and to establish a collaborative relationship with the parents during treatment, recovery, and the aftermath.

The focus of this chapter is on attachment and the care of infants and very young children. Attachment-related issues remain important well beyond infancy and early childhood. A discussion of older children, however, would entail issues about body image, fear of death, and other matters that are largely beyond the experience and cognitive sophistication of infants and very young children; these are beyond the scope of this paper. To define the scope and focus of our presentation further, let us limit ourselves to the domain of "typical" families and children. Child or parent psychopathology or family discord obviously complicates many aspects of case management.

Attachment Defined and Measured

When we speak of attachment in infants and very young children, it is easy to evoke images of warmth, holding, and love. For purposes of assessment and in empirical research, however, it is useful to formalize the concept of attachment in terms of two related criteria: First, attachment refers to children's ability to use their parents as a secure base from which to explore and as a haven of safety; Second, it refers to the children's confidence in the parents' availability and responsiveness.

Both of these criteria have been translated into standardized measures for a wide range of ages. Unfortunately, most are directed at home or laboratory assessment and have not been adapted for the hospital setting. Understanding these measures as they are currently used in research, however, does afford a basis for informal assessments in clinical settings. For example, does the infant or toddler look to or move closer to parents when a new person comes into the room? When the children are hurt or frightened, do they cling to their parents or in other ways indicate a desire to be held by the parents? Can the children play comfortably in their parents' presence when there are no immediate stressors? At times children may appear more upset and angry in the presence of their parents than when alone or with other adults. "Good" behavior when the parents are absent combined with clingy behavior when the parents return is often misinterpreted by staff as a poor parent–child relationship. In many instances, the "good" behavior is really reserved noninteractive behavior, and the "bad" behavior when the parents return is an age-appropriate effort to elicit parental responsiveness and to use the parents as a safe haven. Because psychosocial team members often have the best chance of seeing a child's behavior across the widest range of contexts, they are often best positioned to make these kinds of interpretations. Nonetheless, it is useful even for clinicians who see a child in relatively few settings to be aware of the secure base/safe haven phenomenon and of the fact that attachment behavior is most evident when it is observed across time and situations.

Implications of Attachment in the Hospital Setting

The Attachment Relationship as a Resource

There are several attachment-related issues that may be significant when infants and young children require hospitalization or surgery. First, as noted previously, children's attachment to their parents is a resource that the medical teams can draw upon to assist the children in managing the stresses of the hospital experience and the illness. The parents' presence, support, and comfort to the children are vital. Well-functioning parents are frequently able to suspend their own anxiety in the presence of their children and thereby help decrease the children's anxiety and distress.

As mentioned earlier, at times children may express anger toward their parents or withdraw from them. Parents often interpret this as blame or rejection for allowing or participating in the hospitalization and treatment. This, in turn, makes them feel guilty and is often the starting point for what staff members interpret as overprotective and intrusive behavior. It is quite useful therefore for psychosocial staff to clarify the function of this behavior for parents. Far from rejecting the parents, these responses are classic behavioral responses that have the same predictable effect in both animals and humans. They activate the parents' attachment behavior and bring them closer to their children. Children's anger is not an occasion for guilt or blame. It simply reflects the children's efforts to use the parents for comfort and help. Understood in this light, parents can feel less guilty and are less prone to shift into the modes of "emergency parenting" that staff interpret as needlessly or unreasonably intrusive.

It is important that parents believe in the efficacy and necessity of the medical treatment that their children are receiving. In some cases, there is no alternative, or the alternative is for the children to remain limited or chronically ill for years. As much as parents may find a course of treatment painful to endure with their children, psychosocial teams can help them to see and understand the greater physical and psychosocial costs of chronic illness. By taking an active role in the management of therapy and its aftermaths, parents can substantially reduce its psychosocial costs to their children. If a parent withdraws from participation and supervision of care during treatment, the child may learn that the parent was "unable to protect me." Endorsing, supervising, and participating may be difficult for parents, but it at least shows their children that they have not fallen out of their parents' protective reach. Thus, parents' involvement, even in very difficult courses of therapy, is more likely to sustain than to erode their children's attachment to them.

Impact of Hospitalization on the Attachment Relationship

Separation from parents during hospitalization has long been associated with personality and socialization problems. The best evidence today indicates that these negative effects are not due to separation or medical treatment per se. The attachment effects associated with parental separation or loss arise more from discordant circumstances preceding and surrounding the separation than from the separation itself. Moreover, a wide range of variables related to the quality of substitute care provided, children's health at the time of separation, and the context in which the separation occurs can mitigate the severity of separation-related problems. Nonetheless, in view of the benefits of parent participation mentioned previously, the rooming-in arrangements available in most pediatric units today are clearly beneficial, quite aside from any separation-related effects that may be addressed. Currently, rooming-in, hospital play, and visits to the hospital prior to surgery are common efforts to reduce child and parental anxieties about the hospital. In addition to their efficacy vis-à-vis attachment issues, they take contemporary care a step closer to the ideal of being as humane as possible.

It is useful to place parents' concerns about the effects of hospitalization in context by explaining that attachment has a deep foundation established prior to coming to the hospital, and it continues to develop throughout early and middle childhood. Attachment is generally resilient and robust and responds to improvements in family and parent–child circumstances. Further, it is helpful for parents to hear that later development builds on a wide range of assets such as peer and school experience. In summary, the attachment issues that arise in the context of high-quality medical care are not usually "make or break" factors in a child's later development, especially when weighed against the value of the medical therapy.

Parental Attachment to Children

Infants and young children who need surgery are not only attached to their parents, but their parents are also attached to them. This has significant implications for the team's ability to reach the parents and to establish a collaborative relationship. Parents of children who are gravely ill or who require major medical intervention often react with coping responses very much like the processes of grief and mourning seen when a loved one is lost. The parents may deny problems, become angry, feel guilty, or become passive and withdrawn. These attachment-related responses may be intensified by disruptions in the parent–child interaction because of the demands of the illness, by parental characteristics, or by events in the parents' past that resurface, such as previous losses they have experienced.

Grieflike responses may lead to a variety of behavioral patterns to which the team must be alert. Supportive strategies can then be developed to work with the parents. For example, parents may be overeager or overly dependent on the staff. This can make it difficult for the parents to be responsible in a variety of ways, such as in giving informed consent, in having realistic expectations about the current illness or surgery, or about their children's prognosis. It may become a source of conflict that serves neither the children, the parents, nor the staff.

Case 1

Patty was 20 months old and had been born prematurely and with a cleft lip and palate. She had severe respiratory distress syndrome and required intubation for many weeks. Because of poor weight gain and difficulty in taking food orally following extubation, she had been given a feeding gastrostomy. Surgery for the cleft lip and palate had also been done in her first year of life. The medical staff and her parents wanted her to make the transition from the gastrostomy to a regular diet and eating. She was hospitalized for a number of weeks to work on this problem.

Patty's mother, Mrs. P., was very young, and the family lived far from the hospital. Her young husband was working and visited the hospital only on weekends. She had no other family in the area. Mrs. P. was very affectionate toward Patty and enjoyed playing with her. Nevertheless, the hospital staff found Mrs. P. difficult to work with because of her passivity in taking responsibility for Patty's medical and daily care. She frequently sought the staff's attention, but as much for herself as for Patty. Mrs. P. denied that she felt concerned about Patty's problems. However, she was found several times sleeping in Patty's crib with her daughter. The staff was supportive of Mrs. P. in part because of her obvious fondness for her daughter.

As advances were made in getting Patty to eat, Mrs. P. became increasingly responsible and competent in caring for her daughter. She and her daughter became close to several staff members, and for a number of years after discharge, they visited the unit whenever Patty came to the clinic for a routine checkup.

Parents may also withdraw, become aloof, or feel guilty. These are also attachment-related responses to their children's difficulties. Such parents are similar to overdependent parents in that they are also difficult to share information with, difficult to work with, and may distress rather than comfort their children. One form of aloofness or withdrawal occurs when a parent becomes a child's nurse and becomes the most competent caregiver in terms of the medical problems. This competence may come at the cost of other types of interactions with the child, such as playing, cuddling, and other, more intimate, aspects of the parent–infant relationship. The parent thus maintains an emotional distance from the child while appearing to be very actively involved.

Case 2

Jennifer was a 12-month-old girl with a severe form of glycogen storage disease diagnosed early in infancy because of failure to thrive and an enlarged liver. She had been hospitalized several times in her first year because she frequently became hypoglycemic. Her medical regimen to prevent the hypoglycemic attacks consisted of feedings every 2 hours round the clock. At night Jenny received her feedings via nasogastric tube. The tube was in place at all times and was used during the day when Jenny did not take adequate calories orally.

Jenny's mother, Mrs. M., was 28 years old, and Jenny was her only child. She was quite competent in handling Jenny's medical needs but tended to be emotionally distant from the baby, unlike her husband, who was very involved and also warm and playful with Jenny. In talking with Mrs. M., it was learned that she felt very guilty about having a child with a chronic illness. Although raised a Catholic, she had had an abortion when she was 17 years old. Her current guilt about Jenny was compounded by her earlier guilt about the abortion, making it difficult for her to respond fully to Jenny.

One of the most common problematic parental responses to a child's illness is to become acutely protective of the child. Parents may try to guard their children from the staff. Often their anxiety is based upon events that occurred earlier in the children's or family's experience. In such instances, the parents may avoid contact with or alienate sources of medical care and assistance. They protect their children because they love them, but the protection may be shortsighted.

Case 3

Twenty-four-month-old Amy had been born with a tracheo-esophageal fistula. She had nearly died in the first days of life from aspiration prior to the diagnosis of the fistula. She had been hospitalized on several occasions for surgical repair of the defect and various complications. Like the child in Case 1, Amy had failed to thrive. A feeding gastrostomy had been placed, and she did not take any food orally. She was in the hospital for assessment of chronic vomiting after feedings and also to transition her to taking food by mouth.

Amy's parents, Mr. and Mrs. B., were very protective of their child. Despite her apparent curiosity about the staff, Amy's parents felt that she was afraid of the staff members. It became evident that Amy's vomiting after meals was largely due to the parents' method of feeding her, which involved holding her in a prone position as one would hold a infant to nurse. The parents were very opposed to changing this type of feeding and were angry with the staff for making suggestions about Amy's care.

In talking with the parents, it became evident that they were very fearful of losing their baby. This fear went back to Amy's first days of life, when she was very ill and nearly died. After they spoke about these feelings (which they had not shared before), they became more relaxed with the staff and were able to take suggestions about how to help Amy learn to eat.

Case 4

Brian was a 26-month-old boy who had chronic inflammatory bowel disease of an unusual and severe type. Multiple surgeries had been done to remove segments of bowel as they became necrotic and perforated. He had been hospitalized nearly continuously since age 10 months. Brian's parents were devoted to him, and one of them was with him in the hospital nearly all the time. When he was at his best, Brian's parents would occasionally leave him with his grandparents for a few hours. They strongly resisted attempts by the staff to carry out medical procedures and care, as much as possible preferring to take care of him themselves. Because of their interest and desire to be with him, both of them had become more skilled and knowledgeable about his complex treatment regime than the ever-changing nursing staff. On several occasions, each parent had prevented serious errors by staff. Therefore, in addition to their desire to support him and to be available, they became fearful of leaving Brian and, in particular, fearful that he might die in their absence.

In this case, when the staff was able to understand the parents' behavior, they became more supportive and better able to collaborate with the parents. The treatment plan was changed to allow the parents to do most of his care in the hospital and, ultimately, at home, despite his intensive needs.

Another attachment-related problem that may arise for chronically ill children also comes from the parents' desire to provide for their children's safety and security and the staff's need to maintain a strict medical regimen. The growing toddler may be stifled in his or her need to explore and achieve some degree of independence. This may result in angry and oppositional behavior in the child and affect treatment adversely. This problem played a role for all three children described in our case histories who had feeding problems and was relieved to a great degree by allowing them more freedom in domains where they could exert control, such as in play.

Interference with Normal Parental Responsiveness

Parents may find themselves unhappy with the hospitalization because it interferes with the kind of warm, sensitive parental care and relationship that they want to give to their children and that their children need. The literature on the development of attachment primarily involves nonclinical samples. The emphasis is on the parents' sensitivity to the infants' signals and on timely and appropriate responsiveness. Patterns of parental care are clearly significant in the quality of developing attachments. The type of care idealized in this literature can be very difficult to provide when children are ill, have a birth defect, are hospitalized (perhaps repeatedly), or are recovering. Parents feel this and can be concerned about it.

Sensitivity and warmth, on the one hand, and the parents' role as protector and defender, on the other, are complementary aspects of parenting. They are of equal importance in attachment theory. The focus in much of the literature is on sensitivity and warmth. This focus is often communicated to parents through the popular press. This emphasis on sensitivity has to be understood as a function of the samples being studied. Most attachment research has employed stable middle-class samples in which basic issues of safety, protection, and supervision can be taken for granted. In this context, the focus of research naturally falls on sensitivity and other aspects of care in which the range of individual differences is greatest. But this emphasis should not diminish the importance of the parent as protector.

Insofar as parents have the impression that sensitivity is the critical element in maintaining their relationship with their children, they are likely to find even the most enlightened hospital regimen intrusive and potentially threatening. Thus, it is particularly useful for them to understand that good parenting has many facets and that they can meet their children's needs in important ways even if medical treatments somewhat constrain their usual manner of interacting with their children. Young children have to find the experience of hospitalization and surgery strange and frightening. In this context, the parent's role as secure base often comes down to this: "Do my parents know what is safe and what is right, and can they stop anything that is not safe or right?" Simply by being present, predictable, and confident, parents are doing a great deal to maintain the relationship that both they and their children value so much.

In addition to the advantages of having parents appreciate the importance of their presence, confidence, and endorsement of the treatment, it is useful for hospital staff at every level to understand how important it is to let children continue to believe in their parents' power to protect them. Staff behavior toward parents can confirm and support children's view that the parents are an effective secure base, or it can undermine it. Although the notion of a powerful parent is something of an illusion in the contexts we are discussing, it is an illusion worth preserving, for the children's sake. Insofar as staff treat parents with dignity, respect, and a sense that the parents are indeed potent guardians, children can remain confident and secure in the basic ways, even in the face of surgery of their difficult treatment. Busy staff rarely mean to overlook, demean, "look through" parents, treat the parents as children, or compete with the parents to be the children's friend. Our point is that both staff and parents should look as well to the impressions that their bearing and interactions leave with children, who are ever alert and seeking meaning in what they see and overhear. This should be a matter of concern for every member of the hospital staff, from physicians, to nurses, to housekeepers.

Summary

It is important for all members of the medical team and other staff to recognize the motivations behind diverse parental perceptions of their children's needs and their efforts to maintain their relationship to their children and to protect and comfort. One of the most important contributions of the psychosocial team to children's treatment, attachment status, and later development is to evaluate the parents' potential as collaborators in treatment and to help the medical team monitor and sustain that collaboration.

References

Waters, E., Kondo-Ikemura, K., Posada, G., & Richters, J. (1990). Learning to love: Mechanisms and milestones. In M. Gunner & A. Sroufe (Eds.), *Minnesota Symposia on Child Psychology,* Vol. 23 (pp. 217–255). Hillsdale, NJ: Erlbaum.

Part 3
Social Cognition, Self-Concept, and Social Interaction

8
Individual Differences in Young Children's Self-Concepts: Implications for Children with Cleft Lip and Palate

REBECCA A. EDER

This chapter reflects a belief that a consideration of the emotional basis of self-understanding will lead to a more accurate picture of the development of the self-concepts of children with clefts of the lip and/or palate (CLP). Recently, there has been a great deal of attention paid to the role of emotionality in personality and self-concept development. For example, Watson and Clark (in press) have delineated the emotional core of extraversion in adults. Emde (1983) and Stern (1985) have suggested that early affective experiences form a core around which children organize their representations of themselves and their world.

Emotionality is distinct from emotion and affect in several ways: First, it describes the tendency to experience nonspecific affects (e.g., the presence or absence of positive affects), as opposed to those specific affects (e.g., anger, fear, sadness) that are usually called "emotion." Second, emotionality is relatively long term and is thus distinct from affect, which is often associated with short-term mood fluctuations; Third, the terms *emotion* and *affect* usually describe states, whereas *emotionality* is viewed as traitlike (Tellegen, 1985).

Emotionality is a somewhat primitive feeling of self that exists prior to the ability to assign linguistic labels to these feelings (e.g., Tellegen, 1985; Watson & Clark, in press). A central function of one's self-concept is to explain (and perhaps rationalize) one's emotionality. Whereas emotionality is a direct reflection of emotional experience, one's self-concept is a representation of this experience. Stern (1985) has suggested that the emergence of language, and thus the ability to describe these early feelings of self, radically alter the nature of self-knowledge. For example, children might actually *feel* fearful but describe themselves as "cautious." Hence, one's experience of a personally significant event is related to, but not necessarily identical to, one's construction of that event.

Given the early developmental origins of emotionality, children's and adults' self-concepts should reveal certain organizing constructs in common but on which they may differ. For example, issues of self-acceptance are relevant to everyone, but some people feel more accepted than others. When do these different types of self-representations emerge?

Individual Differences in Young Children's Self-Concepts

Even 3-year-olds demonstrate psychological conceptions of themselves (Eder, 1990). Moreover, there are substantial individual differences in these self-conceptions. We interviewed 180 3-, 5-, and 7-year-olds, using a new self-report measure (Children's Self-View Questionnaire, or CSVQ) that contains 50 items each about the high and low end-points of common personality dimensions (e.g., achievement, aggression). Two puppets were used to present pairs of high and low statements, and children were asked to pick which statement most accurately describes themselves. For example, for the aggression dimension, one puppet would say, "When I get angry, I feel like hitting someone," then the other puppet would say, "When I get angry, I feel like being quiet." A child was then asked, "How about you?" Statements were presented in a random order, with the high and low end-points of each dimension being alternated between puppets.

This procedure was essentially a forced-choice recognition task. Hence, if children selected these randomly presented statements in a nonrandom fashion, they must be referring to an underlying conception of themselves to recognize each new item. Three factor–analytically derived scales were developed for each age group. These scales demonstrate good internal consistencies (coefficient alphas range from .73 to .80), indicating that children's responses were nonrandom. Thus, even very young children possess common dispositional conceptions that they use to organize self-relevant information. Further, the means of these scales are at midpoint with substantial standard deviations, revealing that the scales tap individual differences in children's self-conceptions. Finally, children's self-conceptions were found to be stable over 1 month (mean 1-month test-retest $r = .59$, $p < .001$).

What is the nature of young children's self-concept tested by this measure? First, it is multidimensional. Three different constructs were revealed in each age group. For example, the factors that emerged for 5-year-olds were Self-Control, Self-Acceptance via Achievement, and Self-Acceptance via Affiliation.

What accounts for the grouping and internal consistency in children's responses to these items? Five-year-old children scoring high in Self-

Control, for example, state that they tend to avoid harm, are not aggressive, are polite, and are not upset. They select items such as, "I don't climb up on things that are high," "When I get angry I feel like being quiet [as opposed to hitting someone]," "I never get in trouble for being bad," and "I get mad a little." In contrast, children low in Self-Control state that they take risks (such as climbing things that are high or going down slides head first), are aggressive, naughty, and upset.

At first glance, it might appear that children are simply remembering their day-to-day activities and that the coherence evident in their responses is due to behavioral consistency. Perhaps children hear items about climbing high things, going down slides head-first, and so forth, and indicate whether or not they engage in these activities. Whereas this interpretation might explain the consistency in certain clusters of responses (e.g., those about avoiding harm), it cannot explain why children who state that they engage in these behaviors are also more likely to indicate that they hit people, are naughty, and are upset compared with children who state that they do not engage in these behaviors. A better explanation is that children's memory for past events is organized based on the underlying emotionality. The events described by the items on the self-control scale tap the same emotionality—in this case, self-control versus impulsivity in the face of actual or anticipated distress. Further, each of the three constructs within an age group (e.g., Self-Control, Self-Acceptance via Achievement, and Self-Acceptance via Affiliation for the 5-year-olds) differs in the emotionality that is described.

The validity of these self-reports, then, lies in the extent to which they accurately reflect children's representation of their emotional *experience*. For example, a child may indicate that she *feels* like hitting someone when she is angry but may not actually do so when angered. Five-year-olds who frequently state that they are never naughty (as opposed to being sometimes naughty) are likely indicating that they feel like a good boy or girl. In support of this, such children are also likely to agree with statements reflecting high Well-Being (e.g., "I like myself"). These responses do not necessarily reflect memories for actual behaviors but are probably very accurate accounts of these children's emotional experience.

Whereas the particular self-conceptions differ at different ages, the underlying emotionality is thought to be relatively constant. For example, the dimensions Self-Control (for 3- and 5-year-olds) and Extraversion (for 7-year-olds) are similar in describing the presence vs. the absence of energy and the control of energy. Given this similarity, there should be some coherence between diverse self-conceptions at different ages. Some support for this comes from a longitudinal follow-up to our original study. Children who were low scorers on Self-Control at 3 years of age tended also to score low on Self-Control at 5 years of age when they were tested 2 years later. Five-year-olds who were low on Self-Control tended to develop into 7-year-olds who were high in Extraversion.

This coherence is due to stability in children's energy level and their ability to control their energy. Despite the finding that these self-conceptions change with age, knowing the underlying emotionality enables us to predict meaningful relations across different structures (see also Rutter, 1984). In the following section, we summarize some factors in the development of individual differences in emotionality and self-concept.

The Development of Emotionality and the Self-Concept

Eder and Mangelsdorf (in press) have proposed a model that describes the development of emotionality and self-concept. Whereas some researchers have suggested that adult personality is the *direct* result of individual differences in infant temperament (e.g., Buss & Plomin, 1984), we suggest that emotionality is a complex construct that is derived from the interaction between the following different factors: 1) infant temperament; 2) parental personality; and 3) the nature of the caregiver–infant relationship. We propose that each of these factors is a necessary antecedent of emotionality, but none alone is sufficient.

To illustrate: Activity level is thought to be a temperamental attribute because it is present in very young infants and remains somewhat stable over time. Further, activity level (i.e., energy) is thought to be an important component in the trait of extraversion (Watson & Clark, in press). Whether or not energetic infants develop into extraverted adults depends also on additional experiences that are necessary to acquiring other components of extraversion. For example, positive affect is also a component of extraversion, and this likely grows out of the quality of the infant–caregiver attachment relationship.

Individual differences in temperament are an important component of emotionality, but they *constrain* rather than *determine* this emotionality. For example, one cannot become an extravert without also possessing a substantial amount of energy, but the presence of energy does not guarantee that one will develop into an extravert.

Parental perceptions of and reactions to early temperamental differences likely also influence young children's self-concept. Malatesta and Wilson (1988) suggest that contingent responses to an infant's state (e.g., "You're feeling cranky today") is a central factor in young children's emerging understanding of their emotions. Relatedly, parents' global evaluations (e.g., "You're such a nice girl!") must play a role in children's self-understanding.

It should also be clear that parental personality plays a role in this interaction. For example, a temperamentally active child who is raised by parents who appreciate the child's energetic approach to life and who direct the child's energy into constructive activities will have a different self-view than if he or she is raised by lethargic parents who resent and criticize the child's behavior. Whereas the former treatment may lead the child to view him- or herself as "enthusiastic," "peppy," and "vivacious," the latter treatment may lead to the development of a self-concept in which the child believes him- or herself or to be "naughty," "hyper," and "demanding."

Consistent with the view that parent–child interactions play a role in the emergent emotional self-concept is the notion that infants develop a representation (i.e., an "internal working model") based on the quality of their attachment relationship with their caregivers. That is, children who are securely attached are likely to develop internal working models of themselves as worthy of love, whereas insecurely attached children come to view themselves as unlovable and worthless (e.g., Bowlby, 1980). Individual differences in these internal working models contribute to differences in emotionality. For example, children who state that they like themselves and are esteemed by others have an internal working model of themselves and their world based on their feeling of being valued by others and worthy of love and affection (see also Bretherton, in press).

The different factors involved in emotionality are also likely to be differentially involved in the self-concept. For example, whereas temperamental characteristics such as activity level are likely to be strongly implicated in one's degree (or lack) of self-control, the quality of the caregiver–child attachment relationship is likely to influence one's degree of self-acceptance. In the following section, we consider how the additional factor of being born with a cleft of the lip and/or palate might affect a child's emotionality and self-concept.

The Self-Concepts of Children with Cleft of the Lip and/or Palate

There is some disagreement about whether being born with a cleft of the lip and/or palate results in adjustment problems. On the one hand, researchers have reported that CLP children show adjustment problems such as introversion (e.g., Richman, 1983). On the other hand, adults with CLP are no more likely to demonstrate serious psychological disturbance than are other adults (e.g., Williams, 1982).

In contrast, there seems to be a general consensus that being born with a cleft of the lip and/or palate must exert a negative influence on one's self-concept. For example, in summarizing the effects of being born with a craniofacial birth defect, Day (1985) stated that:

> All birth defects create life problems that produce significant stress for both the affected individual and the family. In particular, craniofacial anomalies cause additional intense emotional disturbance for the infant's family because the defect

alters facial structure and function. Facial appearance is one of the most influential elements of interpersonal social acceptance. Discrepancy between the individual's actual facial appearance and that individual's perceived self-image is a root cause of many significant personality disorders. . . . (p. 352)

Empirical results regarding the impact of being born with cleft of the lip and/or palate are mixed, at best.

There is a paucity of research regarding the self-concepts of children born with cleft lip and/or palate. The few studies that exist have examined older children and adolescents (e.g., Kapp, 1979; Richman, Holmes, & Eliason, 1985). For example, Kapp compared the self-concepts of 34 children (ages 11 to 13) with cleft lip and/or palate to those of 34 matched noncleft children on the Piers-Harris Children's Self-Concept Scale. No significant differences were found for scores on the global self-concept scale. Significant differences were reported, however, between the children with clefts and noncleft children on a subset of physical attractiveness items. Children with CLP were less likely to state that they viewed themselves as attractive than their peers. The researcher concluded that "cleft children report significantly more dissatisfaction with their physical appearance than their noncleft peers" (p. 174). This conclusion must be tempered by the low reliability of the Piers-Harris measure (see Harter, 1983). Furthermore, given that reliability decreases as the number of component items in the aggregate is smaller, by selecting a smaller number of items (i.e., the few attractiveness items), the reliability of the measure was further reduced (see Watson & Kendall, 1983).

Most researchers have failed to demonstrate appreciable differences between the global self-concepts of children and adolescents born with clefts of the lip and/or palate when compared to typical children (e.g., Kapp, 1979; Richman & Eliason, 1982). Clifford (1987) believes that the lack of findings and the discrepancy between research and clinical conclusions about the self-concepts of children with clefts has occurred "because approaches to self-concept measurement have been haphazard" (p. 97). An additional problem may be the lack of a clear theoretical perspective on how being born with a cleft might affect a child's emerging self-concept.

Researchers of the social and emotional development of children with cleft lip and/or palate have generally assumed that children's disfigurement (i.e., unattractiveness) is the cause of their social and/or emotional problems. In one of the first attempts to integrate the findings regarding the social and personality development of children with craniofacial anomalies, Tobiasen (1984; this volume) proposes that work in physical attractiveness offers "a useful framework for conceptualizing the psychosocial issues related to congenital facial clefts." Specifically, she suggests that children's psychosocial problems may be related to their "unattractive or negative physical appearance" (pp. 131–132).

Although Tobiasen does not discuss self-concept, given the relation between attractiveness and self-esteem (e.g., Langlois & Stephan, 1981), it seems reasonable to assume that her model would also extend to the self-concept development of children with CLP. As far as we know, no research has examined the role of attractiveness in the development of the self-concepts of young children with CLP. One study that attempted to relate physical attractiveness of young adults with cleft lip and/or palate found no significant differences in self-esteem in the attractive vs. unattractive groups (Starr, 1982). Several studies have suggested that adolescents with CLP are dissatisfied with their appearance (e.g., Bernstein & Kapp, 1981), but it is not known whether the degree of dissatisfaction differs from what is reported for noncleft adolescents or whether it is related to individual differences in attractiveness or disfigurement.

These findings suggest that a more general theoretical perspective may be useful for predicting and investigating if and how being born with a cleft lip and/or palate impacts on one's self-concept. This model comes from the work on the families of children with chronic illness. Rolland (1984) proposed a categorization scheme for organizing similarities and differences between diseases based on their usefulness to psychosocial rather than biomedical inquiry. Specifically, he suggests that the chronic illness should be grouped by factors such as the type of onset (i.e., acute vs. gradual); whether the disease course is progressive, constant, or relapsing/episodic; the expected outcome; and the type and degree of incapacitation. Furthermore, he suggests that the psychological impact of chronic illness is best understood in the context of the individual and family life cycles. For example, if a young adult becomes ill, it can derail the family from its natural momentum by requiring that the adult return to his or her family for caretaking.

A developmental framework is especially helpful in thinking about the effect of being born with a cleft lip and/or palate in the child's emotionality and emerging self-concept. Recall that emotionality develops out of the interaction between infant temperament, parental personality, and the caregiver–infant attachment relationship. Any impact on these variables as a result of the experiences associated with being born with a cleft lip and/or palate would also affect a child's emotionality and subsequent self-concept. Conversely, if being born with a cleft does not affect these variables, then emotionality and self-concept would show the same degree of variability as would be expected by noncleft children.

The first question is, to what extent is CLP associated with infant temperament? Genetic factors are thought to be primarily responsible for cleft lip (with or without cleft palate) than for cleft palate alone (Moore, 1977). Hence, it is possible that CLP is associated with individual differences in infant temperament. As far as we know, there are no studies on this issue. However, research on the relation between minor physical anomalies and temperament may be relevant here. Halverson and his colleagues have found that infants born with minor physical anomalies are more likely to show problem behaviors (e.g., short attention span, aggressions, and/or impulsivity) in preschool (e.g., Halverson & Victor, 1976; Waldrop, Bell, McLaughlin, & Halverson, 1978). These results suggest that factors associated with physical anomalies are related to individual differences in temperament.

Of interest is whether this would also hold true for those with congenital clefts of the lip and/or palate. If this is not the case, then we would expect that CLP children would reveal the same degree of variability in infant temperament as noncleft children. That is, they would be just as likely to score low (or high) in irritability as noncleft children.

Individual differences in parents' personalities and subsequent reactions to their children's personalities would also play an important role in the emergence of children's emotionality. For example, even if it is the case that all infants with cleft of the lip (and/or palate) are high on irritability, individual differences in parents' reactions will result in different emotional experiences for the child. Researchers have shown, for example, that "fussy" babies whose parents consistently respond with soothing behaviors are less likely to be irritable preschoolers than when parents respond with nervous behaviors (e.g., Thomas & Chess, 1977).

My own research suggests that parents who are high in Negative Affectivity are less tolerant of 3-year-olds' behavior in general. This is illustrated by the finding that regardless of their children's behavior, these parents rate their 3-year-old children as lower in Self-Control than parents who are low in Negative Affectivity. It seems reasonable to assume that children with parents who are high in Negative Affectivity would develop different self-views as a function of their parents' reactions from those self-views of children of low scorers.

Individual differences in the quality of the parent–infant attachment relationship is thought to be related to the interaction between infant temperament and parental personality. Researchers have found that mothers with fearful and rigid personalities (as evidenced by a high score on Constraint on the Multidimensional Personality Questionnaire; Tellegen, in press) and who had infants with a high on "proneness-to-distress" temperament (Matheny & Wilson, 1980) at 9 months were likely to have insecurely attached infants at 13 months (Mangelsdorf, Gunnar, Kestenbaum, Lang, & Andreas, in press). In turn, the quality of the caregiver–infant attachment relationship is expected to affect the emergence of emotionality and self-concept. Recall that the formation of a secure parent–infant attachment relation is thought to be associated with feelings of worthiness and an internal working model or self-concept of oneself as a person deserving of love and affection (e.g., Bowlby, 1980).

If factors associated with cleft lip and/or palate such as stressful interactions during feeding (e.g., Field & Vega-Lahr, 1984; Field, this volume) result in insecure attachment relationships, then we might predict that children with cleft lip and/or palate would be more likely to reveal self-concepts of themselves as undeserving of love and affection as compared to the self-concepts of noncleft children. If, however, children with cleft lip and/or palate do not differ from other children in their interactions with their mothers in the quality of other (nonfeeding) interactions (e.g., Speltz, Armsden, & Clarren, 1990) and thus have the opportunity to develop secure attachment relationships, then we might expect that their global self-worth would not differ from noncleft peers.

Rolland (1987) has suggested that chronic illness affects the family's life cycle, particularly in the family members' ability to complete developmental tasks. For example, whereas young children usually receive socialization from their parents about negative and positive social behaviors, dealing with children's illness can derail usual childrearing practices. A final concern regarding the development of the self-concept is how much of the children's behavior is attributed to the cleft lip and/or palate rather than to the other variables described above.

Researchers have suggested that parents of children with CLP are more lenient about behavior problems than are parents of noncleft children (Tobiasen & Hiebert, 1984). This suggests that they attribute their children's behaviors to experiences associated with CLP (e.g., surgery, social stigma) rather than to other variables (e.g., age, temperament). Hence, it may be that parental reaction to children's dispositions is constrained by these parent attributions. This would mean that cleft children low on self-control, for example, might be less likely to receive socialization regarding impulse control than noncleft children.

In summary, it is predicted that rather than affecting children's global self-evaluations (i.e., their self-esteem), experiences associated with being born with a cleft lip and/or palate will have specific effects on one's self-concept. That is, young children with CLP will differ from their noncleft peers in some but not all of the dimensions on which children appraise themselves. Further, in keeping with some recent findings (Speltz et al., 1990) it is expected that these factors will have more to do with the experience of stressful medical procedure than with appearance at this early age. That is, as compared to noncleft children, children with CLP will score higher on Stress Reaction but should not differ in Well-Being. To address these issues properly, then, researchers need to use a multidimensional self-concept measure.

The Self-Concepts of Children with CLP: A Pilot Study

Children's Self-Reports

We recently tested 17 5-year-olds with cleft lip and palate on our self-concept measure. To ensure that differences between the CLP and noncleft group would not be due to other factors (e.g., Socioeconomic

Status), the CLP children were selected to be very similar to the sample of children on whom the measure was standardized. Hence, they were middle to upper middle class, had good to excellent speech, and were all attending school. All children had their lip closures completed and had very good repairs.

Three of the nine lower-order dimensions revealed differences between the responses of the children with CLP and their non-cleft peers.[1] First, children with CLP scored higher in Alienation than did noncleft children. That is, they were more likely than other children to indicate that they sometimes feel that people want bad things to happen to them, that nobody wants to be around them, and that people always say mean things to them. Second, as compared to their noncleft peers, CLP children scored higher in Aggression by indicating that when they get angry they feel like hitting someone, they sometimes try to push in front of people on line, and sometimes it's fun to scare people. Third, CLP children scored higher on Stress Reaction and endorsed items such as "I get scared a lot," "I get mad a lot," and "A lot of things make me upset."

These differences on the lower-order dimensions resulted in two significant differences for the higher-order dimensions. Children with CLP scored significantly lower on the higher-order dimensions of Self-Control and Self-Acceptance via Affiliation, but they did not differ from the noncleft children on the Self-Acceptance via Achievement dimension.

It should also be noted that there were no significant differences between the responses of the children with CLP and the noncleft children on 6 of the 9 lower-order dimensions: Achievement, Harm-Avoidance, Social Closeness, Social Potency, Traditionalism, and Well-being. It is especially striking that CLP children were just as likely as other 5-year-olds to state that they are usually happy, they like themselves, and they laugh a lot.

In summary, children with CLP are just as likely as noncleft children to state that they work hard, avoid (or seek) risks, have friends, are leaders, and respect rules. Children with CLP differ from noncleft children in feeling a greater degree of upset, rejection by others, anger, and aggression.

Mothers' Ratings of Children with CLP

Given that most research on the emotional experience of young children with medical problems has relied on other people's ratings (e.g., parents, teachers), we were interested in how parents' ratings compared to the children. To address this issue, we asked mothers to rate their children on

[1] These data were analyzed using One-Way Analysis of Variance (ANOVA) tests for the mean responses of the CLP versus noncleft children for each dimension. All significant results are significant at $p < .05$ (two-tailed).

the questionnaire used for the children. The items on the parents' questionnaire were changed from the first to the third person (e.g., "I am usually happy" was changed to "Is usually happy"). The mothers of the 17 children who participated in the self study participated in this study. Their answers were compared to those of 30 mothers of 5-year-olds who were born without any birth defects or major medical problems.

There were significant differences between the two groups of mothers on 5 of the 9 lower-order dimensions. Mothers of children with CLP rated their children as higher on Aggression, Harm-Avoidance, and Stress Reaction, and lower on Social Potency and Traditionalism than did mothers of noncleft children. That is, mothers of children with CLP indicated that their childen were more likely to be upset and hit people and less likely to take physical risks, be leaders, and/or follow rules, than did mothers of other 5-year-olds.

Mothers of CLP children did not differ from other mothers on the dimensions of Achievement, Alienation, Social Closeness, and Well-being. That is, they indicated that their children were just as likely to work hard, feel accepted by others, have friends, and like themselves as was indicated by mothers of other 5-year-old children.

A Comparison of Children's and Mothers' Ratings

Children with CLP rated themselves as higher on Aggression and Stress Reaction than did their noncleft peers, and their mothers rated them as higher on these dimensions than did their noncleft peers' mothers. Mothers rated their children as more likely to avoid risks, be naughty, and less likely to act as leaders as compared to the responses of mothers of noncleft children, but this difference was not found in the children's ratings. Children with CLP also rated themselves as higher on Alienation, but this was not found for the mothers' ratings.

Summary

Implications for Research

The remaining question concerns the origins in differences between the self-concepts of children with CLP and noncleft children. Given the results of the current study, it would seem likely that factors associated with children's self-reported well-being (e.g., secure attachment relationships) likely do not differ between cleft and noncleft children. Indeed, it may be the case that secure attachment relationships act as a buffer against stressful situations (e.g., surgery) to maintain children's well-being (see also the chapters by Petersen, Pawl, & Lieberman; Crowell, Waters, & Szanjnberg, this volume). Further, CLP children are just as likely as noncleft children to state that they seek social relationships and are as successful leaders as their peers. Given that the children in the current study were just beginning to attend school, it may be that such children have not experienced a great deal of social stigma.

Children with CLP state that they are more upset, alienated, bitter, and hostile than do their noncleft peers. Of interest is the origins of this difference. It is possible that the experience is not specific to having a cleft of the lip and/or palate but rather is due to factors associated with the treatment of CLP. That is, the multiple surgeries and visits to health care professionals make these children angry about their own and their parents' inability to prevent and control this discomfort. This so far untested hypothesis could be addressed by comparing children with CLP to other children who have different medical problems but similar treatments.

The children in my pilot study were a special group of CLP children. They had excellent repairs (some with almost imperceptible scars) and no speech problems. Hence, of interest is whether these findings would hold for a wider group of CLP children. For example, how might degree of disfigurement affect children's particular dimensions of self-concept? In addition, how would the children in the current study compare to a group of children with a similar history of medical treatment and but no physical trace (i.e., scar)?

Of interest is how individual differences in self-concept affect children's response to treatment. For example, are children who are high in Stress Reaction more likely to be upset by minor stresses (e.g., slightly painful procedures) than children who are low in Stress Reaction? Are children high in Traditionalism more likely to comply with recommendations (e.g., avoiding rough-and-tumble play following surgery) than low scores? This would be important information in evaluating factors involved in the successful treatment of these patients.

Finally, it would be of interest to know the developmental course of these self-concepts over time. We might expect that whereas 5-year-olds might be given some understanding and latitude for upset and hostile behavior, such behavior may negatively affect their peer interactions over time, for example, leading these children to become rejected by their peer group (see Rubin & Wilkinson, this volume). Furthermore, whereas children may be neither self-conscious nor stigmatized by a small scar at 5 years, this might become more of an issue as children have a diverse number of school experiences or during adolescence. In support of this point, the few effects on self-esteem that have been reported are found in adolescents (e.g., Bernstein & Kapp, 1981).

It is noteworthy that the number of differences between CLP and noncleft children were magnified in the mothers' ratings. This may reflect parental reactions to their children's behaviors. For example, children with CLP scored higher on Aggression as rated by themselves and their mothers compared to noncleft peers others also considered the consequences of children's behaviors, adding that children with CLP were low on Traditionalism (i.e., often "naughty"), compared to noncleft children. Other reasons for the difference between mothers' and children's ratings may reflect mothers' implicit theories and their concerns about the child's future opportunities. For example, mothers may have rated their children as less likely to be leaders because they believe that appearance is an important aspect in popularity (see Berry, this volume).

In summary, these differences suggest that mothers and children use different information when asked to rate children's emotionality and self-concept. Whereas previous research on the adjustment of young children with CLP have often relied on the ratings other people we propose that the best account of these children's emotional experience comes from the child's own self-reports.

Implications for Treatment

The majority of articles written about psychological interventions with children with CLP have emphasized young children's self-esteem. For example, Clifford (1987) has suggested that cleft lip and palate teams should be sensitized to CLP children's self-esteem problems. Although self-esteem seems to be a major focus to health care professionals, little empirical research has revealed differences in self-esteem between CLP children and other children. In addition, the mothers of CLP children in our study did not rate their children differently on the self-esteem dimensions (e.g., well-being) than did other mothers.

It may be that the emphasis on self-esteem reflects an implicit theory about the effects of having a cleft lip and/or palate that is not shared by CLP children's mothers or not reflected in the children's actual self-concept. Perhaps this theory overemphasizes the role of attractiveness and the relationship between attractiveness and self-esteem (see Berry, this volume). Regardless of the reason, it may be the case that CLP teams may be providing a type of psychological intervention that is not needed by the patients or their parents.

In contrast, CLP children rated themselves as more upset and angry (and thus lower on Self-Control) than their peers, and this finding was replicated in the differences between mothers of CLP children and other mothers. This suggests that at least two types of intervention by the CLP team would be useful. First, children need some counseling for their feelings of being upset and hostile throughout the course of their treatment. Second, CLP teams need to take actions that will help prevent children's heightened stress and lack of control during their treatment. Some of these actions might involve giving more control (e.g., on when to schedule surgical procedures or office visits) or the illusion of control to parents and children (see Crowell, Waters, & Szajnberg, this volume).

Given that children who engage in aggressive and hostile behaviors in the classroom are more likely to be rejected by their peers (see Rubin & Wilkinson, this volume), the CLP team needs to address these feelings and behaviors early, not only to help children's current negative emotions but also to circumvent future psychological problems. If the parents are (perhaps correctly) attributing children's aggressive feelings and behaviors to the cleft experience and are thus slow to react, they also need some guidance to help them socialize these behaviors and avoid the negative consequences of such behaviors for their children. Given that both children with CLP and their mothers report children's feelings of anger and upset, these feelings are a good starting point for family intervention.

Cleft palate teams also may help parents understand and respond to those differences between parents' and children's views. For example, CLP children report feelings of alienation that are not reflected in the mothers' ratings. It is clear that these feelings must be brought to the parents' attention. Further, parents must learn that some of their concerns (e.g., about their children's leadership potential) are not reflected in their children's self-concepts (or perhaps behaviors). Hence, it might be unproductive for parents to focus on these concerns with their children.

All this suggests that decisions about psychological intervention by the CLP team should be strongly based in current empirical findings. Given that children's psychological health is an important outcome measure of the success of the treatment, whenever possible, other team members (e.g., surgeons, dentists) should take the results of psychological research seriously when performing and scheduling procedures. For example, giving more control (e.g., on when to schedule surgical procedures or office visits) or the illusion of control to parents and children may help families cope with the cleft experience (see Crowells, Waters, & Szajnberg, this volume).

Finally, all members of the CLP team should be aware that individual differences in children's emotionality and self-concept likely result in different reactions to their course of treatment and may be involved in the degree of successful outcome. For example, children high in Stress Reaction will be more likely to be upset by minor stresses (e.g., slightly painful procedures) than will children low in Stress Reaction. Children high in Traditionalism will be more likely to comply with recommendations (e.g., avoiding rough-and-tumble play following surgery) than low scores. Hence, it is important that health care professionals take psychological information seriously when making recommendations for individual children.

In summary, individual differences in young children's self-concept reflect individual differences in emotionality. Emotionality, or the tendency to experience certain nonspecific affects (e.g., high positive affect), develops out of the interaction between infant temperament, parental personality, and the caregiver–infant attachment relationship. I have suggested that any factors associated with being born with a cleft of the lip and/or palate (e.g., feeding problems, multiple surgeries) that affect either infant temperament, parental personality, or the caregiver–infant attachment relationship will influence a young child's emerging self-concept. Data from a pilot study of the self-concepts of 17 5-year-olds with CLP reveals that these children differed from noncleft children in the extent to which they report feelings of alienation, stress, anger, and aggression. These findings have important implications for both future research and treatment of children with clefts of the lip and/or palate.

Acknowledgments. I would like to thank Leigh Berry, Ph.D. for her assistance on all aspects of the pilot study on CLP children's self-concepts. Thanks also to Ian Munro, M.D., for his cooperation and generous help in recruiting subjects for this study. Finally, the space and resources of the Craniofacial Institute at the Humana Advanced Surgical Institutes in Dallas, Texas, are gratefully acknowledged. Thanks to Norah Feeny, M.A. for helpful comments on an earlier manuscript and to Betsy Wood, Ph.D. for several interesting discussions about psychological issues in chronic illness.

References

Bernstein, N.R., & Kapp, K. (1981). Adolescents with cleft palate: Body image and psychosocial problems. *Psychosomatics, 22,* 679–703.

Bowlby, J. (1980). *Attachment and loss. Vol. 3: Loss, sadness and depression.* New York: Basic Books.

Bretherton, I. (in press). A new look at the social self. In M. Gunnar & L.A. Sroufe (Eds.), *Minnesota symposium of child psychology* (Vol. 23). Hillsdale, NJ: Erlbaum.

Buss, A.H., & Plomin, R. (1984). *Temperament: Early developing personality traits.* Hillsdale, NJ: Erlbaum.

Clifford, E. (1987). *The cleft palate experience.* Springfield. IL: Charles C. Thomas.

Day, D.W. (1985). Craniofacial birth defects. In N. Hobbs & J.M. Perrin (Eds.), *Issues in the care of children with chronic illness.* San Francisco: Jossey-Bass.

Eder, R.A. (1990). Uncovering children's psychological selves: Individual and developmental differences. *Child Development, 61,* 849–863.

Eder, R.A., & Mangelsdorf, S.C. (in press). The emotional basis of early personality development: Implications for the emergent self-concept. In S. Briggs, R. Hogan, & W. Jones (Eds.), *Handbook of personality psychology.* Orlando, FL: Academic Press.

Emde, R.N. (1983). The prerepresentational self and its affective core. *Psychoanalytic Study of the Child, 38,* 165–192.

Field, T.M., & Vega-Lahr, N. (1984). Early interactions between infants with craniofacial anomalies and their mothers. *Infant Behavior and Development, 7,* 527–530.

Halverson, C.F, & Victor, J.B. (1976). Minor physical anomalies and problem behavior in elementary school children. *Child Development, 47,* 281–285.

Harter, S. (1983). Developmental perspectives on the self-system. In E.M. Hetherington (Ed.), P.H. Mussen (Series Ed.), *Handbook of child psychology: Vol. 4. Socialization, personality, social development* (pp. 275–385). New York: Wiley.

Kapp, K. (1979). Self-concept of the cleft lip or palate child. *Cleft Palate Journal, 16,* 171–176.

Langlois, J.H., & Stephan, C.W. (1981). Beauty and the beast: The role of physical attraction in peer relationships and social behavior. In S.S. Brehm, S.M. Kassin, & S.X. Gibbons (Eds.), *Developmental social psychology: Theory and research* (pp. 152–186). New York: Oxford University Press.

Malatesta, C.Z., & Wilson, A. (1988). Emotion cognition interaction in personality development: A discrete emotions functionalist analysis. *British Journal of Social Psychology, 27,* 91–112.

Mangelsdorf, S., Gunnar, M., Kestenbaum, R., Lang, S., & Andreas, D. (in press). Infant proneness-to-distress temperament, maternal personality, and mother-infant attachment: Associations and goodness of fit. *Child Development.*

Matheny, A.P., & Wilson, R.S. (1981). Developmental tasks and rating scales for laboratory assessment of infant temperament. *JSAS Catalog of Selected Documents in Psychology, 11* (MS. No. 2367).

Moore, K.L. (1977). *The developing human: Clinically-oriented embryology* (2nd Ed.). Philadelphia: Saunders.

Richman, L.C. (1983). Self-reported social, speech, and facial concerns and personality adjustment of adolesents with cleft lip and palate. *Cleft Palate Journal, 20,* 108–112.

Richman, L.C., & Eliason, M. (1982). Psychological characteristics of children with cleft lip and palate: Intellectual, achievement, behavioral, and personality variables. *Cleft Palate Journal, 19,* 251–257.

Richman, L.C., Holmes, C.S., & Eliason, M. (1985). Adolescents with cleft lip and palate: Self-perceptions of appearance and behavior related to personality adjustment. *Cleft Palate Journal, 22,* 93–96.

Rolland, J.S. (1984). Toward a psychosocial typology of chronic and life-threatening illness. *Family Systems Medicine, 2,* 245–262.

Rolland, J.S. (1987). Chronic illness and the life cycle: A conceptual framework. *Family Process, 26,* 203–221.

Rutter, M. (1984). Continuities and discontinuities in socioemotional development. In R.N. Emde & R.J. Harmon (Eds.), *Continuities and discontinuities in development* (pp. 41–68). New York: Plenum Press.

Speltz, M.L., Armsden, G.C., & Clarren, S.S. (1990). Effects of craniofacial birth defects on maternal functioning postinfancy. *Journal of Pediatric Psychology, 15,* 177–196.

Starr, P. (1982). Physical attractiveness and self-esteem ratings of young adults with cleft lip and/or palate. *Psychological Reports, 50,* 467–470.

Stern, D.N. (1985). *The interpersonal world of the infant: A view from psychoanalysis and developmental psychology.* New York: Basic Books.

Tellegen, A. (in press). *Multidimensional Personality Questionnaire.* Minneapolis, MN: National Computer Services.

Tellegen, A. (1985). Structures of mood and personality and their relevance to assessing anxiety, with an emphasis on self-report. In A.H. Tuma & J.D. Maser (Eds.), *Anxiety and the anxiety disorders* (pp. 681–706). Hillsdale, NJ: Erlbaum.

Thomas, A., & Chess, S. (1977). *Temperament and development.* New York: Brunner/Mazel.

Tobiasen, J.M. (1984). Psychosocial correlates of congenital facial clefts: Conceptualization and model. *Cleft Palate Journal, 21,* 131–139.

Tobiasen, J.M., & Hiebert, J.M. (1984). Parents' tolerance for the conduct problems of cleft palate children. *Cleft Palate Journal, 21,* 82–85.

Waldrop, M.F., Bell, R.Q., McLaughlin, B., & Halverson, C.F. (1978). Newborn minor physical anomalies predict short attention span, peer aggression, and impulsivity at age 3. *Science, 199,* 563–565.

Watson, D., & Clark, L.A. (in press). Extraversion and its positive emotional core. In S. Briggs, R. Hogan, & W. Jones (Eds.), *Handbook of personality psychology.* Orlando, FL: Academic Press.

Watson, D., & Kendall, P.C. (1983). Methodological issues in research on coping with chronic disease. In P.E. Kendall & D. Watson (Eds.), *Coping with chronic disease* (pp. 39–81). New York: Academic Press.

Williams, B.J. (1982). Social and psychological problems associated with cleft palate. *Clinics in Plastic Surgery, 9,* 317–326.

9
Peer Rejection and Social Isolation in Childhood: A Conceptually Inspired Research Agenda for Children with Craniofacial Handicaps

KENNETH H. RUBIN AND MARGARET WILKINSON

Most child development theorists and researchers today would agree that children's peer interactions and their acceptance by others are crucial for normal social and emotional development. Although such views were expressed by psychologists early in this century, it has not been until recent years that researchers have reached some consensus concerning the significance of peer interaction for later development.

One of the earliest theoretical perspectives on the developmental role played by peers can be found in the writings of Piaget (1926, 1932). In one of his first books, Piaget (1932) suggested that children's relationships with their peers should be distinguished from their relationships with adults. The latter relationships were characterized as being dominated by adults, whereas the former were portrayed as being more balanced and egalitarian. As such, it was within the peer context that Piaget believed that children could experience opportunities for conflict, negotiation, and compromise that might result in positive outcomes for them. One hypothesized consequence of such experiences in this egalitarian milieu of multidirectional influence was the development of perspective-taking skills and the decline of egocentrism. These social-cognitive developments were thought to result in positive and productive social interactions in which children could learn from the ideas and opinions of their peers.

Like Piaget, Sullivan (1953) believed that the concepts of mutual respect, equality, and reciprocity developed from peer relationships. Sullivan emphasized the importance of special relationships, chumships and friendships, for the emergence of these concepts. In the early school years, whether friends or not, Sullivan thought children were basically insensitive to their peers. During the juvenile years (late elementary school), however, children were thought to be able to recognize and value one another's personal qualities; as a consequence, peers gained power as personality shaping agents. Peers were thought to help children understand the constructs of cooperation, competition, and social roles such as deference and dominance. During preadolescence, Sullivan suggested that children gained a more complex understanding of social relationships as the concepts of equality, mutuality, and reciprocity became central to their own close friendships. Once acquired between friends, these concepts were thought to be extended to other relationships.

For Mead (1934) peer interaction, especially playing games, was thought to be crucial to the development of the child's perceptions of the self in relation to others. To play games well, Mead thought that one must take into perspective the attitudes of all other participants and to understand the interrelations of each role in order to best carry out one's own role. The child's personality was thought to be shaped by the organization of other's attitudes toward him or her and by the shared social activities of peers.

Empirical evidence for the importance of peer interaction indicates that children have an effect on one another's behavior from as early as infancy. Distress often follows the fussing and crying of an infant peer, and babies display some reciprocal touch during interaction (Hay, Pedersen, & Nash, 1982). In toddlerhood interpersonal influence is indicated by similar form and frequency of communication within peer dyads, reflecting both cooperation and resistance to the other's overtures (Ross, Lollis, & Elliot, 1982).

Research demonstrates also that opportunities for communication, conflict, and role playing in early and mid-childhood can improve perspective-taking skills and lead to decreases in aggression (for a review, see Shantz, 1983). In addition, peers have been found to serve as behavior control agents, decreasing inappropriate behavior by punishing or ignoring it and increasing desirable activities through reinforcement (e.g., Lamb & Roopnarine, 1979). For example, altruism has been shown to increase as a result of peer tutoring (Staub, 1975). Moreover, several studies illustrate the modification of prosocial, aggressive, or sex-typed behaviors, *indirectly,* by mere exposure to peer models (for a review, see Hartup, 1983).

The theoretical and empirical perspectives described here are suggestive of the significance of peer interaction for socioemotional and social-cognitive development; they imply also that a relative lack of relationships with peers may prove detrimental. Children who experience few opportunities for positive peer social contact have fewer opportunities to learn appropriate social behaviors than their more sociable peers. Children who do not, for various reasons, interact with their peers in normal ways, quantitatively and qualitatively, may be at risk for problems in the social-cognitive, social-behavioral, and even academic domains.

In a recent review, Parker and Asher (1987) noted that peer rejection, an index of the quality of children's peer relationships, has been found to be a significant predictor of school dropout and delinquency in adolescence and of psychopathology in adulthood. They noted also that childhood aggression, itself a known cause of peer rejection in childhood (Coie & Kupersmidt, 1983; Dodge, 1983), is predictive of later criminality. Hostility, aggression, and violent crime are often referred to as externalizing (or acting out) problems. Thus, the data extant suggest that *qualitatively* negative aspects of children's peer relationships are associated with negative "outcomes" of an externalizing nature.

Whether *quantitative* features of children's social interactive behavior are predictive of negative outcomes has, heretofore, remained an understudied area (Parker & Asher, 1987). Recently, Rubin and colleagues have distinguished between social isolation by the peer group (i.e., peer rejection) and social isolation from the peer group (i.e., social withdrawal). In a series of programmatic studies, they have shown that children who are socially withdrawn may be at risk for difficulties associated with social-cognitive development, social relationships and the self system. In the Waterloo Longitudinal Project, it has been demonstrated that social withdrawal (i.e., not interacting frequently or at a normal rate with peers) is stable from early through late childhood (Rubin, Hymel, Mills, & Rose-Krasnor, 1991; Rubin, Hymel, & Mills, 1989). These data have corroborated earlier reports of the stability of social withdrawal in childhood (Bronson, 1966; Younger, Schwartzman, & Ledingham, 1986). Moreover, social withdrawal was found to be associated concurrently with perspective-taking and interpersonal problem-solving difficulties (LeMare & Rubin, 1987; Rubin, Daniels-Beirness, & Bream, 1984; Rubin & Krasnor, 1986) and with deference and submission to peers (Rubin, 1985; Rubin & Borwick, 1984) in early and mid-childhood. In mid- and late childhood, social withdrawal was reported to be associated concurrently with negative self-perceptions of social competence (Rubin, 1985; Rubin & Mills, 1988). Furthermore, social withdrawal at both 5 and 7 years of age was shown to be predictive of depression and/or loneliness and anxiety (i.e., internalizing disorders) at 11 years of age (Rubin, Hymel, & Mills, 1989; Rubin & Mills, 1988). These latter findings concerning withdrawn children's negative self-perceptions, and their subjective expressions of loneliness, anxiety, and depression may be characterized as psychological difficulties of an internalizing (or "acting in") nature.

Although the Waterloo Longitudinal Project has demonstrated links between early social withdrawal or isolation from the peer group and later difficulties of an "internalizing" nature on the one hand, and between early rejection (isolation by the peer group) and early aggression and later difficulties of an "externalizing" nature on the other (Hymel,

Rubin, Rowden, & LeMare, 1990), the mechanisms or processes by which these associations are developed require elaboration. Recently, Rubin and colleagues have suggested two developmental models that may account more specifically than the early theories (Piaget, Sullivan, Mead) for the predictive and possible causal associations between early social isolation (by and from the peer group) and later psychological difficulty. Our first pupose, in this chapter, is briefly to present these conceptual models in which we describe pathways to and from peer rejection and social withdrawal/isolation in childhood. Second, we examine how existing research fits these models. Third, we suggest how children with craniofacial handicaps might find themselves on a pathway to rejection and/or social withdrawal. Finally, we indicate several research possibilities concerning the long-term, socioemotional effects for children who are handicapped, in general, and who suffer from facial and cranial anomalies, in particular.

Pathway 1 to Rejection and Isolation

In our developmental models (Rubin, LeMare, & Lollis, 1990; Rubin & Lollis, 1988), we have taken as our starting point the birth of the child. We could, of course, have begun earlier and have considered whether the baby was planned, whether the mother is single or married, whether she has been depressed, has been taking drugs, is poor, is voluntarily or involuntarily unemployed, whether she has available to her a support network, etc. Drawing from the work of Bronfenbrenner (e.g., Bronfenbrenner & Crouter, 1983), we have labeled all of the above-mentioned factors as "setting conditions." These conditions include ecological and psychological factors, and they probably play a critical role in development throughout the life-course. Thus, our choice to begin our developmental models at the point of the infant's birth is actually quite arbitrary. One could easily imagine how negative setting conditions could have some impact on the early parent–child relationship.

The first developmental pathway begins with an infant who is perceived by his or her parents as being of difficult temperament. We do not suggest that all such babies are at risk; however, one might predict that babies who are viewed by parents as fussy and overactive and who are born into less than desirable situations may be recipients of less than optimal care. Consistent with this position are findings reported by Spieker and Booth (1988) and Egeland and Farber (1984). These researchers have indicated that temperamentally difficult infants often have mothers who are more aggressive, less nurturant, more anxious, and less responsive than are mothers of nondifficult babies. The setting conditions noted above may be critical mediating factors; for example, Crockenberg (1981) has reported that mothers of temperamentally difficult babies who have social and financial support are less negative in their interactions with their infants than are "high risk" mothers. For some families, then, the interaction between infant dispositional characteristics and ecological setting conditions may promote parental socialization practices that result in the establishment of insecure, perhaps even hostile, early parent–child relationships (Engfer, 1986).

The data extant do suggest that there is a group of insecure babies who have already established hostile relationships with their primary caregivers by 12 or 18 months. Interestingly, researchers have found that when these insecure babies reach preschool age, they often direct hostility, anger, and aggression to their peers (Sroufe, 1983). Furthermore, as noted earlier, aggression is a highly salient determining cause of peer rejection or dislike (Coie & Kupersmidt, 1983). It follows logically and empirically that children who are initially sociable but, at the same time, aggressive will be rejected by their peers and not be allowed to play with them (Dodge, 1983). Thus, one pathway to social rejection and social isolation may be determined by the display of anger and hostility in the peer group.

Pathway 2 to Isolation and Peer Rejection

In Pathway 1, social solitude could best be construed as imposed by others. Our second pathway begins with newborns who may be biologically predisposed to have a low threshold for arousal when confronted with social (or nonsocial) stimulation and novelty. Recent research by Kagan and colleagues (e.g., Kagan, Reznick, & Snidman, 1987) and others supports this perspective. During infancy, when faced with uncertainty, these babies may experience physical and physiological changes that may make them extremely difficult to soothe and comfort. It is possible that some mothers (and fathers) may find such infantile responses aversive (Kagan, Reznick, Clarke, Snidman, & Garcia-Coll, 1984); consequently, they may react to their babies with hostility, insensitivity, lack of affection, nonresponsivity and/or neglect. Interestingly, each of these parental variables is predictive of insecure attachment relationships at 12 and 18 months. Furthermore, many of these negative socialization practices are associated with environmental and personal stressors such as poverty, unemployment, premature birth of the infant, marital satisfaction, and maternal depression (e.g., Engfer & Gavranidou, 1987). Consequently, it is not simply the interaction between parent and child behaviors that may contribute to the development of a negative primary relationship; the broader context within which the relationship is formed would appear to be important as well.

The interplay of endogenous, socialization, and early relationships factors described above, in addition to negative setting conditions, may lead to a sense of felt insecurity in toddlerhood and early childhood

(Belsky & Rovine, 1987). In temperamentally inhibited children, this felt insecurity may further exacerbate behavioral wariness and inhibition in novel social and impersonal settings. Behavioral wariness and inhibition in the face of novelty is clearly consistent with the description of the play behaviors of many insecurely attached babies. It also describes the behaviors of toddlers who have been identified as "behaviorally inhibited." In novel settings, these babies cling to their parents and refrain from exploring both persons and objects. One can speculate that these children will avoid the peer milieu when they first enter school, and, as such, they may be those who psychologists eventually come to identify as socially withdrawn.

Reticence to explore novel, out-of-home settings precludes: 1) the possibilities of establishing normal social relationships; 2) the experience of normal social interactive play behaviors; and 3) the development of those social and cognitive skills that are supposedly encouraged by peer relationships and social play. Thus, it is easy to imagine a developmental sequence in which an anxious, insecure child withdraws from his or her social world of peers, fails to develop those skills derived from peer interaction and, because of this, becomes increasingly anxious and isolated from the peer group.

It is important to note also that during the early years of childhood, solitary or nonsocial activity is actually quite normal (Rubin, Fein, & Vandenberg, 1983); consequently, there is little reason for nonsocial players to be singled out *by their peers* as displaying behaviors deviant from age-group play norms. Children do, however, become increasingly sociable with age (Greenwood, Todd, Hops, & Walker, 1982; Parten, 1932). This increase in sociability and concomitant decline in solitary activity with age may account for the finding that during the mid- and late years of childhood, children who are socially withdrawn become increasingly salient to their age-mates (Younger & Boyko, 1987; Younger, Schwartzman, & Ledingham, 1986). Their deviance from age-appropriate social norms may well result in the establishment of negative peer reputations. Indeed, by the mid- to late years of childhood, social withdrawal and anxiety are as strongly correlated with peer rejection and unpopularity as is aggression (Hymel & Rubin, 1985; Rubin, Hymel, LeMare, & Rowden, 1989). Thus, this second developmental pathway, like the first described previously, concludes with a child who is socially isolated and rejected by his or her peers.

Conceptually Relevant Outcomes of the Pathways

The two developmental pathways described earlier suggest that the sources of behavioral isolation and social rejection can vary. It is likely that the prognoses for children who follow these pathways probably differ as well. For example, it is well documented that hostility and aggression in childhood, if not intervened with, are predictive of juvenile delinquency and adult criminality (e.g., Olweus, 1979; Parker & Asher, 1987).

But what about children who follow the second pathway? Conceptually, one might predict that when these children are able, cognitively, to make social comparisons, they will come to realize that they are failing in their social worlds, and they may become distressed with the conditions of their lives. One might predict, therefore, that the logical outcomes for the highly sensitive, anxious, withdrawn child will be problems of an internalizing nature (e.g., anxiety and depressive disorders). Indeed, as noted earlier, this is exactly what we have found in the Waterloo Longitudinal Project; early indices of withdrawal and anxiety, especially when combined with negative self-appraisals of social competence, are predictive of internalizing difficulties in early adolescence (Rubin, Hymel, & Mills, 1989; Rubin & Mills, 1988).

From our perspective, then, children who are rejected by their peers and who are found to spend much, if not most, of their time alone probably comprise a rather heterogeneous group. The causes and the consequences of their "condition" vary. Needless to say, there are likely more than two pathways to peer rejection and social isolation. Yet, given our description of these two particular pathways, we now ask which of them is more probable for craniofacially handicapped children. One possibility is outlined in the following section.

Developmental Anomalies, Peer Rejection, and Social Isolation

Parent–Infant Relationships

As we have noted, social and ecological stresses are likely to have an impact on parental belief systems about normal development and on parenting behaviors (e.g., Rubin, Mills, & Rose-Krasnor, 1989). Needless to say, the birth of a handicapped child is an enormous source of stress for a family. Parents of infants who are mildly deformed or mentally handicapped are often shocked and disappointed by the arrival of their less than perfect baby (Odom, 1983). Moreover, they are likely to have stereotyped beliefs about developmental "norms" and "outcomes" for their physically and/or mentally handicapped infants. As such, it would not be surprising if these strong reactive parental emotions and beliefs interfere with caretaking behavior. It has been shown, for example, that mothers of atypical infants often demonstrate disorganized parenting patterns such as poorly organized play, stereotypic and fixed facial expressions, and interrupted feedings. In addition, these mothers often overstimulate their infants (Greenberg, 1971). It is unlikely that any or all of these parenting behaviors are conducive to the establishment of normal and secure primary attachment relationships in infancy.

Parents, however, are not the sole contributors to the development of abnormal primary relationships. The characteristics of particular handicapping conditions in an infant may disrupt attachment in different ways. For example, Down Syndrome infants cry and exhibit less attachment behavior during separation, initiate less physical contact after reunion, and vocalize less frequently across most episodes of the strange situation attachment paradigm than age-matched nonretarded controls (Cicchetti & Serafica, 1981; Serafica & Cicchetti, 1976). Furthermore, signals indicating infants' needs may not exist or may be "mixed" due to physiological, sensory, or cognitive deficits. In a study of infants handicapped with either Down Syndrome, brain injury, blindness, or multiple disabilities (any or all of which may be accompanying features of a craniofacial handicap), Stone and Chesney (1978) found disturbances in one or more attachment behaviors for *all* infants. Communicative signals such as vocalizations and smiling occurred rarely or were late in developing in most of the infants studied. Thus, under such circumstances, the caretakers' task of *understanding* the infants is extremely difficult. In addition, caregivers are likely to receive less positive reinforcement for their actions if smiling is delayed or infrequent. Failure by the infants to stimulate their mothers may lead to a lessening of quantity and quality of mother–infant interaction. Given this set of circumstances, it is not surprising that infants with Down Syndrome or multiple handicaps have been found to exhibit disturbances in almost every attachment behavior measured.

As mentioned previously, the communication cues (e.g., cries and smiles) of handicapped infants are difficult to interpret under ordinary circumstances; one might expect, therefore, that they would be less well attended to and more often misinterpreted by parents who are experiencing many negative life circumstances in addition to the stress evoked by the birth of a handicapped child. It is known, however, that various situational and personal characteristics may help parents adapt to handicapped infants. For example, parents with good support systems, including physicians who provide frank and detailed information about the child's handicap (Pueschel & Murphy, 1976) and agencies that can provide assistance for parent–child interaction problems (e.g., Bromwich, 1976, 1981), are likely to accept their infants' handicapping conditions earlier than those without these supports.

Nevertheless, the presence of social and other forms of support may be necessary but insufficient to preclude the development of difficulties in early parent–child relationships. Given the communication styles noted briefly above, it is not surprising that researchers have indicated disruptions in the attachment process between handicapped infants and their mothers.

While it is likely that disruptions in attachment will have similar developmental consequences for handicapped and nonhandicapped children, the risk for disruptions, and therefore for later difficulties, appears to be greater for handicapped infants. Given interactions between initial parental grief and feelings of guilt, possible parental beliefs that handicapped children are less responsive to socialization attempts (e.g., Kogan, 1980), and possible deficiencies in handicapped or disfigured infants' abilities to communicate affect and to respond normally to stimulation, handicapped infants appear at high risk for developing insecure attachment relationships with their parents.

Toddler and Preschool Relationships

Beyond the family, interaction with infant and toddler peers is likely to be disrupted as well. Although very little research exists, it is probable that other infants or toddlers, who respond less contingently and appropriately than adults to begin with, may find that interaction with a handicapped age-mate puts a strain on their own newly developing communicative and cognitive skills. For example, it has been found that developmentally delayed toddlers engage in more solitary play and interact less often than do nondelayed toddlers in previously unacquainted integrated play settings. Furthermore, normal toddlers indicate a preference for interacting with other normal toddlers, seeking them as partners and more often rejecting social initiations from handicapped children (Guralnick & Groom, 1987). As a consequence, handicapped toddlers may gain a very early sense of peer rejection, a perception that may make already insecure toddlers feel even less secure. Moreover, limited opportunities to interact with nonhandicapped peers precludes the possibility of experiencing initial exchanges of either cooperative or conflictual natures. As such, handicapped youngsters are placed at risk for not developing those skills that are derived from social exchanges of conflict, communication, and cooperation.

It is important to note, however, that a supportive adult environment can provide a buffer against these risk possibilities. For example, if encouraged by adults, nonhandicapped preschool age children will increase levels of interaction with handicapped children (Guralnick, 1978; Guralnick & Paul-Brown, 1980). Nonhandicapped children have been observed, for example, to adapt their communication to the appropriate cognitive "level" of their peers (mild, moderate, or severely retarded), thereby increasing the likelihood of being understood and eliciting a response (Guralnick & Paul-Brown, 1980). It is possible, therefore, that adaptive communications and relatively frequent social interaction with nonhandicapped peers will help lessen the risk status of handicapped children.

Nevertheless, it is the case that during the preschool years, children begin to be aware of themselves as social beings who can have an impact on others. Public self-awareness leads to acute self-conscious shyness in some children. Labeled "late developing shyness" by Buss (1986), this acute self-consciousness may be caused by a lack of or too much attention from others. In the case of children with craniofacial deformities, a feeling of conspicuousness may result with the realization of the differences between self and others. The experiences of being stared at and teased by peers are hypothesized to increase the likelihood of children withdrawing from social situations (Buss, 1986).

In addition, parents, fearing social failures for their children, may contribute to the inhibition of social development by being overprotective of their handicapped children (Wallander & Hubert, 1987). In addition to protecting their children from outside interaction, parents may also impede social development by their style of interaction. Terdal, Jackson, and Garner (1976) found mothers of developmentally delayed children to be more directive, to receive less response to social behavior from their children, and to provide more poorly differentiated consequences to compliant and noncompliant behaviors than were mothers of "normal" children at similar developmental levels. Wasserman, Allen, and Solomon (1985) also found mothers of orthopedically handicapped toddlers to be less responsive and more directive than mothers of normal toddlers. When children were 24 months old, mothers ignored their handicapped children during free play at a much greater rate than did mothers of premature or normal toddlers. Although the number of handicapped children in this latter study was fairly small (n = 12), significantly, the 5 most ignored handicapped children all had facial, rather than orthopedic, anomalies (Wasserman & Allen, 1985). Given that early parent–child relationships and interactions may be less than optimal, it is not surprising that social competence of physically disabled children has been rated by parents as being below the 30th percentile on a distribution for all children (Wallander & Hubert, 1987).

In summary, it would appear as if craniofacially handicapped infants are at risk for developing insecure attachment relationships with their primary caregivers. Parental feelings of guilt concerning the infant handicap may lead to "overcontrol" or overstimulation as noted above. Such overcontrol may preclude infants and toddlers from opportunities to become appropriately independent. That is, craniofacially handicapped infants or toddlers may be shielded from or overprotected in new situations; as a consequence, when finally left to fend for themselves in novel situations, the infants or toddlers may prove neither willing nor able to explore and interact with the social and nonsocial stimuli that are encountered therein. The lack of such opportunities may, in turn, preclude experiences to develop the confidence and skill necessary to overcome wariness and insecurity in early peer encounters. Finally, such wariness, in concert with the recognition of one's own facial handicap, may result in exacerbated anxious withdrawal in the peer milieu. In keeping with this scenario, Rubin and Mills (1990) have discovered that the parents of extremely anxious and withdrawn nonhandicapped preschoolers are highly directive and authoritarian (i.e., overcontrolling) in their relationships with their children. Furthermore, it is known that extremely anxious and withdrawn youngsters come to develop negative self-perceptions with age (Rubin, 1985). Thus, the scenario suggested above for young craniofacially handicapped children appears plausible.

The Social Relationships of Elementary Schoolers

As children reach elementary school age, even if they have been previously shielded from other children, many will have increased opportunities for peer interaction and modeling within educational mainstreaming. However, unless a child's handicap is mild, little peer attention may be given handicapped children by nonhandicapped peers. Indeed, in the case of facially deformed children, attention may be bimodally distributed—that is, some peers may ignore them while others may tease them mercilessly. Thus, the social interactions of handicapped children may remain limited to those involving similarly handicapped peers (Guralnick, 1986; Wallander & Hubert, 1987). Unfortunately, these associations are less likely to promote advanced forms of social and communicative development than interaction with nonhandicapped peers.

Children without developmental delays tend to exhibit low acceptance of mentally retarded peers and children with learning disabilities or attention deficit disorders (Wallander & Hubert, 1987). Taylor, Asher, and Williams (1987) found that 77% of mainstreamed educable mentally retarded (EMR) third- to sixth-grade children were rejected by their peers, and these children were perceived as less cooperative and more shy than other children. Teachers also perceived EMR students as less friendly and cooperative, more avoidant and withdrawn. The EMR children expressed more dissatisfaction with their social relationships than did non-EMR students.

Less research has been done on the peer status of children with physical disabilities; however, recent work investigating children's preferences for pictures of disabled and nondisabled children indicates a similar pattern to that described above. Harper, Wacker, and Seaborg-Cobb (1986) found that nondisabled children were consistently preferred by nondisabled children over disabled children or those who exhibited some observable physical difference such as a facial cleft or obesity. When the children were asked who would be a preferred activity partner, social preferences ratings varied with the necessary mobility for an activity. For the general question, "Who do you like best?" and for those contexts requiring little mobility, children in a wheelchair or with braces and crutches were preferred to children depicted with a facial deformity or as obese.

The data described above may be taken as preliminary evidence that, if anything, handicapped elementary school-aged children are likely to be described by teachers and peers as withdrawn (not aggressive) and that they *are* at risk for peer rejection or unpopularity. These data may be contrasted with those found in studies linking physical attractiveness and peer acceptance. It is known, for example, that young children perceive attractive children as possessing many positive social qualities, while unattractive children are thought to exhibit negative social behaviors (Dion, 1973; Dion & Berscheid, 1974).

In more recent studies, Langlois and Downs (1979) have reported that behavioral differences exist between attractive and unattractive children and that these differences match stereotypic beliefs. Unattractive 3- and 5-year-old children of both sexes were found to be more aggressive, and to engage in more male sex-stereotyped activities than attractive children. They were, however, just as sociable as their attractive counterparts. Furthermore, both attractive and unattractive children displayed more affiliative behaviors when paired with a child of similar attractiveness than when with a partner of greater or lesser attractiveness. These data suggest that the behavioral characteristics of facially handicapped children may be rather different from those who are rated as physically unattractive on some continuum of attractiveness. As such, it may be inappropriate to conceptualize, as similar or identical, the developmental prognoses for craniofacially handicapped and unattractive children.

As noted earlier, handicapped children are rated by teachers and peers as more anxious and withdrawn than are their nonhandicapped age-mates (Taylor, Asher, & Williams, 1987). More germane to issues concerning facial handicaps, Richman and Harper (1978) found that children with a cleft palate were significantly more withdrawn than children without observable disabilities and that they avoided others to reduce teasing and the lack of positive social response from their peers. In addition, social inhibition appeared to extend to academic competitiveness as these children also exhibited lower educational achievement than controls matched to sex, age, grade, socioeconomic status, and intelligence.

Physical unattractiveness, in contrast to facial deformity, appears to be a stronger correlate of aggression than of withdrawal. Moreover, Coie, Dodge, and Coppotelli (1982) and Dodge (1983) have reported substantial correlations between social preference and attractiveness in middle childhood. Physical attractiveness, however, predicted social preference significantly less well than social behaviors such as aggression. These latter findings may reflect support for the hypotheses of Dion and Berscheid (1974) and Langlois and Downs (1979) that unattractive children come to behave in manners that fulfill the social expectations of their peers who negatively evaluate them. The findings also suggest, however, that even if a child's attractiveness changes, the production of aggressive social behaviors will not preclude him or her from maintaining a negative reputation among peers.

In summary, it would appear as if children with craniofacial handicaps should not be regarded simply as a group whose members fall at some extreme of an attractiveness continuum. The behavioral correlates of unattractiveness and facial deformity differ, and probably the processes by which these two groups become rejected by their peers differ as well. Whereas anxiety, negative self-perceptions, withdrawal, and physical deformity may predict peer rejection for craniofacially handicapped youngsters, aggression may be the primary determinant of rejection for unattractive children.

All in all, children who have a craniofacial handicap appear at high risk for developing negative self-perceptions, social inhibition and anxiety, and peer rejection and their sequelae, but only under certain conditions. First, if they form insecure primary attachment relationships with their mothers due to a breakdown in early mother–infant communication and responsivity, these children may be placed immediately in a high-risk category (Belsky & Nezworski, 1988). Second, if they are rejected by peers early in life and if they withdraw from social contacts, their risk status increases significantly (Parker & Asher, 1987). Third, if parents and teachers do not intervene in some way to lend support for these insecure and potentially anxious/withdrawn children, their prognosis would appear to be quite negative.

Needless to say, much of what we have described stems from conceptual leaps and jumps through a widely varying research literature that rarely deals with the problem of craniofacial handicap per se. Thus, our developmental prospectus at this time is, admittedly, pure conjecture. Researchers have yet to study the causal relations between handicapping conditions, parent–infant/child interaction, the availability of social support, cognitive prowess, and the development of extrafamilial relationships and social skills. We would predict that craniofacial anomalies, because of their extreme salience to parents and peers, are likely to place children at high risk for the development of socioemotional difficulties.

Research Recommendations

In the remainder of this chapter, we suggest a research agenda for those interested in the developing relationships and social skills of those children who suffer from craniofacial handicaps. Our primary concerns stem from our own basic research biases. Over the years, we have investigated the long-term correlates and consequences of social withdrawal and negative self-perceptions in childhood. As previously mentioned, these phenomena, as evidenced in childhood, collectively predict the development of internalizing problems in early adolescence (Rubin, Hymel, & Mills,

1989). The research agenda is described simply by a set of currently unanswered questions in the literature extant concerning children with craniofacial handicaps. It would seem to us that any and all of these questions deserve serious attention.

1. Is it the case that, relative to their nonfacially handicapped agemates, children with craniofacial anomalies are more socially withdrawn when in peer group situations? Given our reading of the available literature, as described earlier, we would expect an affirmative answer to this question.

2. If children with craniofacial handicaps are less socially interactive, is it because they are rejected by peers (i.e., isolated by the peer group) as a function of their physical appearance or because of a lack of social skills, or are they less interactive because of negative self-perceptions and felt insecurities that lead to self-imposed isolation from the peer group? Might it be that some combination of a lack of skills, negative self-perceptions and insecurities, and physical anomaly conspires to produce social withdrawal and peer rejection? Needless to say, the optimal research strategy would be to follow longitudinally a group of facially handicapped children. This would allow the *prediction* of rejection in the peer group. It would also allow an analysis of the timetabling of sequences leading ultimately to rejection. Finally, it would allow a test of whether the causes of rejection in facially handicapped children differ from those for nonhandicapped children.

3. Are there protective factors that serve to prevent the development of negative social and emotional outcomes for craniofacially handicapped children? For example, do parents of handicapped children who are neither withdrawn from nor rejected by the peer group provide a socialization context for their children that is different from parents of children who are withdrawn and/or rejected? Does the former group of parents differ from those whose *nonhandicapped* children are neither withdrawn nor rejected? That is, is there something particularly special about these parents and their relationships with their handicapped children?

4. If social inhibition is determined partially by negative self-perceptions, how early can these negative self-perceptions be identified? What are the causes of these negative self-perceptions?

5. If peer rejection and social isolation are, to some extent, determined by a child's craniofacial anomalies, what can be done to prevent or ameliorate these negative outcomes and their hypothesized sequelae? Is social skills training directed at the child, his or her peers, and his or her parents enough to prevent or alter the course of rejection and isolation?

6. Can different social and emotional outcomes be predicted for children with different craniofacial handicaps?

7. Finally, and perhaps most significantly for readers of this volume, what is the impact of craniofacial surgery on children's development of

self-regard and social relationships and skills? What timetable should surgical procedures follow? Does surgery have differential impact for children with varying craniofacial handicaps? Should data concerning the development of the self-concept and the development of familial and extrafamilial relationships in childhood help direct the schedule and course of surgery? Needless to say, we would suggest that questions 1 through 6 be addressed prior to conducting research on the impact of surgery.

Acknowledgments. Preparation of this manuscript was aided by a Killam Research Fellowship to author Rubin and by a Social Sciences and Humanities Research Council of Canada doctoral fellowship to author Wilkinson. The research described herein concerning The Waterloo Longitudinal Project was supported by grants from Health and Welfare Canada and The Ontario Mental Health Foundation.

References

Belsky, J., & Nezworski, T. (Eds.). (1988). *Clinical implications of attachment.* Hillsdale, NJ: Erlbaum.

Belsky, J., & Rovine, M. (1987). Temperament and attachment security in the strange situation: An empirical rapprochement. *Child Development, 58,* 787–795.

Bromwich, R.M. (1976). Focus on maternal behavior in infant intervention. *American Journal of Orthopsychiatry, 43,* 439–446.

Bromwich, R.M. (1981). *Working with parents and infants: An interactional approach.* Baltimore, MD: University Park Press.

Bronfenbrenner, U., & Crouter, A.C. (1983). The evolution of environmental models in developmental research. In W. Kessen (Ed.), *Handbook of child psychology: Vol. 1. History, theory and methods.* New York: Wiley.

Bronson, W.C. (1966). Central orientations: A study of behavior organization from childhood to adolescence. *Child Development, 37,* 125–155.

Buss, A.H. (1986). Two kinds of shyness. In R. Schwarzer (Ed.), *Self-related cognitions in anxiety and motivation* (pp. 65–75). Hillsdale, NJ: Erlbaum.

Cicchetti, D., & Serafica, F.C. (1981). Interplay among behavioral systems: Illustrations from the study of attachment, affiliation, and wariness in young children with Down's syndrome. *Developmental Psychology, 17,* 36–49.

Coie, J.D., & Kupersmidt, J.R. (1983). A behavioral analysis of emerging social status in boys' groups. *Child Development, 54,* 1400–1416.

Coie, J.D., Dodge, K.A., & Coppotelli, H. (1982). Dimensions and types of social status: A cross-age perspective. *Developmental Psychology, 18,* 557–570.

Crockenberg, S.B. (1981). Infant irritability, mother responsiveness, and social support influences on the security of mother-infant attachment. *Child Development, 52,* 857–865.

Dion, K.K., & Berscheid, E. (1974). Physical attractiveness and peer perception among children. *Sociometry, 37,* 1–12.

Dion, K.K. (1973). Young children's stereotyping of facial attractiveness. *Developmental Psychology, 9,* 183–188.

Dodge, K.A. (1983). Behavioral antecedents of peer social status. *Child Development, 54,* 1386–1389.

Egeland, B., & Farber, E.A. (1984). Infant-toddler attachment: Factors related to its development and change over time. *Child Development, 55,* 753–771.

Engfer, A. (1986). Antecedents of behaviour problems in infancy. In G.A. Kohnstamm (Ed.), *Temperament discussed: Temperament and development in infancy and childhood* (pp. 165–180). Amsterdam, the Netherland: Swets & Zeitlinger.

Engfer, A., & Gavranidou, M. (1987). Antecedents and consequences of maternal sensitivity: A longitudinal study. In H. Rauh & H. Steinhausen (Eds.), *Psychobiology and early development* (pp. 71–99). Amsterdam: Elsevier/North Holland.

Greenberg, N.H. (1971). A comparison of infant-mother interactional behavior in infants with atypical behavior and normal infants. In J. Hellmuth (Ed.), *Exceptional Infant* (Vol. 2). New York: Brunner/Mazel.

Greenwood, G.R., Todd, N.M., Hops, H., & Walker, H.M. (1982). Behavior change targets in the assessment and treatment of socially withdrawn preschool children. *Behavioral Assessment, 4,* 273–297.

Guralnick, M.J. (1978). Integrated preschools as educational and therapeutic environments: Concepts, design, and analysis. In M.J. Guralnick (Ed.), *Early intervention and the integration of handicapped and nonhandicapped children* (pp. 115–145). Baltimore, MD: University Park Press.

Guralnick, M.J. (1986). The peer relations of young handicapped and nonhandicapped children. In P.S. Strain, M.J. Guralnick, & H.M. Walker (Eds.), *Children's social behavior: Development, assessment, and modification* (pp. 93–140). Orlando, FL: Academic Press.

Guralnick, M.J., & Groom, J.M. (1987). The peer relations of mildly delayed and nonhandicapped preschool children in mainstreamed playgroups. *Child Development, 58,* 1556–1572.

Guralnick, M.J., & Paul-Brown, D. (1980). Functional and discourse analyses of nonhandicapped preschool children's speech to handicapped children. *American Journal of Mental Deficiency, 84,* 44–454.

Harper, D.C., Wacker, D.P., & Seaborg-Cobb, L. (1986). Children's social preferences toward peers with visible physical differences. *Journal of Pediatric Psychology, 11,* 323–342.

Hartup, W.W. (1983). Peer relations. In E.M. Hetherington (Ed.), *Handbook of child psychology: Vol. 4. Socialization, personality, and social development* (pp. 103–198). New York: Wiley.

Hay, D.F., Pedersen, J., & Nash, A. (1982). Dyadic interaction in the first year of life. In K.H. Rubin & H.S. Ross (Eds.), *Peer relationships and social skills in childhood* (pp. 11–39). New York: Springer-Verlag.

Hymel, S., & Rubin, K.H. (1985). Children with peer relationships and social skills problems: Conceptual, methodological, and developmental issues. In G.J. Whitehurst (Ed.), *Annuals of child development*, Vol. 2 (pp. 251–297). Greenwich, CT: JAI Press.

Hymel, S., Rubin, K.H., Rowden, L., & LeMare, L. (1990). Children's peer relationships: Longitudinal predictions of internalizing and externalizing problems from middle to late childhood. *Child Development, 61,* 2004–2021.

Kagan, J., Reznick, S.J., Clarke, C., Snidman, N., & Garcia-Coll, C. (1984). Behavioral inhibition to the unfamiliar. *Child Development, 55,* 2212–2225.

Kagan, J., Reznick, S.J., & Snidman, N. (1987). The physiology and psychology of behavioral inhibition in children. *Child Development, 58,* 1459–1473.

Kogan, K.L. (1980). Interaction systems between preschool handicapped or developmentally delayed children and their parents. In T.M. Field, S. Goldberg, D. Stern, & A.M. Sostek (Eds.), *High-risk infants and children: Adult and peer interactions* (pp. 227–247). New York: Academic Press.

Lamb, M.E., & Roopnarine, J. (1979). Peer influences on sex-role development in preschoolers. *Child Development, 50,* 219–222.

Langlois, J.H., & Downs, A.C. (1979). Peer relations as a function of physical attractiveness: The eye of the beholder or behavioral reality? *Child Development, 50,* 409–418.

LeMare, L.J., & Rubin, K.H. (1987). Perspective taking and peer interaction: Structural and developmental analyses. *Child Development, 58,* 306–315.

Mead, G.H. (1934). *Mind, self, and society.* Chicago: University of Chicago Press.

Odom, S.L. (1983). The development of social interchanges in infancy. In S.G. Garwood & R.R. Fewell (Eds.), *Educating handicapped infants: Issues in development and intervention* (pp. 215–254). Rockville, MD: Aspen.

Olweus, D. (1979). Stability of aggressive reaction patterns in males: A review. *Psychological Bulletin, 86,* 852–875.

Parker, J.G., & Asher, S.R. (1987). Peer relations and later personal adjustment: Are low-accepted children at risk? *Psychological Bulletin, 102,* 357–389.

Parten, M.B. (1932). Social participation among preschool children. *Journal of Abnormal Psychology, 27,* 243–269.

Piaget, J. (1926). *The language and thought of the child.* London: Routledge & Kegan Paul.

Piaget, J. (1932). *The moral judgement of the child.* Glencoe, IL: Free Press.

Pueschel, S.M., & Murphy, A. (1976). Assessment of counseling practices at the birth of a child with Down's syndrome. *American Journal of Mental Deficiency, 81,* 325–330.

Richman, L., & Harper, D. (1978). School adjustment of children with observable disabilities. *Journal of Abnormal Child Psychology, 6,* 11–18.

Ross, H.S., Lollis, S.P., & Elliot, C. (1982). Toddler-peer communication. In K.H. Rubin & H.S. Ross (Eds.), *Peer relationships and social skills in childhood* (pp. 73–98). New York: Springer-Verlag.

Rubin, K.H. (1985). Socially withdrawn children: An "at-risk" population? In B. Schneider, K.H. Rubin, & J. Ledingham (Eds.), *Peer relationships and social skills in childhood: Issues in assessment and training.* New York: Springer-Verlag.

Rubin, K.H., & Borwick, D. (1984). The communication skills of children who vary with regard to sociability. In H. Sypher & J. Applegate (Eds.), *Social cognition and communication.* Hillsdale, NJ: Erlbaum.

Rubin, K.H., Daniels-Beirness, T., & Bream, L. (1984). Social isolation and social problem solving: A longitudinal study. *Journal of Consulting and Clinical Psychology, 52,* 17–25.

Rubin, K.H., Fein, G., & Vandenberg, B. (1983). Play. In E.M. Hetherington (Ed.), *Handbook of child psychology: Socialization, personality and social development.* New York: Wiley.

Rubin, K.H., Hymel, S., LeMare, L.J., & Rowden, L. (1989). Children experiencing social difficulties: Sociometric neglect reconsidered. *Canadian Journal of Behavioural Science, 21,* 94–111.

Rubin, K.H., Hymel, S., & Mills, R.S.L. (1989). Sociability and social withdrawal in childhood: Stability and outcomes. *Journal of Personality, 57,* 238–255.

Rubin, K.H., Hymel, S., Mills, R.S.L., & Rose-Krasnor, L. (1991). Conceptualizing different pathways to and from social isolation in childhood. In D. Cicchetti & S. Toth (Eds.), *Rochester Symposium on Developmental Psychopathology,* Vol. 2., New York: Cambridge University Press.

Rubin, K.H., & Krasnor, L.R. (1986). Social cognitive and social behavior perspectives on problem-solving. In M. Perlmutter (Ed.), *Minnesota Symposia on Child Psychology,* Vol. 18. Hillsdale, NJ: Erlbaum.

Rubin, K.H., LeMare, L.J., & Lollis, S. (1990). Social withdrawal in childhood: Developmental pathways to rejection. In S.R. Asher & J.D. Coie (Eds.), *Peer rejection in childhood.* New York: Cambridge University Press.

Rubin, K.H., & Lollis, S. (1988). Peer relationships, social skills and infant attachment: A continuity model. In J. Belskey (Ed.), *Clinical implications of infant attachment* (pp. 219–252). Hillsdale, NJ: Erlbaum.

Rubin, K.H., & Mills, R.S.L. (1988). The many faces of social isolation in childhood. *Journal of Consulting and Clinical Psychology, 56,* 916–924.

Rubin, K.H., & Mills, R.S.L. (1990). Maternal beliefs about adaptive and maladaptive social behaviors in normal, aggressive, and withdrawn preschoolers. *Journal and Abnornal Child Psychology, 18,* 419–435.

Rubin, K.H., Mills, R.S.L., & Rose-Krasnor, L. (1989). Parental beliefs and children's social competence. In B. Schneider, G. Atilli, J. Nadel-Brulfert, & R. Weissberg (Eds.), *Social competence in developmental perspective.* Dordrecht, Netherlands: Kluwer International Publishers.

Serafica, F.C., & Cicchetti, D. (1976). Down's syndrome children in a strange situation: Attachment and exploration behaviors. *Merrill-Palmer Quarterlty, 22,* 137–150.

Shantz, C.U. (1983). Social cognition. In J.H. Flavell & E.M. Markman (Eds.), *Handbook of child psychology: Vol. 3. Cognitive development* (pp. 495–555). New York: Wiley.

Spieker, S.J., & Booth, C.L. (1988). Maternal antecedents of attachment quality. In J. Belsky & T. Nezworski (Eds.), *Clinical implications of attachment* (pp. 95–136). Hillsdale, NJ: Erlbaum.

Sroufe, L.A. (1983). Infant-caregiver attachment and patterns of adaptation in preschool: Roots of maladaption and competence. In M. Perlmutter (Ed.), *Minnesota Symposia on Child Psychology* (Vol. 16). Hillsdale, NJ: Erlbaum.

Staub, E. (1975). To rear a prosocial child: Reasoning, learning by doing, and learning by teaching others. In D. DePalma & J. Foley (Eds.), *Moral development: Current theory and research.* Hillsdale, NJ: Erlbaum.

Stone, N.H., & Chesney, B.H. (1978). Attachment behaviors in handicapped infants. *Mental Retardation, 16,* 8–12.

Sullivan, H.S. (1953). *The interpersonal theory of psychiatry.* New York: Norton.

Taylor, A.R., Asher, S.R., & Williams, G.A. (1987). The social adaptation of mainstreamed mildly retarded children. *Child Development, 58,* 1321–1334.

Terdal, L, Jackson, R.H., & Garner, A.M. (1976). Mother-child interactions: A comparison between normal and developmentally delayed groups. In E.J.

Marsh, L.A. Hamerlynck, & L.C. Handy (Eds.), *Behavior modification and families* (pp. 249–264). New York: Brunner/Mazel.

Wallander, J.C., & Hubert, N.C. (1987). Peer social dysfunction in children with developmental disabilities: Empirical basis and a conceptual model. *Clinical Psychology Review, 7,* 205–221.

Wasserman, G.A., & Allen, R. (1985). Maternal withdrawal from handicapped toddlers. *Journal of Child Psychology and Psychiatry, 26,* 381–387.

Wasserman, G.A., Allen, R., & Solomon, C.R. (1985). At-risk toddlers and their mothers: The special case of physical handicaps. *Child Development, 56,* 73–83.

Younger, A.J. & Boyko, K.A. (1987). Aggression and withdrawal as social schemas underlying children's peer perceptions. *Child Development., 58,* 1094–1100.

Younger, A.J., Schwartzman, A.E., & Ledingham, J. (1986). Age-related differences in children's perceptions of social deviance: Changes in behavior or perspective? *Developmental Psychology, 22,* 531–542.

10
Reactions to Craniofacial Disfigurement: Lessons from the Physical Attractiveness and Stigma Literatures

Harry T. Reis and Holley S. Hodgins

Many idioms of the English language attest to the importance of the human face for the presentation of self to others. An interaction in which both parties are physically present, for example, is termed "face to face." Appearing in public is described as "showing one's face," whereas "falling flat on one's face" implies failure. Accusations and criticism are considered most frank and unvarnished when offered "to one's face," and problems should be "faced up to." Many types of contests, such as sporting events and political debates, begin with a "face-off."

If the face is such a common metaphor for various aspects of social interaction, it should not surprise us that facial attractiveness exerts a marked and pervasive influence on judgments about and reactions to others. After all, although faces vary along many dimensions, aesthetic differences represent one of the simplest, but at the same time consensually shared, schemes for categorizing and comparing one face to another. Even children as young as 3 months of age are capable of distinguishing attractive from nonattractive faces (Langlois, this volume), and reliability estimates in adult ratings tend to be high. Furthermore, the face that we bring to different interactions is essentially constant, varying much less than the time, energy, and ego invested in cosmetics, hairstyling, grooming, and even surgery would seem to indicate.

Research on the impact of facial attractiveness began in earnest during the late 1960s, spurred in large part by the dramatic early experiments carried out by Ellen Berscheid, Elaine Walster (Hatfield), and their colleagues. By now hundreds of studies have been conducted, so that the phenomenon itself has become part not just of the standard social psychological curriculum but of popular culture as well. Excellent and timely reviews of this literature are available (Bull & Rumsey, 1988; Hatfield &

Sprecher, 1986; Patzer, 1985), and we will not duplicate those efforts in this chapter. Instead, our goal will be to consider the relevance and implications of this work for individuals with craniofacial abnormalities.[1] To preview a distinction we will feature, extensions of the attractiveness literature to this specific handicap might begin with either of two assumptions: 1) Because such faces are generally considered unattractive, the problems typically faced by unattractive but structurally normal individuals should apply with equal or perhaps greater weight to persons with craniofacial abnormalities; or 2) Because they embody significant disturbances of normal facial structure, and because they are generally considered stigmatizing, craniofacial anomalies might engender fundamentally different reactions, involving different processes, than normal unattractiveness does. Each of these positions, as we shall see, suggests different implications about the psychological, social, and developmental experiences of facially disfigured individuals. Thus, although they share a common core of principles and conclusions that can be extrapolated from the attractiveness literature, many of the more interesting and complex possibilities await future research.

What Do We Know about the Impact of Unattractiveness?

It is telling that most research in this area is nominally concerned with the effects of physical *attractiveness* rather than *unattractiveness*. (Witness the popular designation for appearance-based stereotyping: What is beautiful is good.) More often than not, studies have simply contrasted reactions to attractive and unattractive stimulus persons, making it impossible to determine the relative impact of deviations from the norm in either direction; in other words, from these studies we cannot tell whether beauty is an advantage or ugliness is a disadvantage. A few experiments do permit disentangling these alternatives, and we will highlight them in this chapter. Our review encompasses the broader literature, however, emphasizing studies that permit generalizations about the impact of relative unattractiveness in everyday life. We group existing work into three categories: studies of social perception based exclusively on judgments of photographs, slides, or videotapes; studies of actual social participation and interaction; and studies of nonsocial competencies.

---

[1] Our analysis will focus on craniofacial abnormalities in general. Since cleft lip and palate are such irregularities, our arguments should apply to them in particular. For pedagogical reasons, we will occasionally refer to cleft lip and palate as a specific instance that is intended to exemplify the more general case of craniofacial abnormalities.

Social Perception

An extensive and well-developed literature demonstrates that unattractive individuals are perceived more negatively than their attractive peers on a cornucopia of traits, behaviors, and skills. For example, physically unattractive persons are perceived to possess less desirable personality characteristics (Dermer & Thiel, 1975; Dion, Berscheid, & Walster, 1972; Miller, 1970), have their work evaluated more negatively (Clifford & Walster, 1973; Landy & Sigall, 1974), are rated as poorer employment choices (Dipboye, Arvey, & Terpstra, 1977; although there are exceptions, see below), are judged more harshly for misbehavior or criminal acts (Dion, 1974; Sigall & Ostrove, 1975; Solomon & Schopler, 1978; again, exceptions will be described), and are seen as more psychiatrically disturbed (Cash, Kehr, Polyson, & Freeman, 1977). They are also felt to be less desirable dating and working partners (Feingold, 1989; Stroebe, Insko, Thompson, & Layton, 1971; Walster, Aronson, Abrahams, & Rottmann, 1966).

Although the breadth and ubiquity of this phenomenon is firmly established, important exceptions suggest that derogation of the unattractive may be more contextually bound than is typically assumed. For one thing, stereotypic bias against unattractive faces is relatively stronger on dimensions that tap social activity and competencies than on those concerned with nonsocial characteristics or moral behavior (Ashmore, 1988). Perhaps this finding indicates subjects' implicit understanding of the comparatively stronger role that appearance and beauty play in heterosexual attraction, for both culturally prescribed and evolutionary reasons, than they do in other endeavors. Moreover, although nonsocial judgments were clearly affected by attractiveness in Ashmore's review, a few very specific measures tended to show no difference or even derogation of attractive persons (e.g., perceived parental competence, Dion et al., 1972; perceived vanity and egotism, Dermer & Thiel, 1975). This represents in part an awareness that under certain conditions, attractiveness can be detrimental. In simulated jury studies, for example, when the crime is likely to have been facilitated by beauty, such as a swindle, unattractive people receive *lighter* sentences. Similarly, unattractive women are preferred for high status, traditionally masculine jobs (Heilman & Saruwatari, 1979), presumably because attractiveness in women is associated with femininity (Jackson, 1983). These qualifications indicate that attractiveness stereotyping may not be as totally one-sided as is often thought; in a few (and, admittedly, very limited) circumstances, beauty is a liability and unattractive persons may be judged more favorably.

From the standpoint of generalizing established physical attractiveness findings to craniofacial abnormalities, it is important to determine whether the relationship between attractiveness and positive social perception is monotonic and linear—that is, whether the benefits of beauty are roughly equivalent to the disadvantages of ugliness. Hatfield and Sprecher (1986) proposed that although "what is beautiful is good" may be true, "what is ugly is bad" is more true. Research explicitly testing this hypothesis is scarce, however; most studies use two levels of stimulus attractiveness, precluding the necessary contrasts. We identified 16 studies that included at least three levels of attractiveness, allowing comparison of mean differences on both sides of "average." Those articles generally do not report formal tests of this proposition, but it is apparent that the deviation from monotonicity was not significant in any of them. Nonetheless, 10 of 16 studies revealed a slight tendency for negative ratings of unattractive targets to deviate more from ratings of average stimuli than positive ratings of attractive targets did; in only three studies was the reverse true.

Problems of scaling plague such comparisons, of course; it is not at all clear how well trichotomous splits map onto lay impressions of "attractive," "average," and "unattractive" (Berscheid, 1986). Minimally, if attractiveness is normally distributed, it should be expected that more than one-third of the population would fall into the middle category. It may also be that the phenomenological threshold for attractiveness is different from that of unattractiveness. We are currently conducting a meta-analysis to determine whether this trend is reliable across studies and, if so, to compare relative effect sizes on both sides of the norm. Still, to the extent that informal inspection can be trusted, in studies of first impressions, the detriments of ugliness are at most only slightly more substantial than the benefits of beauty.

Social Participation

A great many studies demonstrate that attractive persons, regardless of their sex, are preferred to the unattractive as dating partners (Brislin & Lewis, 1968; Feingold, 1989; Hatfield & Sprecher, 1986; Tesser & Brodie, 1971; Walster et al., 1966). The generality of this finding, especially because it coincides with folk wisdom, suggests that ugly individuals may be at a considerable disadvantage insofar as dating and romantic preferences are concerned. Furthermore, studies have shown that beauty "radiates"—that is, people are evaluated more positively when accompanied by attractive partners of either sex (Kernis & Wheeler, 1981; Sigall & Landy, 1973). It seems likely, then, that unattractive persons would also be disadvantaged in same-sex socializing.

Although the role of beauty in first impressions, especially of potential interaction partners, is well established, it is not as clear how attractiveness influences the broader scope of social activity in everyday life. Most studies deal with initial judgments about others who are not known to the subject and about whom limited information is available. In contrast, the vast majority of social events involve partners who have met previously and know something about each other. The evidence from studies that examine ongoing patterns of interaction in naturalistic contexts is mixed. Krebs and Adinolfi (1975) found that sociometrically accepted and rejected individuals of both sexes were more attractive than isolates were; unattractive persons, in other words, were more likely to be ignored than liked or disliked.

In our own research (Reis, Nezlek, & Wheeler, 1980; Reis, Wheeler, Spiegel, Kernis, Nezlek, & Perri, 1982), we have had college students complete detailed diaries about their daily social activities. Subsequently, their physical attractiveness was rated from still photographs. Less attractive males and females reported lower levels of satisfaction and intimacy in same-sex and opposite-sex interaction, spanning both close and superficial partners. The results for interaction quantity were qualified by sex in an unexpected way. Unattractive males socialized less often with the opposite sex and more often with the same sex. Among females, surprisingly, for whom the same pattern might have been anticipated, no significant correlations occurred. It is important to note that these findings were obtained in two separate samples, one of first-year college students and one of college seniors, so they do not depend on age-linked dating restrictions that inhere in a college environment. At least for females, then, unattractiveness may not presage less social access to males.

Why might this be? One reason is males' tendency to anticipate rejection by attractive females. Presumably because common folklore indicates that attractive women's attention is dominated by the most desirable men, most males may approach less attractive women simply to avoid a painful rejection (Glenwick, Jason, & Elman, 1978; Huston, 1973). Indirect evidence for this position is provided in a clever study conducted by Bernstein, Stephenson, Snyder, and Wicklund (1983). Through variations in the experimental scenario, some male subjects were given a plausible extrinsic motive for approaching an attractive female (needing to watch a specific movie), whereas other males had no such excuse. Plausible-extrinsic-motive subjects were more than twice as likely to approach the female (72% vs. 33%), even though there were no differences in how attractive or positive she was perceived, suggesting that no-excuse subjects anticipated rejection if the woman were to think their approach was a "come-on." On the other hand, when the woman was low in attractiveness, plausible explanations had little impact on males' willingness to approach. Fear of rejection might therefore steer men away from very attractive women to those of average attractiveness. No firm evidence suggests that this benefit extends to unattractive women, however, although several studies (e.g., Morse, Reis, Gruzen, & Wolff, 1974) imply that males with low self-esteem might seek relatively unattractive female partners.

A second line of reasoning also suggests that the social reality of unattractive persons is not as dire as some writers intimate. Although, when asked, subjects consistently express preferences for more attractive dating partners, matching of attractiveness levels describes reality more accurately. Many studies have demonstrated such matching in dating and married couples. In a meta-analysis of 27 samples, for examples, Feingold (1988) found a correlation of .39 between romantic partners' levels of attractiveness. The processes responsible for this phenomenon are unclear. Whereas some theorists suggest it represents an intrinsic desire for equity (Hatfield, Traupmann, Sprecher, Utne, & Hay, 1984), others (e.g., Kalick & Hamilton, 1986) propose a "marketplace" explanation: Because attractive partners are most desirable, they select each other sooner and are removed from the pool of available partners. As this pool shrinks, partners of diminishing attractiveness levels are accepted, thereby producing de facto matching as people "take what they can get." Irrespective of underlying explanations, however, the point is that despite more negative first impressions, unattractive persons apparently are not as restricted in their heterosexual interaction as is often thought; they manage to form intimate relationships with similarly attractive partners, just as attractive people do.

The influence of physical appearance on attraction may in part reflect the circumstances of interaction. Berscheid (1985) distinguished between open fields, in which affiliation is voluntary and selective, and closed fields, in which tasks or environments constrain interaction choices (e.g., coworkers, teammates, roommates). She notes that in open fields, individuals are most likely to pursue interaction with those partners perceived to be most desirable on the basis of readily available information. In closed fields, in contrast, interaction is induced and maintained by situational requirements, circumventing the channeling effects of first impressions and allowing partners to acquire more in-depth information about each other. Closed fields, in other words, provide a setting in which first impressions may play a less significant determining role.

These findings therefore suggest that although unattractive people may be perceived more negatively in still photographs and in initial interactions, especially along social dimensions, they may nonetheless develop satisfying close relationships by choosing partners of comparable appearance or by developing other capacities, such as intelligence or good listening skills, that, in different contexts, will make them desirable partners (Berscheid, 1986).[2] Perhaps because friendship and romance often grow out of task-oriented or incidental contact, the decided disadvantage that unattractive individuals face in initial social judgment and in group-oriented superficial contexts may not predestine them to

[2] As the fictional detective Kate Fansler once said, "I sometimes think homely women have a fine start in life: they know the rules, and how the game will be played. The early pain, the early lack of that marvelous ego satisfaction when all the men are gathered around like peacocks is well repaid later in life with accomplishment. But what young girl will believe that if you tell her?" (From Cross, A. (1981). *Death in a tenured position* (pp. 105–106). New York: Ballantine Books.)

isolation or unsatisfying relationships. In this vein, Bull and Rumsey note that "no consistent relationship between facial appearance and marital adjustment has been found" (1988, p. 39). Further, there are known individual differences in the importance of attractiveness as a selection criterion in heterosexual dating. Snyder, Berscheid, and Glick (1985) found, for example, that although high self-monitors (i.e., people very much concerned with managing social impressions) selected dating partners on the basis of looks, low self-monitors (i.e., people more concerned with personal standards) relied on personality information.

Competence

Numerous studies have undertaken to determine whether attractive and unattractive persons differ in various nonsocial competencies. Unfortunately, most of those studies utilize variations of the social perception paradigms mentioned earlier—for example, having judges rate the quality of an attractive and unattractive person's performance. Such studies cannot identify true performance differences with certainty, in that judges are aware of the target's appearance and might therefore be influenced, be it with or without awareness, by beauty. One must look, instead, to studies that assess competencies absent of possible confounding by attractiveness levels.

Several studies have found positive correlations between attractiveness and grade-point average or standardized testing scores (e.g., Felson, 1980; Singer, 1964; Udry & Eckland, 1982). This should not seem surprising in view of teachers' tendencies to respond more positively to attractive students (Clifford, 1975; Clifford & Walster, 1973; Lerner & Lerner, 1977); a lifetime's experience with more favorable treatment in educational settings would likely enhance learning and motivation. It is probably the a priori reasonableness of this position that has prematurely led some researchers and commentators to accept it as fact. Nonetheless, many studies have failed to find significant correlations between beauty and academic performance (e.g., Maruyama & Miller, 1981; Murphy, Nelson, & Cheap, 1981; Reis et al., 1982; Udry & Eckland, 1982), and others (e.g., Holmes & Hatch, 1938) have supported an inverse relationship. Furthermore, studies using grade-point average as a criterion should be discounted, in that teachers are obviously aware of their students' looks when grading them and might therefore be swayed by appearance. Thus, despite its inherent plausibility, the link between attractiveness and academic performance has not been established empirically (cf. similar conclusions by Bull & Rumsey, 1988; Sorell & Nowak, 1981).

Research within other performance domains has been scant, partially because objective criteria (i.e., independent of potential attractiveness confounds) are difficult to define and assess in naturalistic settings. In a review of studies on workplace performance, for example, Bull and Rumsey concluded that "although aspects of appearance (e.g., attractiveness) may enhance ratings or expectations, there is little evidence that actual behavior is affected" (1988, p. 79). Thus, at least insofar as existing studies indicate, it is difficult to conclude that attractiveness relates clearly or consistently to objective measures of nonsocial abilities or performance. This conclusion is necessarily narrow and circumspect, however. For one thing, many important performance judgments are made by judges with full awareness of attractiveness levels: a supervisor's evaluation, a teacher's grade, a critic's review. For another, many tasks require interpersonal contact, either as part of the work itself or in the act of sharing those efforts with others. To the extent that attractiveness influences social skills and the reactions of others—as we have already seen—performance effectiveness is implicitly affected by the actor's appearance.

Unattractiveness vs. Stigma

The literature discussed to this point indicates clearly that unattractive individuals are disadvantaged relative to attractive persons, most notably in terms of their perceived desirability as social partners and in terms of people's expectations and judgments about their traits and capacities. It is not necessarily appropriate, however, to generalize these findings unconditionally to children and adults with craniofacial abnormalities. Empirical studies of unattractiveness invariably utilize faces with essentially normal structure—that is, without disfigurement, scars, or striking imperfections other than relative unattractiveness. The sorts of features that characterize what we will call "normal" unattractiveness have been described by Cunningham (1986), among others. Such faces differ mostly in degree from the norm, and they tend not to stand out dramatically in social contexts. Craniofacial disfigurement typically involves more severe abnormalities, at least until corrective surgery has been performed, so that the usual structure and symmetry of the face is intensely and vividly disrupted. Thus, clefts and other craniofacial anomalies are salient and stigmatizing markers in a way that ordinary unattractiveness may not be, and consequently may differ fundamentally from "normal" unattractiveness, rather than reside at the low end of the standard ugly-to-beautiful continuum. In other words, the stigmatizing nature of facial disfigurement may invoke different processes and hence different outcomes than simple unattractiveness does.[3]

---

[3] The question arises as to whether we are proposing that attractiveness and facial abnormalities are independent dimensions or whether "normal" and "disfigured" are two subtypes of unattractiveness. For several reasons, we prefer the latter

For this reason, we find it useful to examine the literature on stigmatization. Many researchers have attempted to identify the central variables underlying stigmatizing conditions. Jones, Farina, Hastorf, Markus, Miller, and Scott (1984) outlined six dimensions that they believed most critical for understanding the impact of a given stigma on social interaction. These are: 1) concealability, or the extent to which the stigmatizing condition can be hidden voluntarily; 2) the course of the stigma over time; 3) disruptiveness, or the extent to which a stigma strains or adds to the difficulty of interpersonal relations; 4) aesthetic factors, or how pleasing or repulsive the stigma is to the senses; 5) origin (whether the stigmatized person is responsible for the condition, and whether it is congenital); and 6) peril posed to others by the condition.

These six dimensions suggest a mixed picture for equating "normal" unattractiveness and craniofacial disfigurement. For one thing, facial abnormalities are not only unconcealable, they are visually omnipresent, owing to the centrality of the face in human communication. The face is an important channel for expressing emotions and recognizing them in others (Ekman, 1973; Izard, 1977) and as such plays a critical role in social interaction. Facially disfigured individuals therefore have the disadvantage of an unconcealable stigma, in that they are unable to choose if and when to reveal their condition to others (see Goffman's [1963] discussion of "passing"). People who are normal but unattractive, on the other hand, have numerous techniques for at least partially veiling and enhancing their appearance (e.g., cosmetics, hairstyles, beards, moustaches, false eyelashes, etc.). These concealment strategies may also be used by facially disfigured persons, but unless their defect can be hidden completely, it is unlikely that the condition will go unnoticed.

The expected course over time of facial disfigurement is less clear, depending to a large extent on modifiability of the defect in question. Corrective surgery for clefts, for example, usually produces positive, albeit incomplete, improvements (Lefebvre & Munro, 1986), although Edwards and Watson estimate "a stubborn residue of 20 to 30 percent of bad results" (1980, p. 281). Nonetheless, in the eyes of potential interac-

---

view. For one, most cases of noticeable craniofacial disfigurement are judged to be significantly unattractive. Perhaps this is because symmetry is one important standard of beauty, and many facial abnormalities are asymmetric. Moreover, attractive faces tend to resemble prototypical, or "average," human faces (Langlois, this volume), whereas disfigured faces are stigmatizing precisely because they deviate from the norm. Some individuals with craniofacial abnormalities may nevertheless be rated as average or even high in attractiveness. We suspect that this occurs when their disfigurement is relatively minor or not visibly salient. (Indeed, many people have minor facial blemishes that probably play little, if any, role in their appearance.) In this instance, we would expect social reactions to be influenced more by attractiveness than by facial defects. Our analysis in this chapter refers largely to persons with conspicuous and substantial facial flaws.

tion partners, the likelihood that clefts can be surgically ameliorated is probably greater than the likelihood that ugliness can be transformed into beauty. Therefore, on the dimension of expected future course, the impact of craniofacial abnormalities on social interaction may be somewhat less severe than the effect of homeliness.

As for disruptiveness, we would expect facial deformities to be quite distracting and disturbing. Not only is the face central in human communication, but it is "the single most distinguishing physical feature of any person" (Munro, 1981, p. 171). Langlois (this volume) suggests that symmetry and similarity to facial norms determine which faces are pleasing and which are not. In contrast to facially disfigured persons, normal but unattractive persons would probably have smoother interactions simply because their faces deviate less from normal and are consequently less distracting to the observer.

There can be little doubt that facial deformity and normal ugliness are both aesthetically displeasing. But although unattractive people may be at the low end of an aesthetic dimension, they are still perceived as belonging on the normal continuum. People with clefts and other facial anomalies may be categorized on an altogether different scale, one that, we would imagine, is considered qualitatively less appealing than the normal scale.

Derivations for Jones et al.'s (1984) final two dimensions, origin and peril, are less clear. We suspect that neither ugly nor facially disfigured persons are generally perceived to be responsible for their plights in lay perceptions. Research on the belief in a just world (Lerner, 1980) suggests that perceivers sometimes hold victims accountable for their misfortunes in order to protect their own sense of personal security. It seems plausible to us that facial abnormalities might produce such reactions in some observers or in certain circumstances, although we know of no empirical evidence to substantiate this point. Regarding peril, although severe facial defects sometimes provoke fearful responses (which normal unattractiveness rarely does), these reactions are probably slight as compared to other stigmas, such as AIDS or mental retardation.

When contrasted on the dimensions proposed by Jones et al. (1984), then, facial disfigurement appears to have potentially more pronounced negative effects on social interaction than normal ugliness does. This would seem to imply that the predictions of the attractiveness literature for the social interaction of unattractive people would apply even more strongly to facially deformed individuals. In other words, people with craniofacial abnormalities would be perceived more negatively in initial encounters and stereotypic judgments and would possess less desirability as potential interaction partners.

Alternatively, it might be the case that because these anomalies are significantly more stigmatizing than normal ugliness along several of Jones et al.'s dimensions, different processes would apply. Such a perspective suggests that individuals with facial irregularities may have inherently different social experiences than normally unattractive people do. One important aspect of this divergence is ambivalence, a reaction that Katz (1981) posits as a common human reaction to all forms of stigmatization. In his framework, stigma is thought to engender feelings of threat, fear, or hostility. But simultaneously, the observer is aware of strong social norms to be kind to disadvantaged or handicapped people. The combination of these contradictory attitudes creates conflict and ambivalence in the observer. Katz proposes that this ambivalence produces behavioral amplification, that is, exaggeration of positive or negative response tendencies, whenever specific input (i.e., thoughts, feelings, or new information) discredits one of the conflicting attitudes that the self holds toward the stigmatized other. The self then acts to defend or deny the discredited attitude by compensatory over- or undervaluation of the stigmatized person, depending on which attitude has been discredited.

Katz (1981) presents several studies operationalizing stigma in terms of race and physical handicaps that provide support for this theory. These studies demonstrate, first, that when white subjects were given a chance to derogate someone whom they had harmed during an experiment, they were more likely to derogate a black or handicapped confederate than a white, nonhandicapped one. On the other hand, when given an opportunity to assist victims of a similar harm, white subjects were more likely to help black or handicapped confederates than white, nonhandicapped confederates. In addition, when given a second opportunity to help, subjects were more willing to help handicapped than nonhandicapped confederates. Taken together, these studies suggest that tendencies to both help and hinder were stronger when subjects encountered stigmatized others than nonstigmatized others.

In another study, Katz (1981) examined individual differences in ambivalence by observing response latencies in ratings of handicapped people. He assumed that those with greater ambivalence toward the handicapped would take longer rating the targets. Subjects with longer response latencies, and presumably more ambivalence toward handicapped people, did evaluate socially desirable handicapped people more positively, but they rated socially undesirable handicapped people more negatively. This was interpreted as evidence of the exaggeration of simultaneously experienced positive and negative attitudes by ambivalent subjects.

Research carried out within other frameworks provides additional evidence that stigmatized others are avoided (Kleck, 1969; Kleck, Ono, & Hastorf, 1966; Langer, Fiske, Taylor, & Chanowitz, 1976). In particular, facially disfigured children are ranked lower in likability than normals (Richardson, Goodman, Hastorf, & Dornbusch, 1961), are rejected more often (Landsdown & Polak, 1975), are less likely to be chosen as a friend (Tobiasen, 1984), are rated less accurately on intelligence by teachers (i.e., both the most and least intelligent facially disfigured children are rated more toward the scale midpoint than objective criteria imply; Richman, 1978), and marry less often and later than their siblings or matched normal controls (Peter & Chinsky, 1974).

One especially relevant study used an unobtrusive measure to demonstrate avoidance of the facially disfigured. Rumsey, Bull, and Gahagan (1982) assessed the distance between pedestrians and confederates waiting for a streetlight on a busy noontime corner. The confederates appeared to be temporarily (with a bruise and abrasion) or permanently (with a "strawberry" birthmark) facially disfigured or nondisfigured. Pedestrians stood further away from the permanently disfigured confederate than the temporarily disfigured confederate, but they stood further away from both disfigured confederates than from the nondisfigured confederate. In addition, they more often stood on the nondisfigured side of the disfigured confederates.

Thus, evidence for the social avoidance and rejection side of ambivalent reactions to handicapped and facially disfigured individuals is plain. Other studies provide support for overvaluation or preferential treatment of the handicapped—that is, the other side of the ambivalent reaction proposed by Katz (1981). For example, subjects sometimes rate handicapped confederated more positively (Kleck, 1969); shock handicapped confederates for a shorter duration (Farina, Sherman, & Allen, 1968); distort their own opinions to be consistent with the expected opinions of a handicapped confederate (Kleck, 1968; Kleck et al., 1966); give money more often and in larger amounts when the confederate is handicapped (Levitt & Kornhaber, 1977); comply with requests to fill out a questionnaire more often when the confederate wears an eyepatch (Doob & Ecker, 1970); and are less distressed when treated inequitably by handicapped confederate than nonhandicapped confederates (Feldman, Barbaresi, & Caiola, 1983). To sum up, nonstigmatized persons appear to react to stigmatized others with a parcel of seemingly inconsistent positive and negative attitudes best characterized as ambivalence.

Katz's theory (1981) suggests several intriguing speculations regarding differences between cranoifacial abnormalities and normal unattractiveness. For one, facially disfigured individuals may experience greater rejection than the nondisfigured, but simultaneously they may enjoy enhanced prosocial behavior from others. In contrast, the large literature on physical attractiveness indicates that the unattractive person's experience is predominantly one of disadvantage in social situations and of negative perception by others (excepting the special circumstances cited earlier). We would speculate therefore that the social norm of "kindness to the disadvantaged," which underlies Katz's theory, does not extend to normal but unattractive people, in spite of the demonstrated disadvantages of ugliness. Perhaps this is because in our culture, ugliness is not considered a stigmatizing condition requiring medical intervention, whereas facial disfigurement is.

Unattractive people may therefore experience the social disadvantage of being at the low end of a normal scale in terms of the various outcomes that relate to attractiveness, whereas the facially disfigured may have the social disadvantage of being on a different scale altogether. Being on a different scale connotes both more rejection and more help, however. Because facial defects elicit both positive and negative reactions from others, whereas ugliness elicits only negative reactions, disfigured individuals may experience more conflict and ambivalence from others than ugly persons do.

A hypothetical example may highlight this distinction. Were people with severe clefts to canvas a neighborhood soliciting donations for the Foundation for Craniofacial Deformities, we would expect a reasonable level of contributions. In contrast, were ugly individuals to request donations for the Association for Homely Persons, our guess is that they would be largely unsuccessful. Further illustrating this point is the fact that the aforementioned Foundation for Craniofacial Deformities actually exists, providing valuable information and direct assistance to patients and their families and funding research. We know of no organizations whose primary purpose is to provide help or information to homely individuals or to parents of homely babies, even though the pervasive negative impact of this factor is well documented.

Further support for our assertion that facial disfigurement and normal unattractiveness differ qualitatively to some extent can be extrapolated from several studies of child behavior problems. In general, unattractive children tend to be more aggressive and more likely to engage in high-activity play than are attractive children (e.g., Langlois & Downs, 1979). In contrast, children and adults with cleft palates tend toward problems associated with excessive impulse inhibition (Richman & Harper, 1978) and withdrawal from social interaction (McWilliams, 1982). This deduction must remain speculative, in that we are aware of no controlled studies directly comparing facial disfigured and normally unattractive individuals. Nevertheless, inhibition and withdrawal seem to us natural responses to ambivalence, whereas active hositility seems an understandable reaction to antipathy.

In conclusion, we have suggested that unattractive but nondisfigured individuals may experience exclusively negative outcomes because of their appearance, whereas craniofacially disfigured individuals may receive both advantages and disadvantages. True, disfigured individuals may experience these "advantages" as patronizing reminders of their differentness; nevertheless, their interactions sometimes include positive features that normally ugly persons are less likely to enjoy. Therefore, predictions from the attractiveness literature may not map isomorphically onto facial disfigurement (cf. Tobiasen, 1984), even though disfigured people are generally rated as less attractive than nondisfigured people (Richardson et al., 1961; Tobiasen, 1987).

Implications for Research

Although the research findings described earlier suggest several fruitful applications of the physical attractiveness literature to the specific circumstances of children and adults with craniofacial deformities, they nonetheless reveal substantial gaps that preclude drawing these generalizations with confidence. On the most superficial level, the parallelism of unattractiveness and craniofacial problems seems straightforward; there can be little doubt that most craniofacial abnormalities are considered unattractive by conventional standards. Thus, the better-established effects of unattractiveness, such as negative stereotypic ratings and first impressions, would seem to apply. But closer examination reveals several important questions and potential qualifications that await additional research.

Chief among them is the question of whether craniofacial abnormalities are isomorphic with "normal' unattractiveness. In that they involve significant disturbances of the usual facial characteristics and symmetries, it seems likely to us that reactions to craniofacial disturbances are more complex, in the sense of involving additional processes, than are reactions to "normal" unattractiveness. These processes might temper the impact of unattractiveness, so that typical effects are attenuated, exacerbated, or otherwise moderated in these individuals. It will be important, therefore, to examine in considerable detail the comparability of facial disfigurement and normal unattractiveness.

Notions about stigma, as described earlier, suggest several directions such research might take. Using the Jones et al. (1984) framework, when compared to "normal" but unattractive persons, facial defects are less concealable, more disruptive to social interaction, and more aesthetically repelling. This would seem to presage stronger reactions than to normally unattractive persons, essentially magnifying the effects described earlier and perhaps extending the domain of activities and inferences to which they apply. At the same time, Katz's (1981) conception of ambivalence amplification connotes an alternate state of affairs. The very stigmatizing nature of craniofacial flaws may simultaneously evoke norms of helpfulness, sympathy, and charity, along with the expected prejudices. Thus, we might propose that stereotypically negative reactions to such persons will be paired with prosocial behavior (which, incidentally, has never been demonstrated as a response to normal unattractiveness).

If this prediction is correct, it will be particularly important to determine the conditions that elicit positive and negative reactions—that is, to identify the circumstances under which people with craniofacial abnormalities can expect helpful or undermining responses from others. Several possibilities come to mind: 1) the relative salience of conflicting norms toward helpfulness and antipathy in that setting; 2) distance and degree of involvement (i.e., we would expect that situations requiring close contact with disfigured strangers will engender distancing and avoidance, whereas situations permitting less involvement will foster altruism); 3) self-presentation pressures (we assume here that avoidant responses to craniofacial disfigurement are considered socially undesirable and that helpfulness is considered desirable); 4) the nature of the relationship between subject and partner (we expect less avoidance in closer relationships); 5) concern with external appearance and social impressions, as opposed to inner characteristics and personal impressions; and 6) various attitudinal and personality predispositions.

From the standpoint of researchers interested in the attractiveness phenomenon per se, the special case of craniofacial disfigurement offers several new research directions. We have already mentioned the need to determine whether "what is beautiful is good" or whether "what is ugly is bad" or both. Even more intriguing is the possibility that attractiveness and unattractiveness may not be unidimensional phenomena. That is, if it is the case that facial disfigurement produces qualitatively different reactions than normal ugliness does, then it follows that there may be various types of attractiveness and unattractiveness, each with distinct stereotypes and behavioral consequences. "What is beautiful is good" and "what is ugly is bad" may be overly generalized conclusions, in other words, in the sense that different types of attractiveness might provoke different judgments and social reactions. Wheeler (Wheeler & Eghrari, 1986; Wheeler & Lesko, 1984) has already identified three types of attractiveness within each sex. The female types are "sophisticated," "wholesome," and "sexy"; the male types are "pretty boy," "rugged boy," and "wholesome." Importantly, although the best exemplars within each type were rated as quite attractive, the specific stereotypic traits ascribed to each type varied. For example, sophisticated females were seen as more assertive and stronger of will, whereas the wholesome type was described as kinder and more sincere. Similarly, pretty boys were pictured as artistic, whereas rugged boys were perceived as masculine and active in team sports.

It seems likely that several types of unattractiveness exist, one of which involves craniofacial disfigurement, and that their attendant social consequences diverge in meaningful ways. If so, to speculate further, these different appearance categories might be organized within a hierarchical prototype structure (Mervis & Rosch, 1981; Rosch, 1978), such that the mid-level category, attractiveness, represents the more abstract general features of the various subtypes. We would then expect there to be a few general characteristics that accrue to all forms of attractiveness and unattractiveness as well as more particular consequences that depend upon the specific type. Regardless, the special case of craniofacial abnormalities suggests that researchers move beyond a unidimensional view of attractiveness toward a more differentiated typology.

Implications for Treatment

We have seen from the attractiveness literature reviewed earlier that the primary disadvantages of unattractiveness occur in first impressions, stereotypic judgments, and dating desirability. We see no compelling reasons not to generalize these findings to the specific instance of craniofacial abnormalities. Thus, one implication of our review for people with facial disfigurement is that they seek friends and lovers in closed fields—that is, from interaction partners already well known, such as work colleagues, superficial acquaintances, and neighbors. Alternatively, they might try to develop strategies for continuing new acquaintanceships beyond first meetings, since others are relatively less likely to pursue these relationships on the basis of appearance-based cues (cocktail parties and singles' bars are clearly not the best environments for them). A social life organized around shared interests and activities would permit acquaintanceships to develop beyond first impressions and should effectively highlight personal qualities not directly dependent on appearance (numerous studies have demonstrated that the impact of stereotypes diminishes once partners acquire more information about each other). Unattractive and facially disfigured persons who have cultivated such capacities would thereby provide reasonable bases for attraction by skirting interaction contexts in which their appearance is most disadvantageous.

These suggestions make little distinction between craniofacial disfigurement and normal unattractiveness. In contrast, Katz's (1981) ambivalence-amplification theory implies that these two groups will have qualitatively different experiences in several ways. Most important, along with aversive reactions, the stigmatizing nature of craniofacial abnormalities should evoke altruistic and charitable social norms, such that interaction partners might find themselves simultaneously sympathetic and repelled. We would therefore expect that people with facial defects will receive more ambivalent, conflict-laden responses from others, especially strangers, than normally unattractive people will. Doubtlessly, the unpredictability and variability of these mixed messages are disagreeable and disconcerting and may even engender learned helplessness in the social domain.

One strategy for coping with this ambivalence is founded on the premise that attributions of causality affect subsequent feelings and behavior. Recognizing that others are uncomfortable when encountering facial disfigurement should permit people with such stigmas to attribute interpersonal difficulties and awkwardness to a relatively natural response to their external physical features rather than to more ego-involving psychological or social characteristics. This type of attribution is probably adaptive, since its connotations for the core self-concept are somewhat weaker. Crocker and Major (1989) have in fact suggested that people may protect their self-esteem by attributing misfortunes to stigmatizing conditions that they possess rather than to more ego-involved abilities or personality traits. Thus, facially disfigured persons have available to them an option for discounting the implications of negative feedback that normal individuals do not.

Having an awareness that others' discomfort stems from ambivalence about disfigurement also permits enactment of proactive strategies for smoothing social interaction. In fact, some clinical observers (e.g., MacGregor, Abel, Bryt, Lauer, & Weissmann, 1953) have suggested that individuals with mild facial deformities who anticipate surgical improvement and take active steps to mask their defects are at greater risk for psychological problems than are individuals with severe abnormalities, who are more likely to be resigned to their fate and consequently may develop interaction skills and strategies to offset or even capitalize on their condition. Goffman's (1963) classic essay on stigma outlines several techniques that stigmatized persons may use to diffuse tension in interactions with "normals." These strategies include: 1) a matter-of-fact approach to the stigma; 2) initiation of the disability as a topic of conversation; 3) acceptance of well-intentioned, though perhaps awkward and unnecessary efforts to help; and 4) humor.

An evocative illustration of these techniques for diffusing tension is cited by Goffman (1963):

> Then there was the cigarette gag. That was invariably good for a laugh. Whenever I'd walk into a restaurant, bar, or party, I'd whip out a pack of butts, open it ostentatiously, take one, light it, and sit back puffing on it contentedly. That almost always attracted attention. People would stare and I could almost hear them saying, My! Isn't it wonderful what he can do with a pair of hooks? Whenever anyone commented on this accomplishment I'd smile and say, "There's one thing I never have to worry about. That's burning my fingers." Corny, I know, but a sure icebreaker. . . . (p. 116)

Goffman viewed these techniques as methods of protecting normals from the unfairness and pain associated with a stigma. But they can also serve as assertive tactics to bypass or overcome negative reactions by focusing attention on one's self-awareness, generosity, or sense of humor, all favorable interaction strategies likely to engender positive regard.

Summary

Craniofacial deformities involve visible and often striking disruptions of the normal symmetry and structure of the human face. Because these abnormalities are invariably considered unattractive by observers, and because facial unattractiveness meaningfully influences social judgment and interpersonal attraction, the person with craniofacial disfigurement is presented with a social reality fraught from the outset with disadvantages. Cosmetic surgery, although beneficial in lessening the degree of disfigurement in many cases, is at best a partial solution, in that visible signs of disfigurement typically remain. It is important, therefore, for those who work with craniofacially disfigured individuals—therapists, physicians, parents, teachers, and especially the disfigured individuals themselves—to be aware of and understand the implications of facial abnormalities for social perception and interaction. At the same time, our analysis suggests several boundary conditions and moderating variables that differentiate the experiences of craniofacial abnormalities and normal unattractiveness. Thus, facial anomalies offer a special case that can be highly informative to theoretically oriented attractiveness researchers. What better justification for bridging theory and clinical application with additional research?

References

Ashmore, R. (1988). *Physical attractiveness: A review.* Unpublished manuscript, Rutgers University, New Brunswick, NJ.

Bernstein, W., Stephenson, B., Snyder, M., & Wicklund, R. (1983). Causal ambiguity and heterosexual affiliation. *Journal of Experimental Social Psychology, 19,* 78–92.

Berscheid, E. (1985). Interpersonal attraction. In G. Lindzey & E. Aronson (Eds.), *The handbook of social psychology* (3rd Ed., pp. 413–484). New York: Random House.

Berscheid, E. (1986). The question of the importance of physical attractiveness. In C. Herman, M. Zanna, & E.T. Higgins (Eds.), *Physical appearance, stigma, and social behavior* (pp. 291–298). Hillsdale, NJ: Erlbaum.

Brislin, R., & Lewis, S. (1968). Dating and physical attractiveness: Replication. *Psychological Reports, 22,* 976.

Bull, R., & Rumsey, N. (1988). *The social psychology of facial appearance.* New York: Springer-Verlag.

Cash, T., Kehr, J., Polyson, J., & Freeman, V. (1977). Role of physical attractivenes in peer attribution of psychological disturbance. *Journal of Consulting and Clinical Psychology, 45,* 987–993.

Clifford, M. (1975). Physical attractiveness and academic performance. *Child Study Journal, 5,* 201–209.

Clifford, M., & Walster, E. (1973). Research note: The effects of physical attractiveness on teachers' expectations. *Sociology of Education, 46,* 248–258.

Crocker, J., & Major, B. (1989). Social stigma and self-esteem: The self-protective properties of stigma. *Psychological Review, 96,* 608–630.

Cross, A. (1981). *Death in a tenured position.* New York: Ballantine Books.

Cunningham, M.R. (1986). Measuring the physical in physical attractiveness: Quasi-experiments on the sociobiology of female facial beauty. *Journal of Personality and Social Psychology, 50,* 925–935.

Dermer, M., & Thiel, D. (1975). When beauty may fail. *Journal of Personality and Social Psychology, 31,* 1168–1176.

Dion, K. (1974). Children's physical attractiveness and sex as determinants of adult punitiveness. *Developmental Psychology, 10,* 772–778.

Dion, K., Berscheid, E., & Walster, E. (1972). What is beautiful is good. *Journal of Personality and Social Psychology, 24,* 285–290.

Dipboye, R., Arvey, R., & Terpstra, D. (1977). Sex and physical attractiveness of raters and applicants as determinants of resume evaluations. *Journal of Applied Psychology, 62,* 288–294.

Doob, A.N., & Ecker, B.P. (1970). Stigma and compliance. *Journal of Personality and Social Psychology, 14,* 302–304.

Edwards, M., & Watson, A.C.H. (1980). Future prospects. In M. Edwards & A.C.H. Watson (Eds.), *Advances in the management of cleft palate* (pp. 279–281). New York: Churchill Livingstone.

Ekman, P. (1973). *Darwin and facial expression.* New York: Academic Press.

Farina, A., Sherman, M., & Allen, J.G. (1968). Role of physical abnormalities in interpersonal perception and behavior. *Journal of Abnormal Psychology, 73,* 590–593.

Feingold, A. (1988). Matching for attractiveness in romantic partners and same-sex friends: A meta-analysis and theoretical critique. *Psychological Bulletin, 104,* 226–235.

Feingold, A. (1989). *Sex differences in the impact of attractiveness on heterosexual relationships: A meta-analysis.* Unpublished manuscript, Yale University, New Haven, CT.

Feldman, M.D., Barbaresi, W., & Caiola, V. (1983). Physical stigma as a variable in perceptions of equity. *Representative Research in Social Psychology, 13,* 46–53.

Felson, R. (1980). Physical attractiveness, grades, and teachers' attributions. *Representative Research in Social Psychology, 11,* 64–71.

Glenwick, D., Jason, L., & Elman, D. (1978). Physical attractiveness and social contact in singles bars. *Journal of Social Psychology, 105,* 311–312.

Goffman, E. (1963). *Stigma: Notes on the management of spoiled identity.* Englewood Cliffs, NJ: Prentice-Hall.

Hatfield, E., & Sprecher, S. (1986). *Mirror, Mirror . . . The importance of looks in everyday life.* Albany, NY: State University of New York Press.

Hatfield, E., Traupman, J., Sprecher, S., Utne, M., & Hay, J. (1984). Equity and intimate relations: Recent research. In W. Ickes (Ed.), *Compatible and incompatible relationships* (pp. 91–118). New York: Springer-Verlag.

Heilman, M., & Saruwatari, L. (1979). When beauty is beastly. *Organizational Behavior and Human Performance, 23,* 360–372.

Holmes, S., & Hatch, C. (1938). Personal appearance as related to scholastic records and marriage selection in college women. *Human Biology, 10,* 65–76.

Huston, T. (1973). Ambiguity of acceptance, social desirability, and dating choice. *Journal of Experimental Social Psychology, 9,* 32–42.

Izard, C.E. (1977). *Human emotions.* New York: Plenum.

Jackson, L. (1983). The influence of sex, physical attractiveness, sex role, and occupational sex-linkage on perceptions of occupational suitability. *Journal of Applied Social Psychology, 13,* 31–44.

Jones, E.E., Farina, A., Hastorf, A.H., Markus, H., Miller, D.T., & Scott, R.A. (1984). *Social stigma: The psychology of marked relationships.* New York: W.H. Freeman.

Kalick, S., & Hamilton, T. (1986). The matching hypothesis re-examined. *Journal of Personality and Social Psychology, 51,* 673–682.

Katz, I. (1981). *Stigma: A social psychological analysis.* Hillsdale, NJ: Erlbaum.

Kernis, M., & Wheeler, L. (1981). Beautiful friends and ugly strangers: Radiation and contrast effects in perception of same-sex pairs. *Personality and Social Psychology Bulletin, 7,* 617–620.

Kleck, R. (1968). Physical stigma and nonverbal cues emitted in face-to-face interaction. *Human Relations, 21,* 19–28.

Kleck, R. (1969). Physical stigma and task-oriented interactions. *Human Relations, 22,* 53–60.

Kleck, R., Ono, H., & Hastorf, A.H. (1966). The effects of physical deviance upon face-to-face interaction. *Human Relations, 19,* 425–436.

Krebs, D., & Adinolfi, A. (1975). Physical attractiveness, social relations, and personality style. *Journal of Personality and Social Psychology, 31,* 245–253.

Landsdown, R., & Polak, L. (1975). A study of the psychological effects of facial deformity in children. *Child: Care, Health, and Development, 4,* 85–91.

Landy, D., & Sigall, H. (1974). Beauty is talent: Task evaluation as function of the performer's physical attractiveness. *Journal of Personality and Social Psychology, 29,* 299–304.

Langer, E.J., Fiske, S., Taylor, S.E., & Chanowitz, B. (1976). Stigma, staring, and discomfort: A novel stimulus hypothesis. *Journal of Experimental Social Psychology, 12,* 451–463.

Langlois, J.H., & Downs, A.C. (1979). Peer relations as a function of physical attractivenes: The eye of the beholder or behavioral reality? *Child Development, 50,* 409–418.

Lefebvre, A., & Munro, I.R. (1986). Psychological adjustment of patients with craniofacial deformities before and after surgery. In C. Herman, M. Zanna, & E.T. Higgins (Eds.), *Physical appearance, stigma, and social behavior* (pp. 53–62). Hillsdale, NJ: Erlbaum.

Lerner, M.J. (1980). *The belief in a just world.* New York: Plenum.

Lerner, R., & Lerner, J. (1977). Effects of age, sex and physical attractiveness on child-peer relations, academic performance, and elementary school adjustment. *Developmental Psychology, 13,* 585–590.

Levitt, L., & Kornhaber, R.C. (1977). Stigma and compliance: A re-examination. *The Journal of Social Psychology, 103,* 13–18.

MacGregor, F.C., Abel, T.M., Bryt, A., Lauer, E., & Weissmann, S. (1953). *Facial deformities and plastic surgery: A psychosocial study.* Springfield, IL: Charles C. Thomas.

Maruyama, G., & Miller, N. (1981). Physical attractiveness and personality. In B. Maher (Ed.), *Progress in experimental research in personality,* Vol. 10. New York: Academic Press.

McWilliams, B.J. (1982). Social and psychological problems associated with cleft palate. *Clinics in Plastic Surgery, 9,* 317–326.

Mervis, C.B., & Rosch, E. (1981). Categorization of natural objects. *Annual Review of Psychology, 32,* 89–115.

Miller, A. (1970). The role of physical attractiveness in impression formation. *Psychonomic Science, 19,* 241–243.

Morse, S., Reis, H., Gruzen, J., & Wolff, E. (1974). The "eye of the beholder": Determinants of physical attractiveness judgments in the U.S. and South Africa. *Journal of Personality, 42,* 528–542.

Munro, I.R. (1981). The psychological effects of surgical treatment of facial deformity. In G.W. Lucker, K.A. Ribbens, & J.A. McNamara, Jr. (Eds.), *Psychological aspects of facial form* (pp. 171–199). Ann Arbor, MI: Center for Human Growth and Development, University of Michigan.

Murphy, M., Nelson, D., & Cheap, T. (1981). Rated and actual performance of high school students as a function of sex and attractiveness. *Psychological Reports, 88,* 103–106.

Patzer, G. (1985). *The physical attractiveness phenomena.* New York: Plenum.

Peter, J.P., & Chinsky, R.R. (1974). Sociological aspects of cleft palate adults. *Cleft Palate Journal, 11,* 295–309.

Reis, H.T., Nezlek, J., & Wheeler, L. (1980). Physical attractiveness in social interaction. *Journal of Personality and Social Psychology, 38,* 604–617.

Reis, H.T., Wheeler, L., Spiegel, N., Kernis, M., Nezlek, J., & Perri, M. (1982). Physical attractiveness in social interaction II: Why does appearance affect social experience? *Journal of Personality and Social Psychology, 43,* 979–996.

Richardson, S.A., Goodman, N., Hastorf, A.H., & Dornbusch, S.M. (1961). Cultural uniformity in reaction to physical disabilities. *American Sociological Review, 26,* 241–247.

Richman, L.C. (1978). The effects of facial disfigurement on teachers' perception of ability in cleft palate children. *Cleft Palate Journal, 15,* 155–160.

Richman, L.C., & Harper, D.C. (1978). School adjustment of children with observable disabilities. *Journal of Abnormal Child Psychology, 8,* 11–18.

Rosch, E. (1978). Principles of categorization. In E. Rosch & B.B. Lloyd (Eds.), *Cognition and categorization* (pp. 27–48). Hillsdale, NJ: Erlbaum.

Rumsey, N., Bull, R., & Gahagan, D. (1982). The effect of facial disfigurement on the proxemic behavior of the general public. *Journal of Applied Social Psychology, 12,* 137–150.

Sigall, H., & Landy, D. (1973). Radiating beauty: Effects of having a physically attractive partner on person perception. *Journal of Personality and Social Psychology, 28,* 218–224.

Sigall, H., & Ostrove, N. (1975). Beautiful but dangerous: Effects of offender attractiveness and nature of crime on juridic judgment. *Journal of Personality and Social Psychology, 31,* 410–414.

Singer, J. (1964). The use of manipulative strategies: Machiavellianism and attractiveness. *Sociometry, 27,* 128–150.

Snyder, M., Berscheid, E., & Glick, P. (1985). Focusing on the exterior and the interior: Two investigations of the initiation of personal relationships. *Journal of Personality and Social Psychology, 48,* 1427–1439.

Solomon, M., & Schopler, J. (1978). The relationship of physical attractiveness and punitiveness: Is the linearity assumption out of line? *Personality and Social Psychology Bulletin, 4,* 483–486.

Sorell, G., & Nowak, C. (1981). The role of physical attractiveness as a contributor to individual development. In R. Lerner & N. Busch-Rossnagel (Eds.), *Individuals as producers of their development.* New York: Academic Press.

Stroebe, W., Insko, C., Thompson, V., & Layton, C. (1971). Effects of physical attractiveness, attitude similarity, and sex on various aspects of interpersonal attraction. *Journal of Personality and Social Psychology, 18,* 79–91.

Tesser, A., & Brodie, M. (1971). A note on the evaluation of a computer date. *Psychonomic Science, 23,* 300.

Tobiasen, J. (1984). Psychosocial correlates of congenital facial clefts: A conceptualization and model. *Cleft Palate Journal, 21,* 131–139.

Udry, J.R., & Eckland, B.K. (1982). The benefits of being attractive: Differential payoffs for men and women. Paper presented at the annual meeting of the American Sociological Association, San Francisco, CA.

Walster, E., Aronson, E., Abrahams, D., & Rottman, L. (1966). The importance of physical attractiveness in dating behavior. *Journal of Personality and Social Psychology, 4,* 508–516.

Wheeler, L., & Eghrari, H, (1986). Sexy, sophisticated, or wholesome: Perceptions of different types of attractive females. Unpublished manuscript, University of Rochester, Rochester, NY.

Wheeler, L., & Lesko, S. (1984). Perceptions of different types of attractive males. Unpublished manuscript, University of Rochester, Rochester, NY.

Part 4
Current Research on Craniofacial Anomalies

11
Persons with Down Syndrome: Facial Characteristics, Self- and Other-Perception, and Social Acceptance

FELICISIMA C. SERAFICA

Persons with Down Syndrome (DS) have, in addition to intellectual deficits, specific dysmorphic facial features. These include small, simply formed ears with overlapping helices, upward slant of palpebral fissures, epicanthal folds, small nose with depressed nasal bridge, mid-face hypoplasia, and a small oral cavity with broadened alveolar ridges and narrow palate (Pueschel, 1982). Such distinguishing physical characteristics, it is believed, make the person with Down Syndrome appear markedly different from others, even physically unattractive to some. There is concern (Olbrisch, 1982) lest the characteristic facial features of persons with DS impede their social integration. This concern suggests an implicit model which assumes that physical appearance mediates others' perceptions of an individual and that these, in turn, influence others' acceptance of and consequent behavior toward thc individual. Proponents of this view also assume that physical appearance mediates the individual's self-perception, which, in turn, influences self-acceptance and consequent behavior toward others.

Guided by these implicit assumptions, a growing number of parents are seeking facial plastic surgery to correct the dysmorphic facial features of their children with DS (Hohler, 1977; Lemperle & Radu, 1980; Olbrisch, 1982). Parents are not alone in hoping that facial surgery will benefit this clinical group. A survey (Pueschel, Monteiro, & Erickson, 1986) that compared the perceptions of parents and physicians indicates that the latter are even more staunch advocates of this surgical intervention. The results showed that 44% of the physicians but only 13% of the parents favored performing facial surgery on children with DS. Furthermore, significantly higher percentages of physicians than parents expected that after plastic surgery, children with DS would be better accepted by society, neighbors, other children. and relatives. Moreover, significantly higher percentages of physicians held the opinion that after facial surgery, the child with DS would accomplish more, emotionally and in self-help skills. Physicians were also more optimistic about the effects of facial surgery on intellectual and social development, although the group difference did not reach the accepted level of statistical significance. Language acquisition was the only area in which parental expectations significantly exceeded those of physicians. Parents and physicians did not differ significantly in their expectations that facial surgery would alter society's preconceived prejudices, increase the employability of persons with DS, or result in unrealistic expectations on the part of parents or society in general.

Facial surgery was initially performed on children with Down Syndrome in Frankfurt, Germany (Lemperle & Radu, 1980). Subsequently, it was introduced in Israel, where it obtained the enthusiastic support of Feuerstein (1982, 1983) who was attempting to extend his concept of cognitive modifiability for developmentally delayed children to physical modifiability. Arguing against a passive approach to children with disabilities that merely encourages the environment to accept them as they are, Feuerstein (1979) advocates a philosophy of active modification. Within his framework, facial surgery is expected to enhance the individual's chances for social integration, not only in the immediate lifespace, but also in the larger society. In turn, integration could provide access to higher-level educational programs, heightened performance expectations in all activities, and a better self-concept and self-acceptance in everyday life. In line with this philosophy, Feuerstein (1982) has designed an intervention program for children with DS that includes facial surgery, speech therapy, parent education, and a systematic cognitive development curriculum.

To date relatively little is known about the efficacy of facial plastic surgery for persons with DS, particularly its psychosocial benefits. Lemperle and Radu (1980) used only self-reports of parent satisfaction. Possible changes in speech articulation, language development, voice quality, dentition, frequent respiratory infection, eating facility, and cognitive development of the children with Down Syndrome in Feuerstein's (1982) intervention program were monitored and measured. However, as described by Feuerstein (1982), the research design would not have allowed for the isolation of the surgical psychosocial outcomes from those of the other intervention methods used concurrently. Subsequent reports from his collaborators (e.g., Wexler, Peled, Rand, Mintzker, & Feuerstein, 1986) also do not mention a control group or other attempts to control for other possible sources of improvement such as speech therapy. Hence, any observed effects cannot be attributed to facial surgery alone.

Katz and Kravetz (1989) reviewed the available studies on effectiveness of facial surgery for children with DS. They synthesized the findings around three areas where expected improvements are often advanced as the rationale for performing the procedure on this population: physical functioning, physical appearance, and social acceptance.

For physical functioning, Katz and Kravetz (1989) noted that when parental evaluations were used to measure effectiveness of partial glossectomy or surgical reduction of tongue size, improved eating skills, less drooling, and fewer infections were reported. However, the studies did not include a comparison group of parents whose children with DS had not undergone a similar operation. A study that did (Kravetz, Weller, Tennenbaum, Tzuriel, & Mintzker, 1987) failed to find a statistically significant difference in children's quality of conversation as rated by their parents. Furthermore, a study that employed speech therapists rather than parents as raters did not yield significant differences between pre- and postoperative speech and articulation (Parsons, Iacono, & Rozner, 1987).

According to Katz and Kravetz (1989), results concerning the effects of facial surgery on physical appearance show a similar pattern. Postoperative ratings are higher than preoperative ones in studies that involve parents and physicians and rely on impressions or ask direct questions about the operation's effectiveness. However, studies that use control groups, ask indirect questions, and employ raters who are either elementary school children (Novoselsky, Katz, & Kravetz, 1988), student teachers (Alkawitz, 1987), or adult lay volunteers (Arndt, Lefebvre, Travis, & Munro, 1986) show less positive results. In one study (Kravetz et al., 1987) that included a control group, the overall test of effect for surgical intervention reached only borderline statistical significance. One study (Strauss, Mintzker, Feuerstein, Wexler, & Rand, 1988) that was not reviewed by Katz and Kravetz (1989) showed a slight but statistically significant change from pre- to postsurgery in normal adolescents' ratings of the attractiveness of facial photographs depicting school-age children with DS. However, there was considerable variability. Significant improvements in appearance ratings occurred only for three of the eight children who had undergone surgery, while no change was perceived in three of them and ratings for two others significantly declined.

Improvements in social acceptance following facial surgery have also been assessed. In one study (Wexler et al., 1986), 74% of the parents reported that after the surgery, their children with DS were stared at by strangers much less. Also following the surgery, DS facial characteristics such as the protruding tongue and slanted eyes disturbed the parents less. In another study (Kravetz et al., 1987), children who had undergone facial surgery were perceived as exhibiting fewer outbursts of aggression than those who had not, and other people's reactions to them were reported to have improved following the operation. However, other investigators (Alkawitz, 1987; Novoselsky et al., 1988) did not find that children who had surgery were perceived as having a more pleasant personality, being better behaved in the classroom, or being a more appropriate playmate than children who had not had surgery. Finally, the expectation that facial surgery might also facilitate the integration of persons with DS into the family and society has also not been fulfilled. Arndt et al. (1986) failed to find significant differences between pre- and postoperation scores on family cohesiveness and adaptability, based on parent responses to the Family Adaptability Cohesiveness Evaluation Scale (FACES II). Furthermore, both before and after surgery, cohesiveness and adaptability scores from parents of children with DS did not differ significantly from the norms.

In summary, research thus far has not yet conclusively demonstrated that facial surgery for persons wtih DS significantly improves their physical functioning, physical appearance, or social acceptance. Even the few positive findings have to be regarded cautiously because of either design and measurement problems or weak statistical significance (i.e., marginal *p* values). In addition to these methodological problems, there is a conceptual issue. The implicit model held by those who advocate facial surgery as a means of improving the social functioning of persons with DS may be inadequate and perhaps even inaccurate. The assumption that perceived attractiveness based upon facial characteristics is the major determinant of both self-concept and social relations may not hold for persons with DS. Even if their facial characteristics are regarded as unattractive, which still has to be proven, the image that they hold of themselves and the success of their social relations may be due ultimately to variables other than facial characteristics. Research on the psychosocial efficacy of facial surgery for persons with DS might benefit from adopting a conceptual framework that takes into account the complexity of self-concept and social relations. More specifically, expected changes in these behavioral systems following surgery could be based on available scientific knowledge about their development in persons with DS. The aims of this chapter are: 1) to review the available research literature on self- and other-perception, as well as social acceptance of persons with DS, with particular attention to the influence of physical appearance on these variables; 2) to suggest directions for research that could yield the requisite database for decision making regarding the potential outcomes, from a psychosocial perspective, of facial surgery for this clinical population; and 3) to propose a conceptual framework for such research.

Self-Perception

Self-Concept

Theorists and researchers who write about the self-system distinguish between the self as subject ("I") and the self as object ("Me"). Lewis and Brooks-Gunn (1979) refer to the former as the existential self and to the latter as the categorical self. Development of the self as subject starts with the development of the self as an active agent, an entity that exists separate from other objects and people in the world. According to Piaget (1954), a correlate of the development of object concept is the development of the self concept. As the infant gains in understanding that an object has substance, exists independent of one's actions upon it, and is endowed with permanence through time and space, he or she also realizes that the self, too, is an active and causal agent, separate and distinct from others. Thus, at the culmination of the sensorimotor period in development, acquisition of the concept of object permanence implies the emergence of the existential self.

Development of the concept of object permanence in infants and young children with Down Syndrome has been investigated in both cross-sectional and longitudinal studies (Cicchetti & Mans-Wagener, 1987; Dunst, 1990; Dunst & Rheingover, 1983; Mahoney, Glover, & Finger, 1981; Mervis & Cardoso-Martins, 1984; Smith & Hagen, 1984; Smith & von Tetzchner, 1986). Their results indicate that development of object permanence in this clinical population follows the same sequence observed in normal infants.

The rate of development, however, is slower and varies with degree of intelligence. Reaching Stage VI, the highest level in development of object permanence, implies attainment of the concept of self as an independent, active, causal agent. It does not, however, constitute direct evidence. More solid proof is offered by studies using the visual recognition paradigm.

The development of the self as subject and as object has also been investigated in studies using the visual recognition paradigm. Based on their findings. Harter (1983) has proposed a sequence characterizing the emergence of the self as subject and self as object during infancy. According to Harter, at 5 to 8 months, there is no featural differentiation between the self and other. Furthermore, the self is not yet perceived as a causal agent, independent of others. Facing a mirror, the infant manifests interest in his or her mirror image, regards, approaches, touches, smiles, and vocalizes but does not respond to self vs. another in the mirror. At 9 to 12 months, the concept of self as an active agent in space emerges as the infant becomes aware of cause-and-effect relationships between body movements and the moving visual image. Before a mirror, the infant behaves as if he or she understands the nature of reflective surface, engaging in contingency play, imitation, rhythmic movements, bouncing, waving, and locating objects in space or attached to the body.

At 12 to 15 months, the infant becomes capable of differentiating his or her own actions from those of another, thereby realizing that the self is an active, independent agent separate from others, who can also cause their own movements in space. In front of a mirror, the infant uses it to locate people/objects in space and reaches for an actual person or object instead of that person's or object's image in the mirror. By 15 to 18 months, the self as an object of one's knowledge begins to emerge. The infant's ability to recognize his or her own features suggests that the child has developed an internal schema of his or her own face that can be compared to the external visual image. Confronting a mirror, the infant demonstrates mark-directed behavior. Seeing an image with rouge on the nose, the infant touches his or her own nose. The infant also points to the self and distinguishes between self and image in the mirror. Last, at 18 to 24 months, the infant acquires an appreciation that one has unique featural attributes that can be verbally labeled as the self. Facing a mirror, the infant can state his or her name and attach the appropriate personal pronoun to his or her image in the mirror.

The first study of self-recognition in the Down Syndrome population was conducted by Mans, Cicchetti, and Sroufe (1978) in a cross-sectional sample of 27 girls and 28 boys ranging in age from 15 to 48 months. Mothers were instructed to place their children before a mirror and, using a behavior checklist supplied by the researchers, to observe the children's behavior for 20 to 30 seconds. Then the children were turned around and the mothers, while pretending to wipe the children's noses, smeared rouge on them, being careful not to let the children see the coloring. Again, the children were positioned facing the mirror and their behavior was recorded.

Previous studies have shown that when their image is altered by rouge on the nose, normal infants as young as 22 months indicate self-recognition by touching their noses while looking in the mirror. Only 22% of the children with DS whose ages fell within 15 to 22 months touched their noses. A higher percentage (56%) of those in the middle age group (23 to 33 months) did so. In the oldest group (34 to 48 months), 89% of the children touched their noses upon seeing the altered image. Failure to exhibit self-recognition in front of a mirror could not be attributed to lack of motor ability to touch their noses, since all the children were capable of doing this. Instead, it reflects level of intellectual development. In the youngest group, those who exhibited self-recognition had a mean Bayley developmental quotient (DQ) of 95, vs. 62 ($p < .05$) for those who did not. Similarly, the mean DQ of children in the middle age group who seemed to recognize themselves was 75, but it was only 62 ($p < .05$) for those who did not. Furthermore, a 16-month-old with mosaic Down Syndrome who had a DQ of 125 touched her nose while viewing the rouge-marked reflection, whereas a 38-month-old with a Stanford-Binet IQ of less than 50 showed no signs of recognizing his image in the mirror.

Loveland (1987a) has further demonstrated that, as compared to normally developing children with chronological ages of 14 to 32 months, children with DS who have mental ages of 16 to 32 months and chronological ages of 18 to 59 months, placed in front of a mirror, can find a rouge mark on the face, find their mothers, find a toy, and engage in free play. She concluded that their ability to solve different mirror tasks paralleled that of the control group. She also hypothesized, however, that their motivation, attention, and exploratory behavior might have differed from the control group. The hypothesis regarding a group difference in exploration was later confirmed.

In a subsequent study, Loveland (1987b) found that children with Down Syndrome differed from control subjects, but only in the number, type, and frequency of exploratory behaviors. Also, for most behaviors examined, mental age and chronological age were not related to amount of exploration. Moreover, in four situations in which the subjects had to find things seen in a large standing mirror, the children with DS used all of the following behaviors: free play, finding a facial mark, making faces, kissing and patting the mirror, comparing a person or object with image, looking behind the mirror, touching own body, and staring at another's image. These findings suggest that despite the differences between children with and without DS in number, type, and frequency of exploratory behaviors, exploration contributes to the acquisition of a concept about self in both groups. More specifically, exploration provides opportunities to experience the self as subject and to perceive the characteristics of the self as object. These events, stored and organized in memory, form the basis of the self-system (Eder, 1988).

The studies just described indicate that at least by the time they attain mental ages of 16 to 32 months, children with DS have acquired an existential self—that is, a concept of self as subject or as active, independent, causal agent. They have also acquired the rudiments of a categorical self—that is, a concept of self as object, at least in the sense that they have formed an internal schema of their own faces and can therefore recognize facial features of the self reflected in a mirror. In other words, the development of both the self as subject ("I") and the self as object ("me") can be inferred by the time that children with DS reached a mental age of 16 to 32 months. Additional studies are needed to demonstrate that at such mental ages they have also attained an appreciation that one has unique featural attributes that can be verbally labeled as the self.

Beyond infancy, the development of both the existential and the categorical self takes on new dimensions. Based on early studies of children's self-descriptions, Harter (1983) has hypothesized a sequence of changes in content and structure. Content-wise, self-perception shifts from a focus on observable physical and behavioral dimensions to more psychological constructs. Structurally, changes in the organization of content dimensions follow a sequence starting with specific characteristics that are subsequently integrated into traits, then into single abstractions, and, later, higher-order abstractions that are finally reintegrated hierarchically. However, the validity of this sequence has been challenged by recent studies (Eder, 1990; Eder, Gerlach, & Perlmutter, 1987) showing that young children make general statements about the self earlier than they do specific ones.

With the onset of adolescence, self-concept development becomes increasingly focused on self-identity and the identity of others, moving toward reciprocal coordination of one's own expectations with those of significant others and with societal expectations, then, finally, to the coordination of one's identities over a lifetime, with those of others and with cultural values so as to form a meaningful whole.

To date the only study of self-concept in children, adolescents, or adults with DS was an attempt to assess the psychosocial impact of facial surgery (Travis, 1987). Although a number of studies have assessed the self-concept of developmentally delayed children (Carroll, Friedrich, & Hund, 1984; Jones, 1985), adolescents (Lund, Carman, & Kranz, 1981; Wright & Cowden, 1986), and adults (Koegel & Edgerton, 1982), none reported the results of a separate analysis of the data from the subjects with DS in their samples. The closest to a study of how adults with DS perceive themselves is one by Greenspan and Delaney (1983). These investigators administered the Personal Competence Profile to 30 23- to 43-year-old white male adults with Down Syndrome and 30 male adults without Down Syndrome matched on age, IQ (mean IQ = 43.1), and years of institutionalization. The adults with DS rated themselves higher on attention, calmness, and niceness but lower on sensation, language, and boldness.

Self-Esteem

An individual's self-esteem is distinct from his or her self-concept. The former reflects an evaluation of the self, while the latter is a description. Four salient issues are hypothesized to comprise the basis of self-esteem: competence, moral worth, sense of control, and acceptability (Harter, 1983). These components of self-esteem are assumed to be hierarchically organized, but the relative weights assigned to each of these dimensions at different developmental levels have yet to be ascertained empirically. Additionally, the child also constructs a sense of global self-esteem, a superordinate construct dependent on but detached from the more discrete self-evaluations of the second-order dimensions.

Given the widespread belief that persons with DS might have low self-esteem because of their distinctive facial features, the dearth of studies on this topic is surprising. Other than the study of facial surgery outcome cited earlier, the only study that we found was one conducted by Rynders, Johnson, Johnson, and Schmidt (1980). This study investigated the effects of cooperative, competitive, and individualistic learning experiences in a bowling class on the self-esteem of 18 nonhandicapped and 12 Down Syndrome trainable retarded junior high school students (13 to 15 years old), assigned to conditions stratified on the basis of handicap and sex.

The class met for 1 hour per week for 8 weeks. Results showed that those in the cooperative condition had higher self-esteem and perceived more personal acceptance from the teacher than did the subjects in the competitive and individualistic conditions. Interestingly, the students with DS reported higher self-esteem than did nonhandicapped students. This finding raises some intriguing questions. How accurate are the self-evaluations of persons with Down Syndrome? What referent groups do they use? Studies of the accuracy and basis of self-evaluation in this population are needed. In summary, for the Down Syndrome population, the emergence of the self-concept during infancy has been empirically documented, but there is hardly any documentation for the development of self-concept and self-esteem during childhood, adolescence, and adulthood. There has been no research on identity formation, including the onset of awareness in the person with DS that he or she belongs to a group with distinctive physical, speech, and intellectual characteristics and how this Down Syndrome identity becomes integrated with other identities (e.g., gender, race).

The relationship between physical appearance and self-concept or self-esteem has been investigated only in facial plastic surgery outcome studies.

Future studies will have to take into account methodological issues that arise when instruments normed for normally developing populations are used with developmentally delayed individuals. Lund et al. (1981) found low to moderate reliability coefficients when the Tennessee Self-Concept Scale was given in a 10-week test-retest situation to 39 educable mentally retarded (EMR) adolescents. These findings suggest that the self-concept of individual EMR adolescents is a more variable psychological characteristic than had been previously indicated in the research literature. This variability needs to be more carefully assessed. Until more extensive normative information becomes available, caution must be exercised in interpreting scores of EMR on the Tennessee Self-Concept Scale. Harter (1982) has issued a similar warning in regard to the Perceived Competence Scale for Children after factor analysis of PCSC scores from a developmentally delayed population revealed loadings different from those found for the normative sample. Available instruments will have to be revised and/or new norms obtained. If existing measures cannot be easily adapted for reliable and valid use with the DS population, perhaps because of their heavy reliance on verbal skills, then new measures will have to be constructed, too.

Others' Perception

Down (1866, 1867) specified four distinguishing characteristics of the clinical group that he identified: mimicry, humor, amiability, and obstinacy. Other clinicians expanded this constellation to include such attributes as cheerful, good-tempered, and submissive to authority (Barr, 1904; Brushfield, 1924; Sherlock & Donkin, 1911). Over time individuals with Down Syndrome came to be viewed as inherently endowed with a high degree of social responsiveness and potential for socialization, at least in comparison to others who also exhibit developmental delay. This positive social image became a stereotype of the individual with Down Syndrome. Early research on social aspects of Down Syndrome was largely directed at validating the social stereotype or to test the hypothesis that retarded individuals with Down Syndrome are more sociable than those without this condition. Since these studies were based on ratings made by parents, teachers, nurses, and other caregivers, their results provide information as to how individuals with Down Syndrome are perceived by others. These clinical and quasi-experimental studies, mostly conducted prior to the 1970s, must be regarded with caution because they often had serious methodological flaws. Despite their limitations, however, they still have implications for the design of future studies. They are presented here lest, not knowing the past, we will be condemned to repeat it (Santayana, cited in Beck, 1980).

The hypothesis that individuals with Down Syndrome are more sociable than their counterparts without this condition has received only partial support from studies of both institutionalized and community-reared samples (Blacketer-Simmonds, 1953; Blessing, 1959; Domino, 1965; Domino, Goldschmid, & Kaplan, 1964). Usually, the findings have been mixed. Persons with Down Syndrome are perceived as more sociable than controls in certain ways, but in other ways they appear less so. Blacketer-Simmonds found that prior to and following institutionalization, higher percentages of persons with DS were rated by nurses as solitary when compared to a group of persons without DS who had similar intellectual and physical status. Although teachers frequently described community-reared individuals with DS as amenable, good natured, gay, happy, cheerful, and independent, they also frequently characterized them as stubborn and attention seekers (Blessing, 1959).

The inconsistent findings from attempts to validate the social stereotype could be due to differences in methodology among the various studies. Studies employing the same measure such as the Sonoma Check List (SCL) might show greater consistency. Constructed specifically for rating mentally retarded individuals, the SCL consists of 210 adjective words. Domino et al. (1964) asked professionals and ward personnel to rate female institutionalized persons with DS on this measure. Descriptive social adjectives such as friendly, sociable, and open correlated significantly and positively with a diagnosis of Down Syndrome. The investigators therefore concluded that their subjects conformed to the social stereotype. They also speculated that persons with DS might appear sociable only in comparison to developmentally delayed persons without

DS who have more neurological problems. Because the sample in this study was limited to females, researchers such as Gibson (1978) have hypothesized that the social stereotype was probably more true for the young female. Gender differences were attributed to variations in institutional and home care practices as a function of sex of child, as well as to early mortality rates that are sex and IQ selective. In a subsequent study, Domino (1965) asked college students to rate males with and without DS on the SCL. Persons with DS were rated significantly more often as cooperative and pleasing, results interpreted as confirming the classical social stereotype. However, they were also rated significantly more often as shy, show-off, unfriendly, and hostile. Hence, the findings are more appropriately interpreted as partial support for the social stereotype. More recently, Gibbs and Thorpe (1983) used a modified version of the SCL to rate 98 noninstitutionalized developmentally delayed children, half of whom had DS (mean age 11.5 years) and half of whom did not (mean age 11.17 years). The two groups could be differentiated on the basis of 23 adjectives from the list. There also emerged the classic personality stereotype of the child with DS as affectionate and outgoing. These studies indicate that when studies employ the same measure, their results are more consistent, although not totally.

Some of the inconsistency might also be associated with gender and age differences in the target population. Gender differences were discussed earlier. As for age, the mean age of the Gibbs and Thorpe (1983) sample was around 11 years, while Domino and his collaborators (1964, 1965) used older samples. Clinical and naturalistic observation studies have consistently revealed age-related differences in perceptions of the sociability of this population. Observers of infants and toddlers (Brousseau & Brainerd, 1928; Tredgold, 1947) have described them as minimally alert and responsive to social stimuli. In contrast, children with DS are perceived as quite sociable (i.e., affectionate, amiable, good-natured, extroverted) during early and middle childhood (Engler, 1949; Rollin, 1946; Wallin, 1949). Adolescents and adults, on the other hand, have not been found to be as sociable (Francis, 1970). Previously, these age differences in sociability were attributed to an early and progressive leveling of intellectual development possibly combined with restrictive care practices (Oster, 1953) or to neurologically based stubbornness (Benda, 1956). It is currently assumed that a variety of somatic factors, including fatigability, heart problems, and neurophysiological disturbances, contribute to the observed decline in sociability.

Another source of inconsistency might be differences among raters. Some of these early studies recognized that respondent familiarity with the target population might influence ratings (e.g., Domino et al., 1964), but none of them examined variations in perceptions of the Down Syndrome population held by different groups. More recently, Pueschel et al. (1986) compared parents' and physicians' perceptions of children with DS along several dimensions: problems, development, teacher expectations, and social acceptance. Significantly higher percentages of physicians than parents perceived the child with DS as having problems with eating or chewing and drooling. Also, significantly more physicians than parents perceived the facial characteristics of the child with DS as negatively affecting the latter's mental and social development as well as acquisition of self-help skills. The two groups did not differ significantly regarding the possible negative effect on language development. Reliably, more physicians thought that teachers have low expectations of the children because of the presence of Down Syndrome characteristics. Finally, physicians were significantly more inclined than parents to perceive children with DS as not well accepted by society, neighbors, other children, or relatives. Like adults, children may perceive a child with DS as more attractive than peers with other congenital facial problems. Lefebvre, Bedard, Arndt, Travis, and Munro (1987) studied the perceptions of two groups of 10-year-olds. Group 1 was a "healthy" group, while Group 2 consisted of children referred to an outpatient psychiatric clinic and children with a sibling who had been referred. Across groups, almost half the females, but not the males, rated the photograph of a girl with DS to be beautiful in contrast to photographs of children with Treacher Collins' or Apert's Syndrome. Similar results were obtained in regard to the characteristics of smartness and goodness. Consistent with the social stereotype, the girls in Group 1 and both sexes in Group 2 were as likely to attribute friendliness to the children with DS as to the normal subjects, but not to those with Treacher Collins' or Apert's Syndrome. However, this lack of a difference between attributions to the child with DS and to the normal child was true only for the characteristic of friendliness. For all other attributes assessed, ratings of the child with DS were lower than those of the child who was normal or had Crouzons Syndrome, albeit higher than those for children with Treacher Collins or Aperts Syndrome. Statistical tests of the significance of these differences in ratings, however, were not reported, so the results must be regarded as suggestive rather than conclusive.

The finding that, as compared to their normally developing peers, children with DS receive lower ratings on a variety of attributes is supported by some results from the Strauss et al. (1988) study mentioned earlier. In that study, adolescents' ratings of the preoperative Down Syndrome face were compared to their ratings of "normal" boy and girl faces. The Down Syndrome face was judged less attractive, less intelligent, less friendly, and less good-hearted than were the faces of the normal children. Judgments of the appearance of children with DS may vary with the age of the perceiver. Graffi and Minnes (1988) reported that the third-grade children in their sample responded with more negative affect to target children presented with Down Syndrome than they did to children without DS. The kindergarten children, however, failed to demonstrate the same pattern. Instead, they responded more positively to target children presented with DS.

To recapitulate, most of the available data on others' perceptions of persons with DS come from studies of personality traits. While some studies confirm the social stereotype, the majority indicate that negative as well as positive characteristics are attributed by others to persons with Down Syndrome. The inconsistent results may be due in part to the use of different measures, different groups of raters, and to age or gender differences in the target population. None of the studies systematically determined the bases of ratings or judgments. The actual contribution of the Down Syndrome facial characteristics to the impressions formed by others remains poorly understood. One study suggests that facial characteristics are believed to exert an influence, but even this study clearly indicates that different groups attribute varying degrees of influence to this variable.

Social Acceptance

The significance of peer relations for psychological development and adjustment, emphasized by theorists such as Adler (1930), Piaget (1932), and Sullivan (1953) has been substantiated by research (for a review, see Hartup, 1983). Clearly, the company of peers, positive interactions with them, and enduring friendships are essential for optimum self-actualization and mental health. The availability of a peer group has been shown to be critical for all children, including the developmentally delayed, such as children with DS. Thus, the participation of these children in a peer group is highly desirable. Such participation is contingent on social acceptance.

In a review of the research literature on the correlates of social acceptance, Hartup (1983) concluded that no single trait is of overriding importance in determining normally developing children's popularity among their peers. His review showed that only modest correlations between child characteristics and peer acceptance have been found in most studies. For this population, popularity has both behavioral and nonbehavioral correlates. However, the correlates of peer acceptance differ from those of peer rejection. According to Hartup, significant amounts of the variance in peer acceptance can be accounted for by positively valued characteristics, such as peer acceptance and intelligence. Being a later-born child, having a name that is not unusual, friendliness, sociability, and academic success are also associated with peer acceptance. In contrast, negatively valued characteristics, such as an endomorphic physique and aggressive and antisocial behavior, account for significant amounts of variance in peer rejection. His review of the research on developmentally delayed children revealed that academic failure was negatively correlated with social acceptance of educable mentally retarded children. In contrast, misbehavior was positively related to rejection and uncorrelated with acceptance. Thus, for developmentally delayed children, the correlates of peer acceptance also differ from those of peer rejection.

The empirical basis of the implicit model held by proponents of facial surgery can be examined through a review of the data bearing on several questions. Are persons with DS socially accepted by peers and adults? What factors facilitate their acceptance by handicapped and nonhandicapped groups? What factors lead to rejection by the same groups? In particular, what is the contribution of their distinctive physical characteristics to social acceptance or rejection?

Social Status

Given the correlates of peer acceptance or rejection among normal children, how do children with DS fare? While they might not meet societal standards for certain characteristics (e.g., physical attractiveness, intelligence, academic success), they might still possess other attributes that could win peer acceptance, such as friendliness, sociability, a name that is not unusual, or later-born status.

In the research literature, peer acceptance is usually operationalized as popularity. It is typically indexed by the number of nominations to be a friend, playmate, workmate, etc., on a sociometric measure. Although sociometric studies of developmentally delayed children have been undertaken (e.g., Gottlieb, Semmel, & Veldman, 1978), none has reported separate results for children with DS. A review of relevant research did not yield any sociometric studies focusing exclusively on peer acceptance or rejection of persons with DS. However, there are other ways of assessing social acceptance. One of these is direct observations of social interactions in naturalistic settings. Social acceptance can also be inferred from whether or not someone is sought out by peers and the frequency of social interactions.

Peer Interactions

The social interaction between children with Down Syndrome and their normally achieving peers has been studied. An exploratory study by Sinson and Wetherick (1981) showed that preschool children with DS who, to the casual observer and even to the playground staff, appeared to be socially accepted and little different from other children in normal playgroups, actually did not engage at all in verbal interaction with normal peers and spent relatively little time in constructive behavior. Instead they spent more of their time in inappropriate or nonconstructive behaviors, including aggressive and attention-seeking ones. When they interacted socially, it was with adults. Furthermore, they established eye contact with adults but, unlike their normal counterparts, had little or no eye contact with any of the other children. This behavior was in contrast to their behavior in a nursery school limited to handicapped children. Within this context, they showed a pattern of eye contact similar to that exhibited by normal children and engaged in constructive as well as imaginative play.

In a subsequent study, Sinson and Wetherick (1986) videotaped same-sex play encounters between a child with DS and a normal child in the normal child's own home and in the presence of both mothers. Children with DS ranging in age from 6 to 13 years and 104 normal children ranging in age from 2½ to 6 years were studied. A small subsample of children drawn from the normal sample also met a normal child of the same sex and age as the DS child they had previously met. The following variables were coded: time spent looking at the face of the guest child (DS or normal), time spent playing with the toy, time spent in cooperative play, and time spent talking either to adults only or to adults and the guest child (DS or normal). When the guest was a child with DS, the normal children spent more time looking at the guest and less time in toy and cooperative play and in conversation.

Unfortunately, the data were not subjected to a statistical test for group mean differences. Nonetheless, the investigators interpreted the looking data as evidence of the exaggerated and prolonged patterns of gaze behavior that are normal between children meeting for the first time but that quickly disappear in the normal/normal encounter. They also noted distortions in patterns of play and vocalization. In addition, they inferred that the children with DS showed themselves able and willing to interact with the normal child, whereas the normal children seemed clearly aware that the child with DS was different, in spite of its being the first time that they had encountered such a child. The investigators also observed that only the 3-year-olds, the youngest children with DS, were acceptable to the normal children, possibly because they were classified as "babies" and treated accordingly. Sinson & Wetherick (1986) concluded that integration of the child with DS is more likely to be achieved if he or she is young enough to benefit from being classified as a "baby," for whom special allowance must be made. This conclusion, they add, is only true provided the child with DS has the benefit of prolonged contact with normal children in the neighborhood and family situations with mothers present.

The Sinson and Wetherick (1981) finding that children with DS interact more frequently with handicapped as opposed to nonhandicapped peers was also observed by Rogers-Warren (1980) in both indoor (i.e., classrom) and outdoor (i.e., playground) settings. In an integrated (40% non-handicapped) early interaction program designed primarily for handicapped children, those with Down Syndrome played with handicapped peers about 1½ times as frequently as they played with nonhandicapped children. The latter played with other nonhandicapped peers twice as often as they played with handicapped children. This group difference in playmate preference was significant for the playground, but not for the classroom, setting.

The playmate preferences of children with and without DS were also studied by Peterson (1982). Social interactions of 4 mild and moderately retarded children with DS (ages 5 to 5 years, 11 months) and 4 normal children (ages 4½ to 5 years, 2 months) were observed during classroom and playground free-play periods. In both classroom and playground, children preferred peers who were more like themselves when all options were possible. Children with DS were selected as sole playmates by their nonhandicapped peers or in combination with other peer types, but certain choice conditions and environments appeared to bias their being picked. Overall, they were more likely to engage in social interactions than in solitary play on the playground.

Social play among children with DS was also found in a follow-up study (Rietveld, 1986) of 8 children with DS (ages 6 to 7 years) who had participated in an early intervention program from birth. A year after they had started at a local school, they engaged in social play for similar amounts of time and continued to acquire new skills at the same rate as during their participation in the intervention program. As compared to a contrast group comprised of 3 low-achieving children drawn from each of 8 classrooms, the children with DS were at least as attentive, compliant, and socially integrated as, and no more disruptive than, the contrast children.

In sum, research on peer interaction indicates that while nonhandicapped children do play occasionally with children who have DS, they seek them out as playmates only under certain conditions. On the other hand, they do not actively reject them. Their initial reaction appears to be one of curiosity manifested through staring. With prolonged exposure, they seem to react with indifference and neutrality.

Determinants of Social Acceptance

Several explanations for the observed group difference in social acceptance as inferred from peer preference have been advanced. Sinson and Wetherick (1981, 1982) suggest that the failure of children with DS to establish and maintain mutual eye gaze with normal children upon initial meeting results in the latter's becoming uneasy and eventually ceasing their attempts to engage in the convention of mutual gaze governing relatively casual interactions between children who are not familiar with each other. Although this explanation seems plausible, it does not explain their subsequent finding (Sinson & Wetherick, 1986) that the youngest children with DS were acceptable to normal children whereas the older ones were not.

Other studies by Rogers-Warren (1980) and by Schlottman and Anderson (1975) explored the possibility that playmate choice of children with and without DS may be linked to their level of play. The results of these studies showed significant group differences in play behavior favoring normal children over children with DS, and the latter over developmentally delayed children with a different etiology.

To recapitulate, the social acceptance of persons with DS has not yet been studied through sociometric studies. It can be inferred, however, from observational studies of their interactions with both normally developing children and developmentally delayed peers without DS. These observational studies do not reveal that children with DS are actively rejected. Neither are they completely neglected. Under certain conditions and environments, they are accepted as playmates by non-handicapped peers. Furthermore, they seem to be unconditionally accepted by developmentally delayed children without DS.

Some studies have revealed group differences in mutual gaze behavior, level of social play, and communication skills that might affect social interaction between children with DS and their normally developing peers. However, none of the studies actually attempted to establish causal linkages between these variables and peer preference or frequency of interaction. The prolonged visual regard that children with DS seem to evoke in initial encounters with normally developing children suggests that they may indeed be perceived as somewhat different from the familiar, but whether this impression is based upon their distinctive facial features alone, in contrast to their facial configuration, body build, or overall physical appearance, has yet to be systematically determined. There is no hard evidence that it is physical appearance, no matter how operationally defined, rather than cognitive, language, and social abilities or behavior, that renders the child with DS less socially acceptable as a playmate.

Finally, there is some evidence suggesting that social acceptance is not determined solely by the characteristics of the person with DS, but also by the characteristics of the other person and the context in which their interaction takes place. An adequate understanding of social acceptance for this population requires a more complex theory and more sophisticated research designs than have been employed thus far.

Implications for Intervention through Facial Plastic Surgery

The preceding review did not reveal conclusive evidence that persons with Down Syndrome perceive themselves as having markedly different physical appearance from persons without DS and, as a result of this perceived difference, have a negative self-concept and low self-esteem.

The only evidence that they are perceived by others as different is indirect, suggested by studies showing that they elicit longer visual fixations upon initial presentation and, occasionally, evoke attributions and evaluations different from those assigned to other groups. There is also no strong evidence linking their facial features or any other aspect of their physical appearance with social acceptance or rejection.

In summary, there is as yet no solid empirical support from either developmental or surgical outcome research for the implicit model that is the psychosocial rationale for facial surgery on persons with DS. On the other hand, the available data do not disconfirm the model. Research on this population has simply not yet addressed the relevant research questions. But what *are* the relevant research questions? Before these can be specified, a critical examination of the model is required.

As noted earlier in this chapter, proponents of facial surgery for persons with DS implicitly assume that physical appearance mediates self and other perceptions of the person with DS. These perceptions in turn influence self-concept, self-esteem, and social acceptance. One of the limitations of this implicit model is its narrow conceptualization of physical appearance. Although physical appearance could refer to facial features, facial configuration, body build, etc., proponents of facial surgery usually use it to mean the distinctive facial features that are a hallmark of Down Syndrome. By focusing on facial features, proponents of facial surgery ignore the potential contributions of other physical attributes to self- and other-perception as well as to social acceptance. For example, attributes such as overall facial configuration might play an even more important role in impression formation. Berry and McArthur (1986) have shown that different craniofacial characteristics influence social perception, particularly if they typically reveal psychological attributes whose detection is important for adaptive functioning. Furthermore, they contend, age-related craniofacial changes affect perceptions of people's psychological attributes. The implication is that perceptions of persons with DS are not based solely on their facial features. Evaluations of facial surgery outcome have to be based on a more complex conceptualization of facial appearance that takes into account the relative contributions of different craniofacial characteristics to judgments of physical attractiveness.

Besides facial characteristics, other physical attributes, such as physique or body build, also influence social perception. For example, it has been shown that normally developing children rate the endomorphic physique less positively than other types (Staffieri, 1967). Finally, each of these different physical attributes rarely act in isolation from one another. Their relative contributions and that of the overall physical appearance to social perception are still unknown. Parents, professionals, and researchers interested in facial surgery for persons with Down Syndrome need to take these issues into account in their theorizing.

Also questionable are the model's assumptions that the characteristic Down Syndrome features are perceived as different or atypical and that atypicality is judged to be unattractive. But *are* these features always perceived as atypical? The ability to perceive any deviations from the norm or typical is probably age-related. Furthermore, the extent to which the Down Syndrome facial features are perceived as atypical may be a function of the normative facial features of the race or ethnic group. Even if they are perceived as atypical, does that necessarily imply unattractiveness? Although Tobiasen (1984) has suggested that this might be the case, Kleck and Strenta (1980) argue that normal vs. atypical facial appearance exist on a different continuum than attractive vs. unattractive facial appearance. Atypicality or deviations from the norm could be regarded as either attractive, unattractive, or neither. From their perspective, the Down Syndrome facial features, if perceived as atypical, will not necessarily be judged as unattractive. Thus far, it has yet to be directly ascertained that the DS characteristics are perceived as different. As mentioned earlier, only indirect evidence is available. More important, we still don't know if the difference is judged to be attractive, unattractive, or neither. Relatedly, little is known about who is likely to rate the DS facial characteristics as attractive vs. unattractive vs. neutral, and the bases of the ratings. Given the current state of our scientific knowledge on these issues, it seems premature to assume that persons with DS are perceived as different and unattractive because of their facial appearance.

Some evidence suggests that the individual with DS is not without some appeal. The young child with DS seems appealing to normally developing children of a certain age (Sinson & Wetherick, 1981), while older females with DS also have appealed to adult raters (Domino et al., 1964). These results suggesting that the Down Syndrome facial appearance might not be regarded as unattractive by certain individuals can be explained by the ecological approach to social perception (McArthur & Baron, 1983). From this perspective, facial characteristics reveal affordances or opportunities for acting or being acted upon. That is, they convey knowledge about a person's behavioral and intellectual propensities that facilitate appropriate expectations and responses or demands from others. For example, "babyfacedness" or a childlike facial appearance will be perceived as affording more warmth and cuddliness, less wisdom, and more naiveté (Berry & McArthur, 1986). Such perceptions may elicit nurturance, patience, and protectiveness from the perceiver. Within the ecological framework, it is highly conceivable that the Down Syndrome facial characteristics may reveal psychological attributes that are important for their adaptive functioning. These adaptive functions have to be weighed against possible maladaptive ones in any decision to alter distinguishing facial characteristics and thereby distort their affordances.

The model's conceptualization of the relationship between physical appearance (i.e., facial features) and self-concept as well as self-esteem does not fully take into account the relative contribution of this variable vs. other determinants of self-concept and self-esteem at different age periods. Research on the self-system in the Down Syndrome population has not yet addressed this issue. Instead, the available data raise issues pertinent to the timing of the initial surgery from a psychosocial perspective which could be considered along with those from medical and other relevant perspectives. If one of the goals to be achieved through facial surgery is preventing the development of a negative self-concept or low self-esteem, should it therefore occur before self-recognition emerges? If surgery is deferred until after the child is more fully aware of his or her facial characteristics and even gained a sense of physical identity, what message regarding the child's worth is conveyed by a decision to alter those distinctive facial features? In order not to raise unrealistic expectations, should surgery be postponed until the person with DS has sufficient cognitive maturity to realize that a change in physical appearance does not necessarily imply significant changes in abilities? In the absence of changes other than appearance (e.g., I.Q.), is facial surgery desirable for the positive feelings that it engenders in the person with DS and his or her family?

It seemed to be for at least one child and her family. Sandahl (1980) reported that when this child looked into the mirror for the first time after the bandages were removed, she sang, "I'm beautiful, I'm beautiful." Her self-image, which was reported to be already good prior to surgery, was enhanced.

The assumption that a change in facial features will lead directly to an increment in social acceptance also seems too simplistic. It ignores the role of other determinants of social acceptance. Assuming that facial surgery significantly alters facial appearance so that it deviates less from the norm (Kuczaj, 1987), the child with DS might be stared at less by others (Wexler et al., 1986). A change in physical appearance could possibly result in an increase of social initiations from peers, but this has yet to be proven. However, the critical question is, will any increment in social acceptance following surgery be maintained over the long term in the absence of concomitant changes in the social and communicative skills or behavior of the child with DS? In other words, is physical appearance the foremost determinant of social acceptance? If it were, other things being equal, nonhandicapped children should prefer developmentally delayed children without DS over those with DS. For the same reason, developmentally delayed children should prefer peers of the same developmental level without DS over those with this condition. However, research indicates that this is not the case.

The available data also suggest that when physical appearance and functioning seem relatively congruent, as in very young children with DS whose babyish appearance may be congruent with their behavior, peer acceptance is more easily won. As appearance and functioning become more incongruent, peer acceptance is less easily gained, possibly because the induced cognitive inconsistency is more difficult for peers to resolve.

Another consideration is that the importance of facial appearance may vary developmentally. For example, it may be less important than the availability of a congenial playmate for the young child, whereas it might be more so for the adolescent girl striving for popularity. Adults who hold certain ethical and/or religious standards might assign less weight to the attractiveness of facial appearance and therefore be more accepting than others who do not hold such standards.

To restate the point, social acceptance is a complex process with multiple determinants. It is influenced by factors other than child characteristics such as the characteristics of the perceiver, the attitudes or behavior of the perceiver's significant others, and the situations in which social interactions occur. This complexity has to be reflected in the conceptual framework underlying decisions about facial surgery for persons with DS and research to evaluate its outcomes.

Finally, even with an appropriate conceptual model, there remains the issue of which procedure for enhancing self-concept or social acceptance would be least invasive. Just as educational placement is guided by the principle of providing the least restrictive environment, the choice of intervention method could be guided by the principle of using the least invasive procedure. Intervention studies suggest that self-esteem and social acceptance of developmentally delayed persons, including those with DS, can be increased by improving communication and social skills, particularly within facilitative situations or environments. Similar enhancements result from manipulating variables other than the known correlates of self-esteem and peer acceptance, including involvement in naturalistic situations such as the Special Olympics (Wright & Cowden, 1986), cooperative learning situations (Johnson, Johnson, & Rynders, 1981; Madden & Slavin, 1982) or a class-wide peer tutoring system (Cooke, Heron, Heward, & Test, 1982; Osguthorpe, Eiserman, & Shisler, 1985). The costs and benefits of facial surgery must be weighed against those of other forms of intervention.

Implications for Future Research

The paucity of data on self- and other perception as well as social relations of persons with Down Syndrome revealed by the above review of research clearly indicates the need for research on these topics. They also show that research thus far has been fragmented, seldom guided by theory, nor oriented toward theory building. The field would benefit from theory-based, programmatic research directed toward building theories about deviant and normal development. There is a need for well-designed studies with appropriate controls. Collaborative and replication studies could surmount the problem posed by small sample sizes due to the limited pool of potential subjects in specific research sites. Just as intervention research would be enriched if it were more informed by developmental findings, explanatory developmental research could benefit from intervention studies.

Self-Perception

Obviously, research on development of the self system has to be extended beyond infancy, although some work also remains to be done even on its emergence during the early years of life.

1. Additional studies of how the self-system evolves during infancy and early childhood are needed to answer some questions raised by prior research. What accounts for the finding that children with DS who apparently recognize their unique featural attributes do not use verbal labels denoting the self despite the co-occurrence of these two behaviors in normal infants at the same level of development? Does this failure reflect a lack of understanding that the unique featural attributes can be abstracted and symbolically represented by a verbal label? Or does it reflect an artificial constraint imposed by limited speech or language skills? If the latter explanation holds, then infants or young children with DS should, in addition to exhibiting visual recognition, behave in their play and social interactions as if they had a sense of self. When do they actually begin using verbal labels denoting the self? Finally, what are the relationships among cognitive, language, and self-system development during infancy and early childhood?

2. Development of self-concept and self-esteem during childhood have yet to be studied systematically in this population. At what chronological or mental ages do these children begin to differentiate between different aspects of the self? Similarly, when do they begin to evaluate these aspects? Do they also acquire a general sense of self-worth over and above their estimates of competence in these specific domains? What are the bases of general self-esteem? Are their self-descriptions characterized by the same sequence observed in their normally developing peers?

When do they begin to develop gender or race identity? When do they become aware that they possess distinctive facial features that are different from those of most children but similar to those of some? When do they associate possession of these facial characteristics with possession of certain other characteristics and behavioral patterns? What, if any, is the impact of such awareness on their self-esteem? When do they realize that facial characteristics can be altered? Will changes in facial characteristics result in a higher sense of physical attractiveness? Will this increment generalize to other aspects of the self and to general self-esteem? What advances in cognitive and language abilities are related to developmental changes in self-concept and self-esteem, including those following facial surgery? What experiences and settings contribute to a positive self-concept and self-esteem during this period? Can the development of self-concept and self-esteem be facilitated systematically? How well do the effects of such interventions generalize across situations? Also, do they remain stable over time?

3. Development of self-concept and self-esteem during adolescence and adulthood in persons with DS also needs to be studied further. Their world has broadened considerably within the last few decades. They are out of institutions or residential schools into mainstreamed school environments. Many are also out of sheltered workshops and into the regular work force, working in stores, restaurants, and other settings requiring unskilled or semiskilled labor. One has even managed to land a job as a page in Congress, while another was an actor in a television series. Some are out of the family residence and living independent lives in group homes or in their own apartments. How do they perceive themselves now? Do they view their lives as half-empty or half-full?

The study of a homogeneous group of developmentally delayed adolescents or adults such as persons with DS has implications for developmental theories. In addition to providing a test for the universality of developmental sequences, it can elucidate continuities and discontinuities in developmental processes. Because their development occurs at a slower rate, it might reveal continuities underlying the discontinuities observed in normal development. It could also deepen our understanding of organism–environment interaction. Is IQ destiny, arresting development beyond childhood? Is an integrated self-identity out of the reach for this clinical group? Do they never come to terms with themselves and their lives? These "new" persons with DS who are out in the community, working and leading independent lives, could inform us.

Other-Perception

What we know about how others perceive persons with Down Syndrome comes mainly from personality research. Studies based on person perception and social cognitive theories and research could enrich the available body of knowledge.

1. Prior research suggests that how others perceive the person with DS is influenced by the characteristics of both the perceiver and the target. Well-designed, appropriately controlled studies that attempt to assess the separate and interaction effects of perceiver and target characteristics on others' perceptions of the individual with Down Syndrome are needed.

2. No research has been done on the bases of people's perceptions of persons with DS. Research to identify these bases and how they change as a function of other variables is needed. In particular, research on the contribution of the Down Syndrome facial characteristics to others'

perceptions, expectations, and behavior would be helpful to families considering facial surgery for the members with DS.

3. Research on how perceptions and attitudes toward persons with DS change is certainly indicated. In addition, the relationships between such changes and behavior have to be explored.

Social Acceptance

Despite the widespread concern about the social acceptance of persons with Down Syndrome, very few studies have actually attempted to document their social status and its correlates. Some very basic research questions remain unanswered.

1. What is the social status of persons with Down Syndrome? Does this status vary with group? Are they more accepted by other persons with DS vs. developmentally delayed without DS vs. nonhandicapped? Are they more accepted by peers than adults? Are children vs. adolescents or adults more accepting of them?
2. Does acceptance vary with characteristics of the Down Syndrome group and/or the group doing the nominating?
3. Does acceptance vary with situation or context?
4. What are the correlates of acceptance or rejection by peers and adults?
5. What is the relative contribution of facial characteristics to social acceptance or rejection of this group?
6. Does social status predict behavioral adjustment in this population?

As Hartup (1983) has suggested, more use should be made of experimental strategies and longitudinal studies in studying the correlates of social acceptance. In time intervention studies may also have to be conducted. But until we have more basic information about the social status of this population, it seems premature to institute different forms of intervention on a large scale.

A Conceptual Framework for Future Research

Given the research agenda, how should we proceed? Here we would like to elaborate on a conceptual framework introduced elsewhere (Serafica, 1990) that emphasizes the following: a life-span perspective, an organizational view of development, and a sociocultural perspective.

Life-Span Perspective

A life span perspective is important, particularly because of the observed deterioration with increasing age in the social relations of this population.

While the results of previous studies must be treated with caution because of their conceptual and methodological weaknesses, the reports of increasing serious medical complications, neurological problems, and even accelerated aging in older individuals with Down Syndrome make the possibility of a decline, at least in sociability, a viable hypothesis. Thase (1982) has reported that the life span of persons with DS has gradually increased since the 1920s. The DS individual now has an average life expectancy of 35 years. However, the overall mortality rate remains elevated despite advances in health and institutional care. Next to infancy, late adulthood is the period of highest risk when Alzheimer-type dementia and declining immunological function appear to be significant factors. Hence, we need to conceptualize processes over a long temporal span, even though, for purposes of in-depth analysis, we may focus momentarily on a single age period such as early childhood.

Organizational View of Development

The organizational view of development (Cicchetti & Beeghly, 1990; Cicchetti & Sroufe, 1978; Sroufe & Waters, 1976) draws heavily from general systems theory (Von Bertalanffy, 1968), organismic developmental theory (Werner, 1948), and cognitive developmental theory (Piaget, 1952). At least four of its major assumptions are particularly relevant to the description, explanation, and prediction of development in the Down Syndrome population. These assumptions deal with a systemic view of the organism, the interrelatedness of biology, development, and behavior, the lawfulness of developmental sequences, and multicolinearity in development. They are pertinent because previous research (Gibson, 1978) strongly suggests that in the Down Syndrome population, perhaps even more so than in others, there is strong interrelatedness among biological variables, development, and behavior. The behavior of persons with DS is heavily influenced by physiological variables, somatic state, and neurological status. Furthermore, research on infants and toddlers with DS has demonstrated the relationships among different developmental domains. Research involving both normal and developmentally delayed children without DS indicates that development in one domain, such as the self-system, is related to sequential changes in other domains, such as cognition and language, particularly during infancy and early childhood. Moreover, contemporary research on social relations has shown linkages between peer relations and other types of interpersonal relationships such as those between parent and child or between siblings (Hartup, 1983). Similar findings might also be found in the Down Syndrome population. This implies that in studying the development of persons with DS, a broad organizational view is required for a proper understanding of systemic relationships at different levels of analysis. The organizational view of development is sufficiently complex to describe and explain the multifaceted ways in which constitutional, organismic, and environmental factors interact in development of persons with DS. Finally, the organizational view that continuity in adaptation is to be found not in the manifestation of specific behaviors, but in patterns of means–ends relations that manifest coherence across situations, contexts, and time suggests that the adaptation of persons with DS can be predicted from organized patterns of behavior directed toward specific goals.

Sociocultural Perspective

Also essential is what we call, for want of a better term, a sociocultural perspective, which acknowledges that persons with DS comprise a distinct clinical population with perhaps their own modes of social interaction and world views. This population, perhaps with its own subculture, is embedded within the larger developmentally delayed population, which in turn exists within the larger society. When professionals have studied persons with Down Syndrome, they have usually done so with the normally achieving group as the referent group. But who does the person with DS consider a peer, and who is his or her referent group?

Studies showing that similarity is also a determinant of peer acceptance (Bak & Siperstein, 1987; Siperstein & Bak, 1985; Siperstein & Chatillon, 1982) suggest that, other things being equal, persons with DS might prefer other members of their clinical group as playmates and friends. Research conducted in mainstream environments (Rogers-Warren, 1980; Sinson & Wetherick, 1982) consistently show that when adults attempt to promote interaction between children with DS and their normal counterparts, such interaction does increase, but, ultimately, the playmate choices of both groups seem to be based on compatibility of developmental status or equality between partners. This is not surprising. After all, the term "peer" refers to a person who is one's equal. While we certainly ought to be investigating how the person with DS relates to others with a developmental delay and to normally developing persons, perhaps our primary focus should be on building a solid scientific database about the Down Syndrome peer culture, including how members relate to one another and acquire a sense of group identity, which can be a source of inner strength. Only then, perhaps, will we know how to assist them adequately in attaining a multicultural adaptation that will enable them to move comfortably within and between the three groups to which they belong.

Acknowledgments. This chapter is an expanded version of a paper presented at the symposium on *The psychosocial aspects of craniofacial problems . . . Surgery is not enough*, held at the International Craniofacial Institute, Dallas, TX November 5–6, 1987.

References

Adler, A. (1930). *The education of children*. New York: Greenberg.

Alkawitz, R. (1987). *Student teachers' evaluations of children with Down Syndrome pre- and post-facial surgery as a function of knowledge and training*. Unpublished master's thesis, Bar-Ilan University, Ramat-Gan, Israel.

Arndt, E.M., Lefebvre, A., Travis, F., & Munro, I.R. (1986). Fact and fantasy: Psychosocial consequences of facial surgery in 24 Down Syndrome children. *British Journal of Plastic Surgery, 39,* 498–504.

Bak, J.J., & Siperstein, G.N. (1987). Similarity as a factor effecting change in children's attitudes toward mentally retarded peers. *American Journal of Mental Deficiency, 91,* 524–531.

Barr, M.W. (1904). *Mental defectives: Their history, treatment, and training*. Philadelphia: Philip Blakiston's Son.

Beck, E.M. (Ed.) (1980). *Bartlett's familiar quotations*. Boston: Little, Brown & Company.

Benda, C.E. (1956). Mongolism: A comprehensive review. *Archives of Pediatrics, 73,* 391–407.

Berry, D.S., & McArthur, L.Z. (1986). Perceiving character in faces: The impact of age-related craniofacial changes on social perception. *Psychological Bulletin, 100,* 3–18.

Blacketer-Simmonds, D.A. (1953). An investigation into the supposed differences existing between mongols and other mentally defective subjects with regard to certain psychological traits. *Journal of Mental Science, 99,* 702–719.

Blessing, K.R. (1959). The middle range mongoloid in trainable classes. *American Journal of Mental Deficiency, 63,* 812–821.

Brousseau, K., & Brainerd, M.G. (1928). *Mongolism: A study of the physical and mental characteristics of mongoloid imbeciles*. Baltimore, MD: Williams & Wilkins.

Brushfield, T. (1924). Mongolism. *British Journal of Children's Diseases, 21,* 240.

Carroll, J.L., Friedrich, D., & Hund, J. (1984). Academic self-concept and teachers' perceptions of normal, mentally retarded, and learning disabled elementary students. *Psychology in the Schools, 21,* 343–348.

Cicchetti, D., & Beeghly, M. (1990). An organizational approach to the study of Down Syndrome: Contributions to an integrative theory of development. In D. Cicchetti & M. Beeghly (Eds.), *Children with Down Syndrome: A developmental perspective* (pp. 29–62). New York: Cambridge University Press.

Cicchetti, D., & Mans-Wagener, L. (1987). Stages, sequences, and structures in the organization of cognitive development in Down Syndrome infants. In I. Uzgiris & J.McV. Hunt (Eds.), *Research with scales of psychological development in infancy*. Urbana, IL: University of Illinois Press.

Cicchetti, D., & Sroufe, L.A. (1978). An organizational view of affect: Illustrations from the study of Down's Syndrome infants. In M. Lewis & L.A. Rosenblum (Eds.), *The development of affect* (pp. 309–305). New York: Plenum.

Cooke, N.L., Heron, T.E., Heward, W.L., & Test, D.W. (1982). Integrating a Down's Syndrome child in a classwide peer tutoring system: A case report. *Mental Retardation, 20,* 22–25.

Domino, G. (1965). Personality traits in institutionalized mongoloids. *American Journal of Mental Deficiency, 69,* 568–570.

Domino, G., Goldschmid, M., & Kaplan, M. (1964). Personality traits of institutionalized mongoloid girls. *American Journal of Mental Deficiency, 68,* 498–502.

Down, J.L.N. (1866). Observations on ethnic classification of idiots. *Clinical Lectures and Reports*, London Hospital, *3,* 259.

Down, J.L.N. (1867). Observations on an ethnic classification of idiots. *Mental Science, 13,* 121–128.

Dunst, C. (1990). Sensorimotor development in infants with Down Syndrome. In D. Cicchetti & M. Beeghly (Eds.), *Children with Down Syndrome: A developmental perspective* (pp. 180–230). New York: Cambridge University Press.

Dunst, C.J., & Rheingover, R.M. (1983). Structural characteristics of sensorimotor development among Down's syndrome infants. *Journal of Mental Deficiency Research, 27,* 11–22.

Eder, R.A. (1988). The self conceived in memory. *Early child development and care: Special Issue on the Self-System, 40,* 25–51.

Eder, R.A. (1990). Uncovering young children's psychological selves: Individual and developmental differences. *Child Development, 61,* 849–863.

Eder, R.A., Gerlach, S.G., & Perlmutter, M. (1987). In search of children's selves: Development of the specific and general components of the self-concept. *Child Development, 58,* 1044–1050.

Engler, M. (1949). *Mongolism.* Bristol, England: John Wright & Sons.

Feuerstein, R. (1979). *The dynamic assessment of retarded performers: The learning potential assessment device, theory, instruments, and techniques.* Baltimore, MD: University Park Press.

Feuerstein, R. (1982, February). Multidimensional aspects of the social integration of Down Syndrome children and adolescents. *Surgical and cognitive intervention to effect the social integration of Down Syndrome children and adolescents.* Symposium conducted at the Hadassah-Wizo-Canada Research Institute and Hadassah Medical Organization Jerusalem.

Feuerstein, R. (1983, March). Down's Syndrome surgery as a part of an active modification approach. Paper presented at a symposium on *The future of seriously impaired infants: Where do professionals and society stand*? Held during the annual meeting of the American Orthopsychiatric Association, Boston, MA.

Francis, S.H. (1970). Behavior of low-grade institutionalized mongoloids: Changes with age. *American Journal of Mental Deficiency, 75,* 92–101.

Gibbs, M.V., & Thorpe, J.G. (1983). Personality stereotype of noninstitutionalized Down Syndrome children. *American Journal of Mental Deficiency, 87,* 601–605.

Gibson, D. (1978). *Down's Syndrome: The psychology of mongolism.* London: Cambridge University Press.

Gottlied, J., Semmel, M.I., & Veldman, D.J. (1978). Correlates of social status among mainstreamed mentally retarded persons. In M.J. Begab & S.A. Richardson (Eds.), *The mentally retarded and society: A social science perspective.* Baltimore, MD: University Park Press.

Graffi, S., & Minnes, P.M. (1988). Attitudes of primary school children toward the physical appearance and labels associated with Down Syndrome. *American Journal on Mental Retardation, 93,* 28–35.

Greenspan, S., & Delaney, K. (1983). Personal competence of institutionalized adult males with and without Down Syndrome. *American Journal of Mental Deficiency, 88,* 218–220.

Harter, S. (1982). The perceived competence scale for children. *Child Development, 53,* 87–97.

Harter, S. (1983). Developmental perspectives on the self-system. In P. Mussen (Ed.), *Handbook of child psychology: Vol. IV. Socialization, personality, and social development* (pp. 275–386). New York: Wiley.

Hartup, W.W. (1983). Peer relations. In P.H. Mussen (Ed.), *Handbook of child psychology: Vol. IV. Socialization, personality, and social development* (pp. 104–196). New York: Wiley.

Hohler, H. (1977). Changes in the facial expression as a result of plastic surgery in mongoloid children. *Aesthetic Plastic Surgery, 1,* 245.

Johnson, R.T., Johnson, D.W., & Rynders, J. (1981). Effect of cooperative, competitive, and individualistic experiences on self-esteem of handicapped and nonhandicapped students. *Journal of Psychology, 108,* 31–34.

Jones, C.J. (1985). Analysis of the self-concepts of handicapped students. *RASE: Remedial and Special Education, 6,* 32–36.

Katz, S., & Kravetz, S. (1989). Facial plastic surgery for persons with Down Syndrome: Research findings and their professional and social implications. *American Journal on Mental Retardation, 94,* 101–110.

Kleck, R.E., & Strenta, A. (1980). Perceptions of the impact of negatively valued physical characteristics on social interaction. *Journal of Personality and Social Psychology, 39,* 861–873.

Koegel, P., & Edgerton, R.B. (1982). Labeling and the perception of handicap among black mildly retarded adults. *American Journal of Mental Deficiency, 87,* 266–276.

Kravetz, S., Weller, A.A., Tennenbaum, R., Tzuriel, D., & Mintzker, Y. (1987). Plastic surgery on children with Down Syndrome: Parents' perceptions of physical, personal, and social functioning. Manuscript submitted for publication.

Kuczaj, S. (1987, November). The effects of surgery on others' perceptions of children with Down Syndrome. Presented at the symposium on *The psychosocial aspects of craniofacial problems . . . Surgery is not enough*, held at the International Craniofacial Institute, Dallas, TX.

Lefebvre, A., Bedard, A.C., Arndt, E., Travis, F., & Munro, I.R. (1987, November). The face and the soul: mirror or illusion. Paper presented at the symposium on *The psychosocial aspects of craniofacial problems . . . Surgery is not enough*, held at the International Craniofacial Institute, Dallas, TX.

Lemperle, G., & Radu, D. (1980). Facial plastic surgery in children with Down's Syndrome. *Plastic and Reconstructive Surgery, 66,* 337–342.

Lewis, M., & Brooks-Gunn, J. (1979). *Social cognition and the acquisition of self.* New York: Plenum Press.

Loveland, K.A. (1987a). Behavior of young children before the mirror: Finding things reflected. *Child Development, 58,* 928–936.

Loveland, K.A. (1987b). Behavior of young children with Down Syndrome before the mirror: Exploration. *Child Development, 58,* 768–778.

Lund, N.L., Carman, S.M., & Kranz, P.L. (1981). Reliability in the use of the Tennessee Self-Concept Scale for educable mentally retarded adolescents. *Journal of Psychology, 109,* 205–211.

Madden, N.A., & Slavin, R.E. (1982). Effects of cooperative learning on the social acceptance of mainstreamed handicapped students. Baltimore, MD: Center for Social Organization of Schools, Report No. 321, John Hopkins University.

Mahoney, G., Glover, A., & Finger, I. (1981). Relationships between language and sensorimotor development of Down Syndrome and nonretarded children. *American Journal of Mental Deficiency, 86,* 21–27.

Mans, L., Cicchetti, D., & Sroufe, L.A. (1978). Mirror reactions of Down's Syndrome infants and toddlers: Cognitive underpinnings of self-recognition. *Child Development, 49,* 1247–1250.

McArthur, L.Z., & Baron, R.M. (1983). Toward an ecological theory of social perception. *Psychological Review, 90,* 215–238.

Mervis, C.B., & Cardoso-Martins, C. (1984). Transition from sensorimotor stage 5 to stage 6 by Down Syndrome children: A response to Gibson. *American Journal of Mental Deficiency, 89,* 99–102.

Novoselsky, A., Katz, S., & Kravetz, S. (1988). Children with Down Syndrome: Their evaluation by peers before and after plastic surgery. *Special Education and Rehabilitation, 5,* 89–99.

Olbrisch, R.R. (1982). Plastic surgical management of children with Down Syndrome: Indications and results. *British Journal of Plastic Surgery, 35,* 195–200.

Osguthorpe, R.T., Eiserman, W.D., & Shisler, L. (1985). Increasing social acceptance: Mentally retarded students tutoring regular class peers. *Education & Training of the Mentally Retarded, 20,* 235–240.

Oster, J. (1953). *Mongolism.* Copenhagen: Danish Science Press.

Parsons, C.L., Iacono, T.A., & Rozner, L. (1987). Effect of tongue reduction on articulation in children with Down Syndrome. *American Journal of Mental Deficiency, 91,* 328–332.

Peterson, N.L. (1982). Social integration of handicapped and nonhandicapped preschoolers. *Topics in Early Childhood Special Education, 2,* 56–69.

Piaget, J. (1932). *The moral judgment of the child.* Glencoe, IL: Free Press.

Piaget, J. (1952). *The origins of intelligence.* New York: International Universities Press.

Piaget, J. (1954). *The construction of reality in the child.* New York: Basic Books.

Pueschel, S.M. (1982). Biomedical aspects of Down's Syndrome phenotype. In S.M. Pueschel & J.E. Rynders (Ed.), *Down's Syndrome: Advances in biomedicine and the behavioral sciences.* Cambridge, MA: The Ware Press.

Pueschel, S., Monteiro, L.A., & Erickson, M. (1986). Parents' and physicians' perceptions of facial plastic surgery in children with Down Syndrome. *Journal of Mental Deficiency Research, 30,* 71–79.

Rietveld, C.M. (1986). The adjustment to school of eight children with Down's Syndrome from an early intervention program. *Australia & New Zealand Journal of Developmental Disabilities, 12,* 159–175.

Rogers-Warren, A. (1980). *Playing and learning together.* Lawrence, KS: University of Kansas, Early Childhood Institute (ERIC Document Reproduction Service No. ED 231 104).

Rollin, H.R. (1946). Personality in mongolism with special reference to the incidence of catatonic psychosis. *American Journal of Mental Deficiency, 51,* 219–237.

Rynders, J.E., Johnson, R.T., Johnson, D.W., & Schmidt, B. (1980). Producing positive interaction among Down Syndrome and nonhandicapped teenagers through cooperative goal-structuring. *American Journal of Mental Deficiency, 85,* 268–273.

Sandahl, E. (1980). Plastic surgery and a new image for a Down's Syndrome child. In I. Newman (Ed.), *Readings in Down Syndrome* (pp. 72–75). Guilford, CT: Special Learning Corporation.

Schlottman, R.S., & Anderson, V.H. (1975). Social and play behaviors of institutionalized mongoloid and nonmongoloid retarded children. *Journal of Psychology, 91,* 201–206.

Serafica, F.C. (1990). Peer relations of children with Down Syndrome. In D. Cicchetti & M. Beeghly (Eds.), *Children with Down Syndrome: A developmental perspective* (pp. 369–423). New York: Cambridge University Press.

Sherlock, E.B., & Donkin, H.B. (1911). *The feeble minded: A guide to study and practice.* London: Macmillan & Co.

Sinson, J.C., & Wetherick, N.E. (1981). The behavior of children with Down Syndrome in normal playgroups. *Journal of Mental Deficiency Research, 25,* 113–120.

Sinson, J.C., & Wetherick, N.E. (1982). Mutual gaze in preschool Down and normal children. *Journal of Mental Deficiency Research, 26,* 123–129.

Sinson, J.C., & Wetherick, N.E. (1986). Integrating young children with Down Syndrome: Gaze, play and vocalization in the initial encounter. *British Journal of Mental Subnormality, 32,* 93–101.

Siperstein, G.N., & Bak, J.J. (1985). Social behavior: How it affects children's attitudes toward mildly and moderately retarded peers. *American Journal of Mental Deficiency, 90,* 319–327.

Siperstein, G.N., & Chatillon, A.C. (1982). Importance of perceived similarity in improving children's attitudes toward mentally retarded peers. *American Journal of Mental Deficiency, 86,* 453–458.

Smith, L., & Hagen, V. (1984). Relationship between the home environment and sensorimotor development of Down Syndrome and nonretarded infants. *American Journal of Mental Deficiency, 89,* 124–132.

Smith, L., & von Tetzchner, S. (1986). Communicative, sensorimotor, and language skills of young children with Down Syndrome. *American Journal of Mental Deficiency, 91,* 57–66.

Sroufe, L.A., & Waters, E. (1976). The ontogenesis of smiling and laughter: A perspective on the organization of development in infancy. *Psychological Review, 83,* 173–189.

Staffieri, J.R. (1967). A study of social stereotype of body image in children. *Journal of Personality and Social Psychology, 7,* 101–104.

Strauss, R., Mintzker, Y., Feuerstein, R., Wexler, M., & Rand, Y. (1988). Social perceptions of the effects of Down Syndrome facial surgery: A school-based study of ratings by normal adolescents. *Plastic and Reconstructive Surgery, 80,* 843–846.

Sullivan, H.S. (1953). *The interpersonal theory of psychiatry.* New York: Norton.

Thase, M.E. (1982). Longevity and mortality in Down's Syndrome. *Journal of Mental Deficiency, 26,* 177–192.

Tobiasen, J.M. (1984). Psychosocial correlates of congenital facial clefts: A conceptualization and model. *Cleft Palate Journal, 21,* 131–139.

Travis, F. (1987, November). Psychological and demographic profiles related to Down's children. Paper presented at the symposium of *The Psychosocial Aspects of Craniofacial Problems . . . Surgery is Not Enough,* held at the International Craniofacial Institute, Dallas, TX.

Tredgold, A.F. (1947). *A textbook of mental deficiency*. London: Bailliere, Tindall & Cox.

Von Bertanlaffy, L. (1968). *General system theory*. New York: George Baziller Inc.

Wallin, J.E.W. (1949). *Children with mental and physical handicaps*. New York: Prentice Hall.

Werner, H. (1948). *Comparative psychology of mental development*. New York: International Universities Press.

Wexler, M.R., Peled, I.J., Rand, Y., Mintzker, Y., & Feuerstein, R. (1986). Rehabilitation of the face in patients with Down's Syndrome. *Plastic and Reconstructive Surgery, 77,* 383–391.

Wright, J., & Cowden, J.E. (1986). Changes in self-concept and cardiovascular endurance of mentally retarded youths in a Special Olympics swim training program. *Adapted Physical Activity Quarterly, 3,* 177–183.

12
Social Psychological Model of Craniofacial Anomalies: Example of Cleft Lip and Palate

Joyce M. Tobiasen

Since you're asking, I want to tell you a little about Mary. She is kind, helpful and works very hard to keep up her school work. She has a low C average—takes regular classes. She has good study habits and we don't feel she is just being given a grade. In the past month she has started dieting, has become interested in racquetball and has joined the school play. She is very shy and has no close friends in her age group. One problem we have, is our children go to school in a different town than we live in. She gets along with our family and her cousins next door. She got her driver's license last summer, which she is very proud of, and has become a reliable driver. She drives to play practice and on errands.

Her speech teacher at school feels she has gone as far with her as she can and asks for recommendations for helping any corrections necessary.

Any help you can offer for the social slowness will be very much appreciated.

I feel we have a good family, overprotective sometimes, but we are trying to overcome that!

This letter was written by the parent of a child attending a clinic for children with clefts of the lip and palate. Parents and children commonly report problems with peer rejection and self-consciousness. A 16-year-old male patient with a cleft of the lip and palate dropped out of high school because, he said, he could no longer tolerate being teased and stared at by other students. An 11-year-old patient with a cleft reported that he ate lunch alone because he was embarrassed when others observed him eating. A 28-year-old patient with a cleft reported that he had never had a date and still lived at home with his parents.

The anecdotal and clinical evidence are clear: Children and adults with cleft-related facial impairments have problems with social relationships. The purpose of this chapter is to examine the developmental, social psychological, theoretical basis for these problems and to relate the theory to existing research in the area. Four broad topics will be addressed: 1) the nature of a facial cleft; 2) existing developmental social psychological theory in which facial impairment can be conceptualized as a social cue about which people have multiple expectations that they regularly act upon; 3) social psychological research on clefts and how it relates to existing theory; and 4) directions for future research and implications for clinical psychological treatment of facial clefts.

What Is a Facial Cleft?

A child with a cleft of the lip and palate is born with a split or an opening in the roof of the mouth and upper lip. It is possible for a child to have a cleft lip only, a cleft palate only, or both a cleft lip and a cleft palate. Clefts of the lip and palate are among the most common of all birth defects and occur in all racial and ethnic groups. They are also the most common craniofacial defect. It is estimated that 1 out of every 600 to 700 children born alive has a cleft lip and/or palate (Hobbs, 1980).

The types and severity of clefts vary widely from child to child. A cleft lip can range from a slight notch in the colored portion of the lip to a complete separation of the lip extending up and into the nose. When there is a cleft lip, the alveolar ridge or gum may also be separated, resulting in dental deformities. Clefts of the lip may be unilateral or bilateral, occurring on one or both sides of the lip, with varying degrees of severity. A cleft may be incomplete and involve only the uvula or small portion of the back of the palate, which hangs down into the throat and the velum or muscular soft palate. A cleft that is complete may extend the entire length of the palate, from back to front, from the uvula and velum to the alveolar ridge.

Numerous surgeries, extensive dental work, and long-term speech therapy are typical for youngsters with a cleft defect. The primary surgery to close the lip and palate typically occurs within 1 year of birth. Secondary surgical repairs of the lip and nose may occur throughout childhood and early adulthood to improve appearance. Secondary surgical repair may also be needed to repair clefts of the gum and improve dental appearance. Speech–language and dental treatment may be necessary throughout the school years. Even so, a child born with a cleft of the lip may have visible scars and facial distortions throughout life.

Given the nature of cleft lip and palate as a chronic disability associated with facial impairment and speech problems, it is not surprising that psychological issues associated with clefts have been the focus of considerable study (c.f. McWilliams, 1982; Richman & Eliason, 1982; Tobiasen, 1984). The psychological study of clefts, as with the study of many chronic disabilities (Varni and Wallender, 1988), has been atheoretical in nature. Much of the research has been conducted *by* clinicians *for* clinicians. These studies were designed to ask specific questions about the emotional, intellectual, and social sequelae of cleft lip and palate. There exists psychological theory regarding the impact of appearance and other prominent social cues on the development of personality and social behavior (c.f. Adams, 1977; Darley & Fazio, 1980; Langlois & Stephan, 1981). In this chapter, this theory will be reviewed briefly and evaluated in terms of how well it explains existing social psychological research on facial clefts.

Conceptual Model of Facial Impairment

In the last 20 years, social scientists have developed theory and conducted research on the relationships between the expectancies individuals have of others and the effects of those expectancies on the behavior of the perceiver and the behavior of the target of the expectancies. Developmental (Sameroff, 1975), social (Darley & Fazio, 1980; Rosenthal, 1974), and rehabilitation psychologists (Myerson, 1963; Wright, 1983) have proposed that there is a multi causal chain between expectancies, behavior, and personality development. Adams (1977) and Langlois and Stephan (1981) have applied this general model to explain the effects of the expectations about physical attractiveness on the personality and social development of children who are either attractive or unattractive. The theory is based on the concept of "self-fulfilling prophecy" (Merton, 1957), which asserts that people's expectations influence the behavior of others such that the expectations and the behavior are congruent. The interaction between the expectations of people for the behavior of others can set up a closed social interaction feedback system such that expectations influence behavior that feeds back to confirm the expectations.

Darley and Fazio (1980) have described a six-component model of the social interaction sequence underlying the concept of self-fulfilling prophecy. First, a perceiver has expectancies toward a target person. These expectancies are based on past observations of an individual or on stereotypes that the perceiver may hold about specific categories of people. Second, the perceiver's expectancies influence his or her behavior toward the target person. Third, the target person interprets the perceiver's behavior. Fourth, the target person's behavior reflects his or her interpretation of the perceiver's behavior. Fifth, the perceiver interprets the target's behavior as congruent with expectations. Finally, the expectations and behavior may become central to the target person's self-concept.

The concept of self-fulfilling prophecy has been applied to explain effects of teacher expectations on student achievement (Rosenthal & Jacobson, 1968; Zanna, Sheras, Cooper, & Shaw, 1975); sex differences in behavior (Zanna & Pack, 1975); racial stereotypes (Cooper & Fazio, 1979); and in the behavioral enactment of trait inferences regarding physically attractive women (Snyder, Tanke, & Berscheid, 1977). Others have used the concept to explain the pervasive effects on children's and adults' behavior of the physical attractiveness stereotype (Adams, 1977; Langlois & Stephan, 1981).

Researchers in the field of rehabilitation psychology have recognized the importance of people's expectations for individuals with disabilities. Two essential elements of a physical disability are generally distinguished: the functional disability and the disability associated with deviations from regular expectations and potential social rejection (Wright, 1983). The World Health Organization (1980) has carried the classification system one step further. The international classification scheme distinguishes among an *impairment*, as "any loss or abnormality of psychological, physiological, or anatomical structure or function"; a *disability*, as "any restriction or lack of ability to perform an activity in a manner or within the range which is considered normal"; and a *handicap*, or a disadvantage for a given individual, resulting from an impairment or a disability that limits or prevents the fulfillment of a role that is normal (depending on age, sex, social, and cultural factors) for the individuals." This means that an individual may have a relatively minor disability or impairment but a severe social handicap if the expectations associated with the disability or impairment are markedly negative.

Macgregor and her colleagues (Macgregor, 1982; Macgregor, Abel, Brynt, Laver, & Weissman, 1953) have hypothesized that this is especially the case for individuals with facial impairments such as cleft lip and palate. If the expectancy-confirmation model of the social interaction sequence, as outlined by Darley and Fazio (1980), is applied to an analysis of the cleft lip and palate research and clinical literature, then we should be able to identify: 1) specific expectations associated with cleft-related facial impairments; 2) differential behavior toward individuals with clefts; 3) unique interpretations by individuals with clefts of the behavior of others toward them; 4) identifiable behavioral patterns associated with individuals with clefts; and 5) self-concepts that have been molded by the fact that an individual was born with a facial cleft.

Social Psychological Research on Cleft Lip and Palate

Expectations Associated with Facial Impairment

Historically, societal reactions to facial impairments are negative. From the first cave paintings to the present, artistic representations of the human form have associated what is young and beautiful with what is good, and what is distorted and old with evil and terror (Shaw, 1981). Hogarth's eighteenth-century visual depictions of depravity are notorious for the deformed and ugly nature of the human figures (Munro, 1981). Until recently, several American cities had so-called ugly laws as part of vagrancy statutes, which imposed fines on unsightly people who were seen in public places (Chicago Illinois Municipal Code, 1966).

Weinberg and Santana (1978) sampled comic books for cultural stereotypes of good and evil based on physical appearance. They reported that 80% of individuals with no disabilities or impairments were represented as good (45%) or neutral (35%) characters and as evil only 20% of the time. Individuals with irregularities from the neck up (i.e., distorted heads or facial features, scars, and excessive wrinkles) represented evil characters 71% of the time, were never depicted in neutral roles, and were represented as "good" 29% of the time. These findings suggest that the cultural view of facial impairment is ambivalent but that it is dominantly associated with behavioral and moral impairment.

The empirical literature on expectations for the personalities and behavior of individuals with facial impairments consists of studies of ratings by peers from first impressions of photographs and drawings. One of the most famous studies in this area was conducted by Richardson and colleagues (Richardson, 1970; Richardson, Goodman, Hastorf, & Dornbusch, 1961). They asked children and adults to give their preferences for drawings of youngsters with different visible handicaps (e.g., no handicap, a wheelchair, crutches and leg brace, missing hand, obesity, and a labial scar). Subjects, regardless of age or gender, consistently preferred the nonhandicapped photograph. Subjects least preferred the photographs of the facially impaired and obese children. Children's dislike of functional handicaps (e.g., leg brace) decreased with the increasing age of the rater, while dislike for facial impairment increased. Older subjects had a greater preference for drawings depicting abnormalities that were distant from the face. Richardson et al. concluded that by the age of 5 or 6, English and American children had consistent attitudes toward different forms of handicaps.

In a similar study, Landsdown and Polak (1975) asked children 9 to 11 years of age to rank in order of "best liked" drawings of children with a normal face, "bat ears," eyc squint, protruding teeth, cleft lip, and misshapen nose. Drawings of children with a cleft lip or misshapen nose were consistently ranked as least liked. Glass, Starr, Stewart, and Hodge (1981) used Identikit sketches and asked adults to judge which of two sets were most preferred—a set showing faces with clefts of the lip or a set showing faces without clefts of the lip. Impairments of the lip were least preferred by raters.

Podol and Salvia (1976) asked 60 speech pathology students in a double-blind factorial experiment to assess the impact of impaired lips and noses of cleft patients on the evaluation of various speech dimensions. The subjects were randomly assigned to one of four groups. All subjects read identical case studies about a child born with a cleft. One of two photographs was attached to each case study. One photograph was of a patient with a cleft. The second photograph was of the same patient with the cleft impairment artistically removed. Half the subjects in each photographic condition listened to a recording of a normal speaker, while the other half of the subjects listened to a nasal speaker. Subjects in the facial impairment conditions rated the speech as significantly more speech impaired and in need of speech therapy than did subjects in the nonfacial impairment conditions.

Tobiasen (1987) examined personality and ability judgments associated by peers with cleft-related impairments. Children were shown either photographically corrected versions of children with congenital facial clefts or uncorrected versions. Children and adolescents, males and females, ages 7 through 16 years rated individuals with cleft impairments as less popular, less friendly, less smart, and a less likely choice as a friend. Girls with clefts tended to be rated more harshly than boys.

Shaw and Orth (1981) had adult judges select two attractive and two unattractive photographs, one of each gender, from a set of 60 photographs. The natural teeth in each photograph were replaced with photographs of acrylic teeth mounted in wax to represent five different dental arrangements: normal incisors, prominent incisors, missing upper left lateral incisor, severely crowded incisors, and an arrangement representing dental appearance in a unilateral cleft case. In all, 20 test photographs were prepared. Shaw and Orth found that both children and adult raters judged the photographed children with normal dental facial arrangements to be more attractive, more desirable as friends, more intelligent, and less inclined to aggression than those with impaired dental facial appearance. The photograph depicting the unilateral cleft was least preferred of all. Judges in the study were 840 children, ages 11 to 13, and 840 men and women, ages 20 to 65. Significantly, when the background facial attractiveness of the photographs was compared, the high vs. the low attractive faces were preferred regardless of dental facial impairment. This finding suggests that people consider more than one morphological dimension of the face in forming impressions of others. Lucker, Graber, and Pietromonaco (1981) have suggested that while overall facial attractiveness may be a dominant component in first impressions, occlusal malrelations and other focal facial impairments may be "signals" or social cues that influence judgments of facial aesthetics in ways that, as of yet, are poorly understood.

The studies described here are consistent with the person perception effects described for facial attractiveness—that is, that "what is beautiful is good." The person perception effects for facial impairment can be described as "what is facially impaired is bad." However, studies of people's attitudes toward individuals with other disabilities suggest that there are both negative and positive reactions to physically deviant individuals—that there are conflicting norms to reject and to be kind to people with disabilities. In one of the earliest studies (Mussen & Barker, 1944), college students were asked to rate physically handicapped people on 24 personality traits. Handicapped people were rated as more conscientious, persistent, and religious than the average. They were also rated as more unselfish, gentle, reserved, and creative than nondisabled people. In contrast, subjects reported that they believed that people with handicaps felt more inferior and unhappy than everyone else.

Tobiasen (in preparation) conducted a preliminary study to examine the interaction between facial attractiveness and impairment. An individual may have a localized facial cleft in an otherwise attractive face. The attractiveness theory would predict that the more severe the impairment, the less attractive and socially desirable the individual. Stigma theory would predict ambivalent social perceptions for individuals with facial clefts. A third possibility is that the facial dimensions of attractiveness combined with extreme impairment may produce an exaggerated sympathy effect. It may also produce an exaggerated "ugly is bad" effect.

Tobiasen (in preparation) systematically manipulated the severity of the oral-nasal disfigurement and overall facial attractiveness to assess their combined effects on first impressions. Based on preratings by children and plastic surgeons of slides of children with oral facial clefts that had been artistically corrected to remove disfigurements, two sets of slides that varied by degree of attractiveness and facial disfigurement were created. A second sample of children then rated the slides (3 facial disfigurement × 2 facial attractiveness × 2 sets) on facial attractiveness, friendliness, popularity, and smartness. Strong main effects for both disfigurement and attractiveness on all ratings were obtained. Children ages 7 to 16, males and females, rated photographs depicting the most attractive and unimpaired faces as smarter, friendlier, and more popular. The main effects were qualified by statistically significant interactions for facial attractiveness and disfigurement on all measures.

The pattern of the interactions were not entirely consistent (see Figures 12.1 through 12.4). Figures 12.1 and 12.2 show that when the impaired face is attractive, mean ratings of the overall "good looks" and popularity of the photographed individuals decreased as severity of impairment increased. This was not true for the low-attractiveness photographs. They were rated about the same on good looks and popularity *regardless* of severity of impairment. This suggests that people were less willing to negatively rate unattractive individuals who also had severe facial impairments. The effects for low attractiveness were reversed for ratings of friendlines. Severe-impairment–low-attractive individuals were rated as more friendly than no-impairment or moderate-impairment faces of low attractiveness (see Figure 12.3). Finally, moderate-impairment faces of low attractiveness were rated as smarter than either the no-impairment or severe-impairment photographs. The reverse was true for the attractive faces.

These findings, while preliminary, suggest that there is an interaction between degree of attractiveness and facial impairment for ratings of attractiveness and personality attributions. The data also suggest that specific and even contradictory attributions may be associated with oral

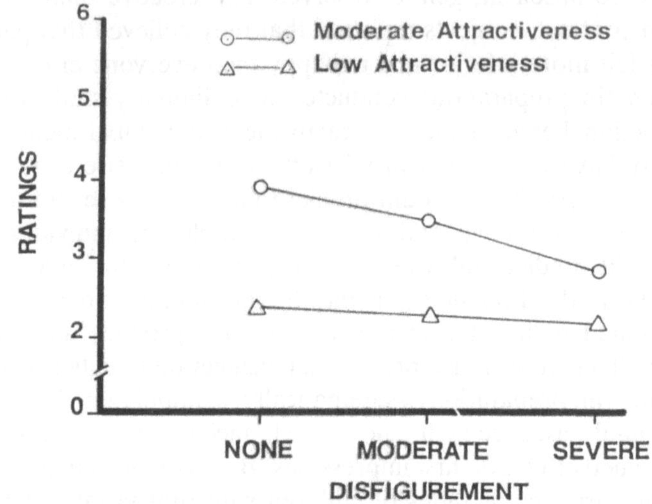

FIGURE 12.1. Ratings of good looks.

facial clefts. For example, individuals with oral facial clefts may be perceived as friendly but probably not popular or intelligent.

Richman (1978) conducted a study of teachers ratings of the intelligence quotients of cleft lip and palate children. He reported that teachers significantly underestimated the intelligence of children with moderate scars but overestimated the intelligence of children with severe scarring

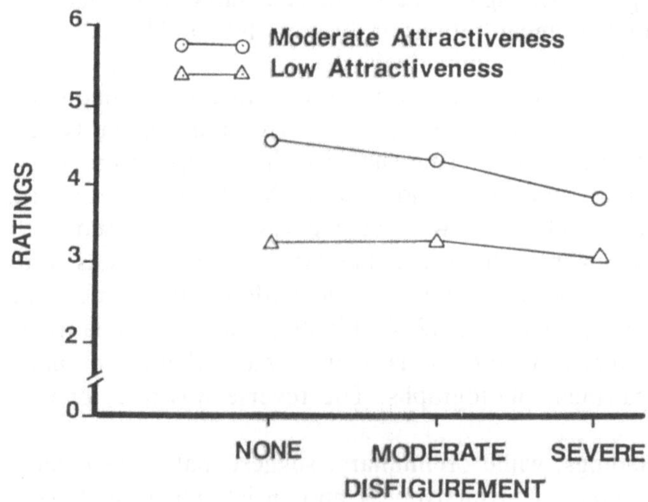

FIGURE 12.2. Ratings of popularity.

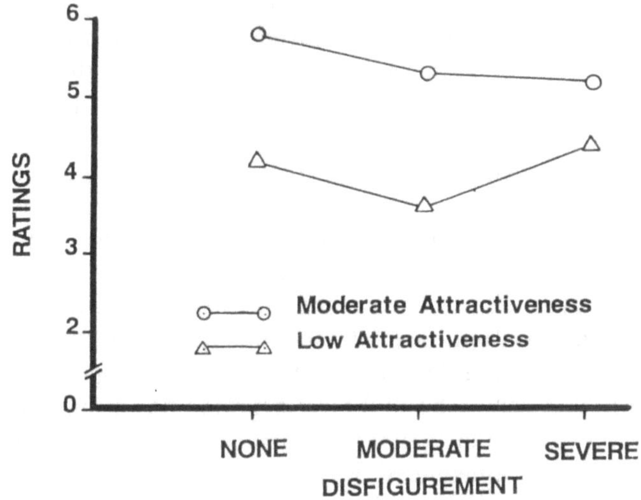

FIGURE 12.3. Ratings of friendliness.

from congenital facial clefts. Richman did not control for global attractiveness. However, the findings suggest a sympathy effect for ratings of intelligence and are consistent with Tobiasen's (in preparation) findings.

These findings have implications for the surgical treatment of clefts. Surgical interventions to revise scars and improve the appearance of children and adolescents with congenital clefts are conducted to improve

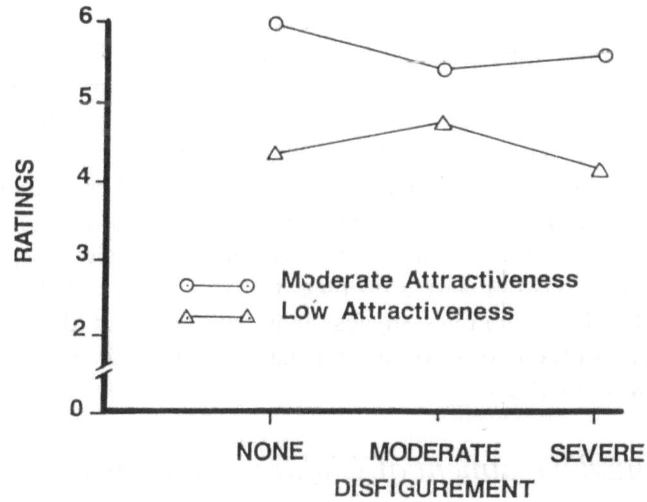

FIGURE 12.4. Ratings of smartness.

the social acceptability of the child's appearance. The facial impairment can be reduced, but rarely is it removed. The research described above (Richman, 1978; Tobiasen, in preparation) suggests that reducing the severity of the impairment may reduce positive and increase negative expectations for behavior and personality in patients who are otherwise unattractive. The sympathy effect associated with impairment may be lost, and the individual may be judged as "simply unattractive." Unfortunately, there are no studies that deal directly with this question.

A related and also unresearched question is if there are specific attributions associated with cleft-type impairments. For example, individuals with clefts often have mid-face retrusion due to bone growth disturbances. They have an elongated flattened area between the upper lip and nostrils and a protruding chin. The mid-face in profile has an inverted "spoon" shape. Macgregor et al. (1953) have suggested that people associate aggressiveness and "toughness" with this facial impairment. Others have suggested that attributions of low intelligence are often associated with facial clefts (Shaw, 1981). The layperson's term for a cleft lip is "harelip." In folklore, individuals with clefts have been associated with lower forms of animal life. The historical, literary, artistic, and legal associations of facial scars with evil and depravity were mentioned earlier. Whether highly specific sets of expectations are associated with facial clefts or whether a simple "ugly is bad" stereotype best applies to social reactions to clefts remains to be studied.

There have been almost no studies of the effects of facial impairment on parents' expectations and no studies of whether expectations change in long-term relationships. There is one study that suggests that parents of children with clefts may have different expectancies for their children than parents of children without clefts. Using the Eyberg Child Behavior Inventory (Robinson, Eyberg, & Ross, 1980), which was designed to measure parents' ratings of the frequency of common behavior problems in children ages 2 to 12 and whether or not the behaviors are bothersome to the family, Tobiasen and Hiebert (1984) found that parents of children with clefts and parents of children without clefts reported comparable frequencies of problem behavior. However, parents of children with clefts were more tolerant of the misbehaviors, reporting that they did not pose a problem in the home. Parents of children without clefts reported that many of the behaviors were a problem for which they might seek professional help. These findings suggest that parents of children with clefts have lower expectations for appropriate behavior than do parents of children without clefts.

Differential Treatment of Children with Facial Clefts

Unfortunately, there are few existing laboratory or naturalistic studies of how children with facial clefts are treated by others. There are several studies of parents' reactions to the birth of a child with a cleft impairment that are suggestive of differential treatment. Brantley and Clifford (1979), Clifford (1969), and Richman and Harper (1978) reported that parents believed that their acceptance of a child with a facial cleft was more difficult than the acceptance of a healthy child. Parents described their reactions as shock, guilt, and anger. Macgregor et al. (1953) described extensive interviews with families of children with various craniofacial anomalies, including clefts. MacGregor noted that many of these families were less likely to take their children on family outings and that they avoided visitors coming to the home to view the new infant.

There is one laboratory study of mothers' early interactions with infants born with cleft lip and palate. Field and Vega-Lahr (1984) studied the social interactions of mothers and their 3-month-old infants. The infants were placed in infant seats on tables at which the mothers were seated in a face-to-face position. A 10-minute play between parent and infant was recorded on video. The results of the analyses revealed that the mothers of infants with clefts, relative to mothers of infants without clefts, smiled and vocalized less frequently. They also engaged in less contingent responsivity and game playing. Field and Vega-Lahr expressed puzzlement with their findings, because typically, mothers of high-risk infants are more active with their less responsive infants. They suggested that mothers of infants with clefts may be depressed because of the long-term nature of the disability. Another interpretation is that mothers of cleft infants may have lower expectations for the social responsivity of their children.

Wasserman, Allen, and Solomon (1985) conducted a longitudinal study of the interactive behavior of mothers and toddlers. There were 3 groups of toddlers: 14 premature infants, 14 healthy infants, and 14 children born with birth defects, including 3 with limb deformities and 11 craniofacial anomalies (6 cleft lip and palate). None of the children in the birth defects group had central nervous system damage. Wasserman et al. studied the children at 9, 12, 18, and 24 months of age. The mothers of the premature and (craniofacial–physically disabled) children treated their children very similarly. Mothers of the high-risk children tended to be more attentive but less responsive than the mothers of the healthy children, but at different ages. They engaged in more attention management, verbal teaching, and physical teaching. They tended to give more orders to their children and use distraction less in managing the behavior of their children. There were subtle differences between the premature and (craniofacial/disabled) groups of mothers. Mothers of (craniofacial/disabled) children tended to use attention-management techniques and encouragement more frequently than the mothers of the premature children as the children became older. Mothers of (craniofacial/disabled) children showed developmental increases in their use of encouragement (e.g., positive reinforcement) and attention-getting activities. The mothers of the (craniofacial/disabled) patients also spent more time ignoring their children at 24 months than did mothers in the other groups. More than one-third of the mothers of handicapped children showed at least one 10-second period of ignoring as opposed to only one mother of a premature and none in the normal sample. These findings suggest that the mothers of the (craniofacial/disabled) children were ambivalent about them—on the one hand, attending closely to their behavior, while on the other hand ignoring and exhibiting behaviors that were nonresponsive to the infants' behavior. The findings reported by Wasserman et al. (1985) and Field and Vega-Lahr (1984) suggest that mothers of cleft infants and toddlers express subtle behavioral cues indicative of avoidance and/or ambivalence. No one has examined the social interactions of older children and their parents.

There are numerous anecdotal reports and correlational studies that suggest that children and adults with facial clefts and related craniofacial anomalies receive differential treatment from strangers and peers. In the pioneer study by Macgregor and her colleagues (Macgregor, 1982; Macgregor et al., 1953), extended interviews with facially impaired patients revealed the serious problems that they faced in daily social interactions. These problems included "staring, remarks, curiosity, questioning, pity, rejection, ridicule, whispering, nicknames, and discrimination" (Macgregor et al., 1953, p. 633). The rejection described by these patients extended to difficulties in obtaining jobs, attracting members of the opposite sex, and making friends.

Rumsey, Bull, and Gahagan (1982) studied the proxemic behavior of 450 people in encounters with a confederate in four different conditions: facial birthmark, facial scarring, facial bruising consistent with a road traffic accident, and nonimpaired facial condition. They reported that people stood significantly farther away from the confederate in the facial scarring condition than the other conditions. Subjects also preferred to stand more often on the confederate's nonfacially impaired side. Subjects stood farther away from the confederate in the birthmark condition than in the acquired facial impairment condition, suggesting that people react more adversely to a permanent congenital facial impairment than to a temporary acquired impairment. Individuals with facial impairments may be correct in their assertion that they are being avoided, at least to the extent that people stand farther away from them than from individuals without impairments or with acquired impairments.

Rumsey (1983) carried out a series of studies of helping behavior toward individuals with facial impairments. Study 1 was designed so that there would be no face-to-face interaction between subjects and the confederates. Completed graduate application forms were left in public telephone booths. Attached to each form were a stamped, addressed envelope; a letter (designed to leave subjects in no doubt that the application had been mistakenly left behind and that it needed to be posted urgently); and a passport-size facial photograph of a disfigured or non-disfigured confederate. Using 248 subjects, high rates of return were found in all conditions, with no significant difference in the level of helping behavior exhibited in the facially impaired and nonimpaired conditions.

The second study (Rumsey, 1983) was designed to provide a low level of face-to-face contact. The facially impaired vs. nonimpaired confederate stood on a busy shopping street holding a collection box for a registered children's charity. Subjects (3,310 passers-by, 90 donors) had to approach the confederate if they wished to donate. There was no significant difference in the number of donors in the impaired and nonimpaired conditions. There was a tendency for fewer people to donate in the impaired condition but for those who did donate to give larger amounts of money.

The third study (Rumsey, 1983) was a situation designed to provide a higher level of face-to-face interaction. The disfigured or nondisfigured confederate approached passers-by and asked if they would be willing to answer questions about television programs. There was no significant difference in the numbers of subjects agreeing to stop in the impaired and nonimpaired conditions. Individuals who stopped in the impaired condition tended to be more helpful.

The findings suggest that adults do not overtly reject individuals with facial impairments. However, there does seem to be a subtle, nonverbal discrimination.

Interpretations of Individuals with Clefts of the Behavior of Others

Individuals with facial impairments, and particularly clefts, tend to make negative interpretations of the behavior of others toward them. The evidence is both anecdotal and experimental.

Abel (1952) reported that all of her sample of 74 patients hospitalized for corrective surgery of facial impairments ranging from clefts to severe acquired traumatic impairments stated that their facial problems often resulted in social and vocational discrimination. Richman and Harper (1978) reported that children with clefts, especially males, believed that their mothers were more controlling and intrusive on their lives than on children with cerebral palsy or healthy children. Clifford (1979) interviewed adolescents with clefts about the impact of the cleft on family life. These children reported that they thought that their parents had negative reactions to them but that their parents nevertheless were accepting and nurturing of them. Heller, Tidmarsh, and Pless (1981) reported that individuals with poor cosmetic repair of clefts believed that they had fewer opportunities to get dates and to make friends as compared to those judged as having a good cosmetic repair.

Several investigators (Davis, 1961; Goffman, 1963; Wright, 1983) have observed that individuals with physical disabilities and impairments often take it for granted that the impairment has a major influence on their social relations. There is some empirical support for this view (Kleck & Strenta, 1980; Strenta & Kleck, 1984). Kleck and Strenta (1980) conducted a series of four laboratory studies with nondisabled and nonimpaired college students that directly examined if individuals with stigmatizing physical characteristics expect that their treatment by others is causally linked to these attributes. The experimental paradigm involved a face-to-face interaction in which college students were given a mental set that involved one of three conditions: a facial scar, epilepsy, and allergy. The set for the scar was implemented with makeup that was removed without the subjects' awareness prior to an interaction with a confederate trained to act in a standard manner and blind to the set given the subjects. Thus, the stigmatizing (facial scar, epilepsy) and nonstigmatizing (allergy) characteristics could, in fact, have no direct impact upon the behavior of others. Nevertheless, participants in the facial scar and epilepsy conditions believed that the behavior of the individuals (confederates) that they interacted with was affected by their presumed impairment, while those in the allergy condition did not.

Strenta and Kleck (1984) conducted a follow-up study in which individuals were given the same three sets described above and then were asked to perform a perceptual segmentation task that required them to mark off each time that they observed a "meaningful action" in the tape. The purpose of the study was to delineate possible perceptual mechanisms that individuals use to distinguish between individuals with and without stigmatizing physical conditions. Strenta and Kleck reported that raters engaged in a significantly finer grain analysis (e.g., more break points) when they thought that they were observing a stigmatized vs. a non-stigmatized individual.

The experimental data and the anecdotal reports support the assertion that physically disabled or impaired persons are prone to interpret social reality in terms of their physical problem. The results of these studies are consistent with the social interaction sequence proposed by Darley and Fazio (1980). However, there is a tenuous leap from these studies to conclusions about people with permanent impairments. Individuals with a long history of physical impairment may learn to evaluate accurately whether or not a specific behavior or social outcome can be attributed to a physical impairment (Kleck and Strenta, 1980).

Behavior of Individuals with Clefts

Academic Performance and Intelligence

In general, individuals with facial clefts tend to score at a significantly lower level than normal children on standardized tests of achievement and teachers' and parents' ratings of achievement (Kommers & Sullivan, 1979; Richman, 1976; Spriestersbach, 1973). However, individuals with clefts finish high school as often as their normal siblings (Demb & Ruess, 1967; Lahti, Rintala, & Soivio, 1974; McWilliams & Paradise, 1973) and obtain jobs of comparable status to their normal siblings (Peter, Chinsky, & Fisher, 1975). However, they do report a significantly lower income, on the average, than their siblings (Peter et al., 1975).

Studies of children with an without clefts suggest that their performance on standardized tests of intelligence is comparable to the normal population of children (Lamb, Wilson, & Leeper, 1972; McWilliams & Mathews, 1979; Pasio & Wilson, 1982; Ruess, 1965; Starr, Chinsky, Carter, & Meier, 1977) except for children who only have clefts of the palate (for a review, see Richman & Eliason, 1982).

In summary, achievement in school does suffer for children with congenital clefts, even though they have average intelligence. These findings suggest that achievement may be affected by what others expect of the children and how they are treated.

Social Behavior

Infants with clefts as young as 3 months old have been observed to be less socially responsive to their mothers than noncleft infants. Cleft infants engaged in less gazing, smiling, and vocalizing than noncleft infants (Field & Vega-Lahr, 1984).

Wasserman et al. (1985) observed toddlers at 9, 12, 18, and 24 months of age. These children performed more poorly on measures of social initiative, focused play, and language production. As they became older, they were increasingly distractable, less compliant, and more reluctant to separate from their mothers.

There are no observational studies of the social behavior of older children with clefts. There are interview and correlational studies that provide some information on the subject. Teachers (Richman, 1978) and parents (Simonds & Heimburger, 1978; Spriestersbach, 1973) rated children with clefts of the lip and palate as more shy than noncleft children. Moreover, individuals with facial clefts tend to marry later and less frequently than their noncleft siblings (McWilliams & Paradise, 1973; Peter & Chinsky, 1974), to participate in fewer social activities, and to depend more on the immediate family for social activities and support (Peter et al., 1975). Investigators have not shown any other consistent behavioral disturbances in cleft lip and palate samples (for a review, see McWilliams, 1982).

The behavioral problems of children with facial clefts seem to be social in nature. They tend to be shy and socially inhibited.

Self-Concept

Self-concept is a complex summary of the multiple views that individuals hold about themselves (Wegner & Vallacher, 1980). It can include views about self-worth, locus of control, evaluation of one's abilities, and body image. Self-concept provides a framework for how individuals relate to others, set goals for themselves, and evaluate personal happiness and satisfaction.

Self-concept of children with facial clefts has been studied. The results of these studies suggest that self-concept is negatively affected in children with clefts as young as 5 years old through adulthood.

Kapp-Simon (1986) compared the responses of 50 5- to 9-years-old with clefts on the Primary Self Concept Inventory (Muller & Leonetti, 1974) with 172 noncleft controls. She reported that children with clefts had a more negative total self-concept and, in particular, a more negative social self-concept. Children with clefts view themselves as lacking the social skills necessary to establish satisfactory relationships.

There have been several studies of the self concepts of older children and adolescents with clefts. Richman (1976) reported that children ages 9 to 14, as compared to matched noncleft controls, described themselves as more anxious, socially withdrawn, less confident, and less socially aggressive using the Quay-Peterson (1967) measure of self-concept.

In a later study, Richman (1983) categorized 30 15- to 18-year-old adolescents into 2 groups depending upon their Minnesota Multiphasic Personality Inventory profiles. One group had individuals with no elevated subscales ($N = 16$; $T \leq 70$) and the other group had individuals with elevated subscales ($N = 14$; $T > 70$). Approximately 47% of the adolescents with clefts had elevations on the three subscales typically associated with anxiety, lack of self-worth, and social avoidance. The greater the adolescents' expressed concern about facial appearance, the higher the score on the social introversion subscale. There was no correlation between severity of cleft impairment (as determined by ratings by peers) and social avoidance. These findings suggest that indivudials who accepted a cleft-related facial impairment as part of their self-concept had fewer concerns about social relationships. Richman, Holmes, and Eliason (1985) reported findings that support the view that the less discrepant individuals' ratings of facial attractiveness were with the ratings of others, the fewer the social adjustment problems.

Similar results for adolescents were reported by Harper and Richman (1978), Kapp (1979), and Starr and Heiserman (1977). Kapp also reported that adolescents with clefts described themselves as less happy in general and expressed dissatisfaction with their success in school. Adolescent females with clefts had a more negative self-concept than males (Kapp, 1979).

The MMPI studies reported above (Harper & Richman, 1978; Richman, 1983) did not uncover significant psychopathology in adolescents with clefts. Rather, many had ongoing problems with anxiety and social concerns.

Brantley and Clifford (1979) reported that children and adolescents with clefts ages 9 to 18, as compared to matched noncleft controls, were significantly more likely to have an external locus of control using the Nowicki-Strickland measure of locus of control (Nowicki & Strickland, 1973) and to be more field-dependent using the rod-and-frame device (Witkin, Lewis, Hertzman, Machover, Meissner, & Wapner, 1954). These findings suggest that not only do children and adolescents view themselves as socially inadequate, but they may also feel helpless and powerless to alter their situation. Moreover, they tend to rely more on internal cues in making social perceptual judgments and therefore may be less likely to perceive social information accurately.

Problems with self-concept have been identified in adult cleft patients. Heller, Tidmarsh, and Pless (1981) conducted a follow-up study of the self-reported social adjustment of 96 adults (ages 18 to 28) born with clefts. Approximately one-third of the respondents reported that they were dissatisfied with their appearance and social life. These individuals reported a dissatisfaction with life in general and in particular with the frequency of their social interactions, social activities, and number of friends. Some degree of dissatisfaction with their current social life was expressed by 56% of all respondents. Only about one-third were "very satisfied." Twenty-four percent felt that they had few friends and reported that they left the house infrequently. Nearly half were dissatisfied with the quality of their leisure activities.

Conclusions and Implications

The expectancy-behavior confirmation theoretical model of the social interaction sequence (Darley & Fazio, 1980) appears to be a useful organizing framework for the diverse social psychological literature related to cleft lip and palate. The model could also serve as a useful conceptual tool to guide clinical practice and future research. Suggestions are given for how the model could be applied to develop clinical interventions and to guide and interpret future research.

Clinical Implications

Changing the Face: Is Surgery an Answer?

Surgery to improve the appearance of facial clefts has been the treatment of choice for decades (Bardach, Morris, Olin, McDermott-Murray, Mooney, & Bardach, 1984). In theory, a reduction of the impairment should modify the negative expectations associated with facial impairment and impact on the social interaction sequence. The rationale for the surgery is dominantly aesthetic—that social psychological benefits are associated with the reduction of the facial impairment. Elliot, Bull, James, and Lansdown (1986) showed children and adults (ages 6 to 35 years old) before- and after-surgery photographs of young adults, several of whom had cleft-related impairments. Subjects were asked to rate photographs for friendliness, happiness, intelligence, social skill, and attractiveness. They reported that children younger than 11 had no differences in their ratings of pre- and postsurgical photographs. Older children and adults rated the "after" faces as more attractive, intelligent, and happy. These findings suggest that surgery may positively alter expectations for individuals with facial impairments in older children and adults. There are no other known studies of the effects of surgery for facial clefts on other aspects of the social interaction sequence.

There are other pre- and postsurgical studies of more severe types of facial impairments that suggest that surgery may not influence social expectations but may positively influence self-concept (Arndt, Lefebvre, Travis, & Munro, 1986; Lefebvre, Travis, Arndt, & Munro, 1986).

Changing the Behavior of People with Facial Impairments: Social Skills Training

Rumsey, Bull, and Gahagan (1986) proposed that good social skills might moderate the negative social reaction to facial impairment. They conducted a preliminary experimental study to test their hypothesis. An actor was trained to conduct interviews in which he was either not made up or was made up with a severe facial port-wine stain. In half the interviews, he used good social skills (e.g., appropriate levels of eye contact, head nods, etc.); in the other half, he demonstrated poor social skills (e.g., monotonous tone of voice, low levels of eye contact, and lack of body tone). Interactants rated the actor more favorable when he used a high level of social skill, regardless of the presence or absence of a facial impairment. The interaction between facial impairment and level of social skill was not significant. Observers of the videotaped interactions rated the interactants in the high social skill group as friendlier, more likeable, interesting, competent, and warm. They also had shorter response latencies and smiled more frequently. These findings seem promising to individuals with cleft impairments who have consistently been reported as socially withdrawn and shy (McWilliams, 1982; Richman & Eliason, 1982; Tobiasen, 1984).

Child and Family Education and Counseling

The clinical management of a child with a facial cleft is typically done by a team of specialists consisting of dentist, speech pathologist, and surgeon. In recent years, clinical psychologists have been added to teams as recognition of the psychological adjustment problems associated with clefts has increased (Broder & Richman, 1987). In addition to the regular assessment, diagnostic, and treatment role of a clinical psychologist on the cleft lip and palate team, the research described above suggests an essential education and counseling role. Parents and children may benefit from preparation for the negative social reactions and education on how to react. For example, parents may see strangers "freezing" in front of their children and feel inhibited in their response to the children. They may need to be encouraged to continue to allow the children to have regular opportunities for social exchange and not restrict the children to the home or other nonthreatening situations. Parents may also benefit in open discussions of how to improve their children's appearance (e.g., clothing, hairstyle).

Parents may need to be encouraged to expose the child as early as possible to regular peer activities. In this way, children may have opportunities to learn age-appropriate social skills, gain self-confidence, and to desensitize themselves as well as others to the socially negative aspects of their appearance and speech. The earlier children develop peer relationships, the sooner they may learn to deal with questions, teasing, and staring. Children can be taught when they are 2 to 4 years old how to answer simple questions about appearance (e.g., "I was born with a split in my lip and the doctors had to fix it when I was a baby").

Not only do children and families need education and counseling about clefts, but teachers and schools often benefit (Mitchell, Lott, & Pannbacker, 1984). Parents can be encouraged to educate teachers about clefts. There are many opportunities to educate classmates about clefts in report writing and science projects. Members of cleft and palate teams can visit classrooms and teacher workshops to provide "expert" support. Education of this kind can promote empathy and sensitivity in an open and honest atmosphere and possibly minimize teasing and gossip.

Implications for Research

There are almost no studies of the actual behavior of children, adolescents, and adults with facial clefts in controlled laboratory situations. Studies similar to the work of Snyder et al. (1977) are badly needed in this area. In the Snyder et al. study, the self-fulfilling nature of the facial attractiveness stereotype was demonstrated in a simple laboratory study. Similar studies need to be done with individuals who have facial impairments to examine if the theory applies to them and, if so, how.

Second, previous research has employed relatively simple approaches to psychosocial adjustment. One or two variables may be manipulated. It is far more likely that a range of psychosocial, medical-surgical, and speech factors mediate adjustment. Researchers should consider factors such as severity of physical handicap, socioeconomic status, social support, developmental delays, coping style, and marital and family factors when studying psychosocial adjustment of children and adults with cleft lip and palate.

Third, there is almost no empirical understanding of the stressors impinging on cleft lip and palate children and adults and their families, how they cope with their stressors, and the social psychological costs and benefits of the stressors. This knowledge is essential for effectively intervening and therefore improving the psychological prognosis for the children and their families.

Fourth, little is known about how the severity of a cleft impairment influences social psychological adjustment. Common sense suggests that the more severe the impairment, the more difficult the social psychological adjustment. However, Macgregor et al. (1953) have observed the opposite to be true, and Tobiasen's (in preparation) experimental work suggests that it may be true for relatively attractive patients but not for unattractive patients. Further research in this area is extremely important because the decision to seek secondary surgical treatment for facial clefts is often the result of concerns about the aesthetic acceptability of appearance. Yet there are almost no data to show that quality of life is improved following secondary surgical repair and long-term treatment of dental and speech problems for children with clefts of the lip and palate (Bardach et al., 1984).

Summary

The purpose of this chapter has been to summarize and interpret the social psychological literature on cleft lip and palate using the expectancy-behavior confirmation theory as a conceptual framework. The results of this analysis support the view that a facial impairment such as a cleft has consistent negative effects on the social interaction sequence. Implications for clinical treatment and research have been discussed.

Clearly, social psychological factors play a central role in the habilitation of patients with facial impairments. The importance of these factors has been relatively neglected by social scientists. Research in this area offers challenging opportunities not only to study the social psychological effects of atypical appearance, but the effects of actually changing an individual's appearance. As such, this area offers overlooked, but nevertheless unique and compelling, opportunities for research in health psychology.

Acknowledgments. The preparation of this article was supported in part by: R.L. Smith Research Center, NIH Grant #HD02528; Sutherland Facial Rehabilitation Endowment Fund #83652: NIDR Grant #R29 DE08153-02.

References

Abel, T. (1952). Personality characteristics of the facially disfigured. *Transactions of the New York Academy of Sciences, 4,* 325–329.

Adams, G.R. (1977). Physical attractiveness research: Toward a developmental social psychology of beauty. *Human Development, 20,* 217–239.

Arndt, E., Lefebvre, A., Travis, F., & Munro, I. (1986). Fact and fantasy: Psychosocial consequences of facial surgery in 24 Down Syndrome children. *British Journal of Plastic Surgery, 39,* 498–504.

Bardach, J., Morris, H., Olin, W., McDermott-Murray, J., Mooney, M., & Bardach, E. (1984). Late results of multi-disciplinary management of unilateral cleft lip and palate. *Annals of Plastic Surgery, 12,* 235–242.

Brantley, H.J., & Clifford, E. (1979). Maternal and child locus of control and field dependence in cleft palate children. *Cleft Palate Journal, 16,* 183–187.

Broder, H., & Richman, L. (1987). An examination of mental health services offered by cleft/craniofacial teams. *Cleft Palate Journal, 24,* 158–162.

Chicago Illinois Municipal Code (1966).

Clifford, E. (1969). Parental ratings of cleft palate infants. *Cleft Palate Journal, 6,* 235–244.

Clifford, E. (1979). Psychological aspects of cleft lip and palate. In K. Bzoch (Ed.), *Communicative disorders related to cleft lip and palate* (2nd Ed.). Boston: Little, Brown & Co.

Cooper, J., & Fazio, R.H. (1979). The formation and persistence of attitudes that support intergroup conflict. In W.G. Austin & S. Worschel (Eds.), *The social psychology of intergroup relations.* Monterey, CA: Brooks/Cole.

Darley, J.M., & Fazio, R.H. (1980). Expectancy confirmation processes arising in the social interaction sequence. *American Psychologist, 35,* 867–881.

Davis, F. (1961). Deviance disavowal: The management of strained interaction by the visibly handicapped. *Social Problems, 9,* 120–132.

Demb, N., & Ruess, A. (1967). High school drop out rate for cleft palate patients. *Cleft Palate Journal, 4,* 327–333.

Elliott, M., Bull, R., James, D., & Lansdown, R. (1986). Children's and adults' reactions to photographs taken before and after surgery. *Journal of Maxillofacial Surgery, 14,* 18–21.

Field, T.M., & Vega-Lahr, N. (1984). Early interactions between infants with craniofacial anomalies and their mothers. *Infant Behavior and Development, 7,* 527–530.

Glass, L., Starr, C.D., Stewart, R.E., & Hodge, S.E. (1981). Identikit model II—A potential tool for judging cosmetic appearance. *Cleft Palate Journal, 18,* 147–151.

Goffman, E. (1963). *Stigma: Notes on the management of a spoiled identity.* Englewood Cliffs, NJ: Prentice-Hall.

Harper, D.C., & Richman, L.C. (1978). Personality profiles of physically impaired adolescents. *Journal of Clinical Psychology, 34,* 636–642.

Heller, A., Tidmarsh, W., & Pless, I.B. (1981). The psychological functioning of young adults born with cleft lip or palate. *Clinical Pediatrics, 20,* 459–465.

Hobbs, J. (Ed.) (1980). *Cleft lip and palate from birth to three years.* Pittsburgh, PA: Cleft Palate Foundation.

Kapp, K. (1979). Self concept of the cleft lip and/or palate child. *Cleft Palate Journal, 16,* 171–176.

Kapp-Simon, K. (1986). Self concept of primary and school age children with cleft lip, cleft palate, or both. *Cleft Palate Journal, 23,* 24–27.

Kleck, R., & Strenta, A. (1980). Perceptions of the impact of negatively valued physical characteristics on social interaction. *Journal of Personality and Social Psychology, 39,* 861–873.

Kommers, M., & Sullivan, M. (1979). Written language skills of children with cleft palate. *Cleft Palate Journal, 16,* 81–85.

Lahti, A., Rintala, A., & Soivio, A. (1974). Educational level of patients with cleft lip and palate. *Cleft Palate Journal, 11,* 36–40.

Lamb, M., Wilson, F., & Leeper, H. (1972). A comparison of selected cleft palate children and their siblings on the variables of intelligence, hearing loss, and visual-perceptual-motor abilities. *Cleft Palate Journal, 9,* 218–228.

Landsdown, R., & Polak, L. (1975). A study of the psychological effects of facial deformity in children. *Child Care Health and Development, 1,* 85–91.

Langlois, J.H., & Stephan, C.W. (1981). Beauty and the beast: The role of physical attractiveness in the development of peer relations and social behavior. In S. Brehm, S.M. Kassin, & F.X. Gibbons (Eds.), *Developmental social psychology: Theory and research.* New York: Oxford University Press.

Lefebvre, A., Travis, F., Arndt, E., & Munro, I. (1986). A psychiatric profile before and after reconstructive surgery in children with Apert's Syndrome. *British Journal of Plastic Surgery, 39,* 510–513.

Lucker, G.W., Graber, L.W., & Pietromonoco, P. (1981). The importance of dentofacial appearance in facial esthetics. A signal detection approach. *Basic and Applied Social Psychology, 2,* 261–274.

Macgregor, F.C. (1982). Social and psychological considerations in plastic surgery. *Clinics in Plastic Surgery, 9,* 283–288.

Macgregor, F.C., Abel, T.M., Brynt, A., Lauer, E., & Weissmann, S. (1953). *Facial deformities and plastic surgery: A psychosocial study.* Springfield, IL: Charles C. Thomas.

McWilliams, B.J. (1982). Social and psychological problems associated with cleft palate. In F.C. Macgregor (Ed.), *Clinics in Plastic Surgery.* Philadelphia: Saunders.

McWilliams, B.J., & Matthews, H.P. (1979). A comparison of intelligence and social maturity in children with unilateral complete cleft and those with isolated cleft palates. *Cleft Palate Journal, 16,* 363–372.

McWilliams, B.J., & Paradise, L.P. (1973). Educational occupational, and marital status of cleft palate adults. *Cleft Palate Journal, 10,* 223–229.

Merton, R. (1957). *Social theory and social structure.* Glencoe, IL: Free Press.

Mitchell, C.K., Lott, R., & Pannbacker, M. (1984). Perceptions about cleft palate held by school personnel: Suggestions for in-service training development. *Cleft Palate Journal, 21,* 308–8312.

Muller, D.G., & Leonetti, R. (1974). *Primary self-concept inventory test manual.* Austin, TX: Learning Concepts.

Munro, I. (1981). The psychological effects of surgical treatment of facial deformity. In G. Lucker, K. Ribbens, & J. McNamara (Eds.), *Psychological aspects of facial form.* Ann Arbor, MI: University of Michigan Press.

Mussen, P.H., & Barker, R.G. (1944). Attitudes toward cripples. *Journal of Abnormal and Social Psychology, 39,* 351–355.

Myerson, L. (1963). Somatopsychology of physical disability. In W.M. Cruickshank (Ed.), *Psychology of exceptional children and youth.* Englewood Clifts, NJ: Prentice-Hall.

Nowicki, S., & Strickland, R. (1973). A locus of control scale for children. *Journal of Consulting Clinical Psychology, 40,* 148–154.

Pasio, J.A., & Wilson, L.F. (1982). Incidence and type of impairment in selected psychological variables in cleft lip and palate children. *Cleft Palate Journal, 19,* 245.

Peter, J., & Chinsky, R. (1974). Sociological aspects of cleft palate adults: I. Marriage. *Cleft Palate Journal, 11,* 295–309.

Peter, J., Chinsky, R., & Fisher, M. (1975). Sociological aspects of cleft palate adults: IV. Social integration. *Cleft Palate Journal, 12,* 304–310.

Podol, J., & Salvia, J. (1976). Effects of visibility of a prepalatal cleft on the evaluation of speech. *Cleft Palate Journal, 13,* 361–366.

Quay, H.C., & Peterson, D.R. (1967). *Manual for the behavior problem checklist.* Champaign, IL: University of Illinois.

Richardson, S.A. (1970). Age and sex differences in values toward handicaps. *Journal of Health and Social Behavior, 11,* 207–214.

Richardson, S.A., Goodman, N., Hastorf, A., & Dornbusch, S. (1961). Cultural uniformity in reaction to physical disabilities. *American Sociological Review, 26,* 241–247.

Richman, L. (1976). Behavior and achievement of cleft palate children. *Cleft Palate Journal, 13,* 4–10.

Richman, L. (1978). The effects of facial disfigurement on teachers' perceptions of ability in cleft palate children. *Cleft Palate Journal, 15,* 155–160.

Richman, L. (1983). Self-reported social, speech, and facial concerns and personality adjustment of adolescents with cleft lip and palate. *Cleft Palate Journal, 20,* 108–112.

Richman, L.C., & Eliason, M. (1982). Psychological characteristics of children with cleft lip and palate: Intellectual, achievement, behavioral, and personality variables. *Cleft Palate Journal, 19,* 251–257.

Richman, L.C., & Harper, D. (1978). School adjustment of children with observable disabilities. *Journal of Abnormal Child Psychology, 6,* 11–18.

Richman, L.C., Holmes, C.S., & Eliason, M.J. (1985). Adolescents with cleft lip and palate: Self-perceptions of appearance and behavior related to personality adjustment. *Cleft Palate Journal, 22,* 93–96.

Robinson, E., Eyberg, S., & Ross, A.W. (1980). The standardization of an inventory of child conduct problem disorders. *Clinical and Child Psychology, 9,* 22–26.

Rosenthal, R. (1974) *On the social psychology of the self-fulfilling prophecy: Further evidence for Pygmalion effects and their mediating mechanisms.* New York: MSS Modular Publications, Module 53.

Rosenthal, R., & Jacobson, C.F. (1968). *Pygmalion in the classroom: Teacher expectations and pupils' intellectual development.* New York: Holt, Rinehart, & Winston.

Ruess, A. (1965). A comparative study of cleft palate children, and their siblings. *Journal of Clinical Psychology, 21,* 354–360.

Rumsey, N. (1983). *Psychological problems associated with facial disfigurement.* Unpublished doctoral thesis, North East London Polytechnic, London.

Rumsey, N., Bull, R., & Gahagan, D. (1982). The effect of facial disfigurement on the proxemic behavior of the general public. *Journal of Applied Social Psychology, 12,* 137–150.

Rumsey, N., Bull, R., & Gahagan, D. (1986). A preliminary study of the potential of social skills training for improving the quality of social interaction for the facially disfigured. *Social Behavior, 1,* 143–145.

Sameroff, A. (1975). Transactional models in early social relations. *Human Development, 18,* 65–79.

Shaw, W. (1981). Folklore surrounding facial deformity and the origins of facial prejudice. *British Journal of Plastic Surgery, 34,* 237–246.

Shaw, W., & Orth, D. (1981). The influence of children's dento-facial appearance on their social attractiveness as judged by peers and lay adults. *American Journal of Orthodontics, 79,* 399–415.

Simonds, J.F., & Heimburger, R.E. (1978). Psychiatric evaluation of youth with cleft lip-palate matched with a control group. *Cleft Palate Journal, 15,* 193–201.

Snyder, M., Tanke, E.D., & Berscheid, E. (1977). Social perception and interpersonal behavior: On the self-fulfilling nature of social stereotypes. *Journal of Personality and Social Psychology, 35,* 656–666.

Spriestersbach, D. (1973). *Psychological aspects of the cleft palate problem* (Vol. 1 and 2) Iowa City, IA: University of Iowa Press.

Starr, P., Chinsky, R., Canter, H., & Meier, A. (1977). Mental, motor, and social behavior of infants with cleft lip and/or palate. *Cleft Palate Journal, 14,* 140–147.

Starr, P., & Heiserman, K. (1977). Acceptance of disability by teenagers with oral-facial clefts. *Rehabilitation Counseling Bulletin, 20,* 198–201.

Strenta, A., & Kleck, R. (1984). Physical disability and the perception of social interaction: It's not what you look at but how you look at it. *Personality and Social Psychology Bulletin, 10,* 279–288.

Tobiasen, J. (1984). Psychosocial correlates of congenital facial clefts: A conceptualization and model. *Cleft Palate Journal, 21,* 131–139.

Tobiasen, J. (1987). Judgments of facial deformity. *Cleft Palate Journal, 24,* 323–327.

Tobiasen, J. (in preparation). *Ratings of facial impairments: Aesthetics or stigma?*

Tobiasen, J., & Hiebert, J. (1984). Parents' tolerance for conduct problems of cleft palate children. *Cleft Palate Journal, 21,* 82–85.

Tobiasen, J., & Hiebert, J. (1988). Reliability of aesthetic judgments of cleft impairment. *Cleft Palate Journal, 25,* 313–316.

Van Demark, D., & Van Demark, A. (1970). Speech and socio-vocational aspects of individuals with cleft palate. *Cleft Palate Journal, 7,* 284–299.

Varni, J.W., & Wallender, J.L. (1988). Pediatric chronic disabilities: Hemophilia and spian bifida as examples. In D.K. Routh (Ed.), *Handbook of pediatric psychology.* New York: Guilford Press.

Wasserman, G.A., Allen, R., & Solomon, C.R. (1985). At risk toddlers and their mothers: The special case of physical handicap. *Child Development, 56,* 73–83.

Wegner, D., & Vallacher, R.R. (1980). *The self in social psychology.* New York: Oxford University Press.

Weinberg, N., & Santana, R. (1978). Comic books: Champion of the disabled stereotype. *Rehabilitation Literature, 39,* 327–331.

Witkin, H.A., Lewis, H.C., Hertzman, M., Machover, K., Meissner, P.B., & Wapner, S. (1954). *Personality through perception: An experimental and clinical study.* New York: Harper.

World Health Organization (1980). *International classification of impairments, disabilities, and handicaps.* Geneva.

Wright, B. (1983). *Physical disability: A psychological approach* (2nd Ed.). New York: Harper & Row.

Zanna, M.P., & Pack, S.J. (1975). On the self-fulfilling nature of apparent sex differences in behavior. *Journal of Experimental Social Psychology, 11,* 583–591.

Zanna, M.P., Sheras, P., Cooper, J., & Shaw, C. (1975). Pygmalion and Galatea: The interactive effect of teacher and student expectancies. *Journal of Experimental Social Psychology, 11,* 279–287.

13
A Developmental Framework for Psychosocial Research on Young Children with Craniofacial Anomalies

MATTHEW L. SPELTZ, HOLLY GALBREATH, AND MARK T. GREENBERG

Young children with craniofacial anomalies (CFA) and their families undergo a succession of extremely stressful events through the first five years of life, beginning with the parents' awareness of and coping with the infants' disfigurement at birth, followed by extraordinary caregiving demands (e.g., feeding problems), multiple diagnostic procedures, and the initial reactions of friends and relatives to the babies' appearance. Next come one or more surgeries with varying and uncertain degrees of restorative outcome and associated hospitalizations. Finally, the family must anticipate and prepare for the children's inevitable exposure to possibly negative peer reactions in daycare or preschool. How do these children and their families react to and cope with these extreme and repeated stressors in early life? What influence do these early events have on the developing parent–child relationship and children's internalization of the caregiving environment? Are such factors predictive of the children's later resilience or vulnerability to negative social responses?

At present there are few answers to questions like these in the literature on craniofacial anomalies. This may be due in part to the very small number of studies of CFA infants or young children and also to the lack of a developmental model for understanding what to look for at this early stage of life. Whereas developmental models applied to other high-risk groups have tended to emphasize individual differences and multifactorial causation (e.g., Belsky, 1984), much of the research on CFA has been organized in relation to the study of *group* differences in psychosocial adjustment and the "main effect" of facial appearance on interpersonal behavior. Although these latter areas of research have contributed strongly to our understanding of the processes by which societal expectations and interactional feedback systems may influence the behavior of older children and adolescents with CFA, the social psychological orientation has not been as helpful in explaining individual differences in young children's initial vulnerability to social expectations.

The primary objective of this chapter is to formulate a developmental model that will serve as a framework for identifying potential "predictor variables" early in life that might explain the range of psychosocial outcomes in the CFA population. This model will emphasize the importance of children's early social relationships on the integration of cognition, behavior, and affect during the first five years of life. Within this model, infants' craniofacial birth defect is viewed as but one factor in a broad range of medical, social, and ecological factors potentially affecting the course of the children's psychosocial development. Research and theory in support of this model will be reviewed, and some of our preliminary research on the application of this model to CFA toddlers and mothers will be presented (Speltz, Armsden, & Clarren, 1990).

A secondary objective of this chapter is to examine closely the evidence for the existence of "internalizing" (or inhibited) types of behavior problems in school-age and older CFA children and the presence of parent–child relationship problems in this population. The description of CFA children as "shy and inhibited" with rejecting or overprotective parents is ubiquitous in research reports and case studies and is commonly cited as a key rationale for the further study of these children. Yet several studies have found no differences between children with CFA and matched controls in adjustment or relationship functioning (see Clifford, 1983); others have found evidence of "externalizing" (or disruptive) behavior problems that are quite inconsistent with the prevailing view of these children. Thus, we have felt the need for a comprehensive and methodologically detailed review of the studies in this area, with the objective of discovering what outcome variables in relation to "adjustment" are important for the longitudinal study of children with CFA. This will be undertaken first, followed by a presentation of the developmental model described above.

Research on the Psychosocial Adjustment of Children with CFA

Among the several procedural and sample variations in studies examining the psychosocial adjustment of CFA children (i.e., age, sex, CFA diagnosis, instrument used to assess adjustment), one important variable is the identity of the "informant"—the person who provided the information used to determine adjustment (i.e., self, parent, teacher, diagnostician, or trained observer). Several factors support the centrality of the informant (or observer) variable in examining the relative adjustment of CFA children. First, in social psychological formulations of "psychopathology" (Ullmann & Krasner, 1975) the *labeling* of undesired or problematic child behavior by caregivers or others is considered to be as important as the behavior itself in defining the construct of maladjustment. Second, in the measurement of child adjustment generally, the reports of different informants (e.g., child, parent, teacher) on checklists or during interviews correlate only modestly (Achenbach & Edelbrock, 1981). In this regard, Richman (1978) found that the parents and teachers of cleft lip children had significantly different perceptions of child adjustment, with parents tending to report more favorable impressions. Third, and perhaps most important, observer biases related to facial appearance (see Langlois, this volume) would be expected to affect the informant's perception of the CFA child as "deviant" or maladjusted. Just as observers are known to attribute undesirable or problematic characteristics to children with unattractive facial characteristics (Adams, 1980), an "observer" of a child with CFA—whether it be self or caregiver—may be inclined to attribute negative affect or problem behavior to such a child regardless of the objective or observed indications of such behavior.

The reported adjustment of children with CFA might then be at least partially "in the eye of the beholder"—that is, dependent upon *who* is doing the observing under *what* conditions of observation. In view of this possibility, we have reviewed the following studies in relation to who is the provider of information, beginning with self- (or child-) assessed behavioral and emotional status, followed by the reports of parents, teachers, professional diagnosticians, and, finally, trained observers watching "live" or videotaped interactions. Throughout the remainder of the chapter, the term "internalizing" will refer to shy/withdrawn or anxious behavior and the term "externalizing" to disruptive, impulsive, or aggressive behavior, these behavior patterns being the most stable and frequently replicated dimensions in factor analytic studies of child behavior adjustment (Achenbach & Edelbrock, 1981; Quay, 1979).

Self-Reported Adjustment

The majority of studies in this area have focused on self-concept measures, but some have also included specific behavior problem checklists or personality measures. Overall, this research has produced few differences between CFA and typical children. Starr (1978), for example, gave a behavior problem checklist and a self-esteem scale to 72 cleft adolescents and 48 controls matched for age, sex, and socioeconomic status (SES). The two groups did not differ in self-esteem; but on the problem behavior checklist, cleft children reported less aggressiveness than did their nonimpaired peers.

Kapp (1979) used the Piers-Harris Self-Concept Scale to measure the self-evaluations of 34 cleft lip and/or palate children (ages 11 to 13) with a matched normative group. No difference in global self-concept (total scores) was obtained, although on specific subscales, girls with clefts reported greater anxiousness and general unhappiness and dissatisfaction than did same-sex controls. In a follow-up study with much younger children (ages 5 to 9), Kapp-Simon (1986) gave the Primary Self-Concept Inventory to cleft lip and/or palate children and a control group consisting of all age mates in two elementary schools. The results were analyzed in terms of the relative frequency of scores falling below the 50th percentile for the norms of this test (defined by the test authors as indicating "undesirably low self-concept"). No sex differences were found in this study. Although a significant group difference was found—with 54% of the cleft children vs. 42% of the control group falling below the 50th percentile—the scores of the cleft group were obviously very close to the norms for this instrument. In another study using elementary school children, Richman and Harper (1979) gave a pictorial personality measure (Missouri Children's Picture Series) to 55 cleft children and a group of children with orthopedic handicaps. Although the cleft children reported more internalizing characteristics than did children in the orthopedic group, their scores also did not differ significantly from the means for this test in normative samples.

Brantly and Clifford (1979) administered their own extensive battery of behavioral adjustment instruments and performance tests to adolescents with clefts, obese adolescents, and adolescents with no identified problems (ages 10 to 18). These groups were not matched, and the nonproblem group contained a relatively higher proportion of high SES families. Of 18 body-image and 15 self-concept variables, significant group differences were found on only 2: cleft children reported a higher degree of self-esteem than the obese children and a lower degree of perceived parental acceptance at birth than did children in either the normal or obese groups. The authors suggested that the experience of having coped successfully with a cleft generated heightened self-esteem in these youngsters.

Finally, the MMPI has been used in several studies to assess self-reported personality functioning in cleft adolescents (e.g., Richman & Harper, 1978). Control groups of typical children were not used in this research; instead, scale scores were compared with norms and with the scores for groups of children with orthopedic impairments. Taken together, these studies found that the responses of cleft children did not deviate significantly from the orthopedic groups nor from the MMPI norms (Richman & Eliason, 1982).

Teacher-Reported Information

Richman and his colleagues have conducted a series of comparative studies employing teacher reports of behavioral adjustment (Harper, Richman, & Snider, 1980; Richman, 1976; Richman & Harper, 1978), all using the Quay and Peterson (1967) Behavior Problem Checklist (BPC). The BPC provides scores on two major factors called Personality Disorder and Conduct Disorder, corresponding to the Achenbach and Edelbrock (1981) internalizing and externalizing dimensions, respectively. In the Richman (1976) investigation, teacher BPC reports were gathered for 44 cleft children (29 cleft palate only; 15 cleft lip and palate) and 44 matched controls ages 9 to 14. Cleft children had significantly higher scores on the internalizing scale than controls but did not differ on the externalizing dimension. These results were replicated by Richman and Harper (1978), who also found that their sample of 39 cleft children (ages 10 to 15) scored significantly higher on the BPC than did children with cerebral palsy. Harper et al. (1980) examined older children (ages 10 to 18) and related their degree of impairment (extent of facial disfigurement or physical immobility) to teacher BPC scores. These findings were inconsistent with the previous studies: Cleft children had significantly *higher* externalizing scores than both the BPC normal standardization group and the cerebral palsy group. The authors attributed this finding to the older age of the subjects in this study.

In another study of teacher-reported behavior, Brantley and Clifford (1979) administered the National Health Survey Questionnaire to the teachers of 44 cleft children and 61 controls. No significant differences were found on two factor scores, one pertaining to general emotional adjustment (an internalizing scale) and the other to the presence of specific behavior problems (an externalizing scale).

Parent-Reported Adjustment

We are aware of only two studies that have gathered systematic parent reports of child adjustment (vs. anecdotal or interview-based information), and these did not reveal reliable group differences. Simonds and Heimburger (1978) gave a 120-item behavior checklist (presumably constructed by the investigators) to assess the adjustment of 114 cleft children (ages 6 to 18). Explicit distinctions were made in CFA diagnostic status by the formation of male and female cleft lip and palate and cleft palate only groups. A control group consisting of children from a primary medical practice, matched for age, SES, and sex, was assessed in the same manner. Analyses of the CFA diagnostic subgroups produced no significant differences. Significant differences between the combined CFA subgroups and controls were found on 4 of the 120 behavior checklist items (e.g., clefts were rated as more "dependent" than controls; controls were reported as verbalizing more negative self-evaluations than clefts). However, this finding is qualified by the statistical procedure used: Since 120 separate analyses were conducted, 6 of these could occur by chance at an alpha level of .05.

In the other parent-report study, Tobiason and Hiebert (1984) gave the Eyberg Behavior Problem Checklist to the parents of 41 cleft lip and palate children, ages 2 to 12. With the exception of two items (cries easily and wets the bed), the Eyberg scale focuses exclusively on externalizing problems (aggressiveness, tantruming, noncompliance). Tobiason and Hiebert compared the parent ratings in the cleft sample with scores from the standardization group of the Eyberg and found no significant differences on total scores or individual items.

Reports of Diagnosticians

In an early and often-cited study involving psychiatric diagnosticians, Gluck, McWilliams, Wylie, and Conkwright (1965) used child mental health clinicians to review the case records of 50 children with unspecified clefts who had been brought to a medical clinic and 292 children who had been seen in a child guidance clinic for various psychiatric symptoms. Case records were compared by using a structured review process that tallied presenting problems and clinicians' identification of behavioral symptoms. Although higher frequencies of shyness and enuresis among the cleft children were reported, this finding is qualified by the lack of comparative statistics and a matched comparison group. In a much better-designed study with matched cleft and nonproblem control groups (Simonds & Heimburger, 1978), child psychiatrists used a semistructured diagnostic interview to evaluate psychiatric status. Chi-square analyses of psychiatric diagnosis frequency indicated that there were no differences between the cleft and control groups, nor were there differences in psychiatric diagnosis between CFA diagnostic subgroups (cleft lip and palate vs. cleft palate only).

Two studies involving cleft infants included a diagnostician's evaluation of infant social and emotional behavior. Starr, Chinsky, Canter, and Meier (1977) administered the Infant Behavior Record (IBR) from the Bayley Scales of Infant Development (as well as the Bayley exam itself) to 75 infants with cleft lip and/or palate at ages 6, 12, 18, and 24 months. The IBR consists of 30 rating scales of examiner-observed infant social and behavioral characteristics during the testing situation (attention, focus, task persistence, sociability, etc.). In this study, two trained observers completed these ratings with 90% interrater reliability. Although the cognitive and motor scores for the cleft infants did not differ significantly from the Bayley normative sample, examiner ratings of passivity were significantly higher than the norms. In a similar study, Fox, Lynch, and Brookshire (1978) gave the Denver Developmental Scale to 24 cleft palate infants and toddlers, ages 2 to 33 months. The study also utilized a matched control group of children from a well-child clinic. Cleft infants and control group infants were found to differ on three of the four subscales of the Denver, including the personal-social scale, which measures play skills, imitation, feeding, dressing, self-care, and ability to separate from mother.

Assessment of Adjustment Through Direct Observation

The use of direct observation in the behavioral study of CFA children and infants is relatively new. In the studies conducted thus far, child or infant behavior during interaction with the mother has been videotaped, with trained observers subsequently using a prescribed coding system to count or rate targeted behaviors. In the first of these, Long and Dalston (1982) examined the gestorial communication skills of 10 1-year-olds with cleft lip and palate and a matched group of nonimpaired infants during interaction with their mothers. Frequency analyses of such behaviors as pointing, showing, giving, reaching, and so on revealed no significant differences between groups. Field and Vega-Lahr (1984) videotaped 12 3-month-old infants with cleft lip and palate and matched controls, in this case rating the infants' activity level, head orientation, gaze behavior, facial expressiveness, fussiness, and vocalizations. The CFA infants were found to show significantly less smiling, turning, and looking at their mothers than the controls. Finally, Barden, Ford, Jensen, Rogers-Salyer, and Salyer (1989) observed the behavior of five infants with wide-ranging craniofacial anomalies (Aperts Syndrome, Crouzons Syndrome, microfacial microsomia, unilateral and bilateral clefts) and five nonimpaired infants during interactions with their mothers. The results of this study were consistent with those of Field and Vega-Lahr: CFA infants were less likely to smile/laugh, vocalize, and show head orientations toward their mothers.

Summary of Psychosocial Adjustment Literature

Of the 18 comparisons reviewed in this section involving a CFA and normative group, half produced differences in the direction of greater internalizing behavior in the CFA group, using the term "internalizing" very broadly in order to accommodate substantial age differences (e.g., interpreting both the passivity/unresponsiveness of infants and the shyness/low self-esteem of adolescents as internalizing). In seven studies, no group differences in behavioral or emotional functioning were evident, and the remaining two comparisons found significant group differences in a direction inconsistent with an internalizing pattern (Brantly & Clifford, 1979; Harper et al., 1980). These very mixed findings are not surprising in view of the tremendous sample and procedural variations across studies, but it is significant that the "shy and inhibited" personality characterization of CFA children is not supported by half the studies in this area.

Can we discern any patterns that might distinguish the studies with positive vs. negative findings? Among the different informants used in these studies, self- and parent-reports were the least likely to indicate behavioral/emotional differences, and trained observers were the most likely to find differences. This can be interpreted in one of two ways: CFA children and their parents might be inclined to minimize their reports of problems as an adaptive response to the social biases and expectations regarding facial appearance described by Tobiason (this volume) and others (perhaps a "defensive" response set). On the other hand, it may be that the influence of negative social attributions is inversely related to the familiarity of the observer with the child and that the number of positive findings involving trained observers is the product of self-fulfilling prophecy effects—that is, student observers may *expect* that CFA children are less emotionally stable or well-adjusted than children with typical appearance and their ratings may reflect this expectation more than any true difference in the overt behaviors or emotions of the children rated.

Age may also be an important factor. Group differences in adjustment were found more frequently in studies of CFA toddlers and infants (four out of five studies reviewed in this age group found differences) as compared to older children. This may indicate that problems in the behavioral/emotional development of CFA children are most prominent during the first five years, dissipating with age. This explanation is probably too simplistic, however, as there may be several changes between infancy and adolescence in the overt display of problem behavior in vulnerable or high-risk children, including those with CFA. The early passivity of infancy may give way to an exaggeration of the preschool tendency for disruptive and noncompliant behavior, followed by a return to behavioral inhibition during the elementary school years, when beginning peer relationships are tenuous. Among vulnerable children, this pattern of behavior may, in turn, change to exaggerated "acting out" during the mid- and late adolescent period (Harper et al., 1980) followed by a return to greater inhibition during early adulthood (Bjornsson & Agustsdottir, 1987; Heller, Tidmarsh, & Pless, 1981; McWilliams & Paradise, 1973). Thus, there may be continuity in certain underlying emotional and cognitive processes (e.g., insecurity, low self-esteem) that are observed in discontinuous forms of overt expression throughout any child's development (Sroufe & Rutter, 1984). Unfortunately, the relative influence of age and type of informant cannot be discerned from the studies conducted thus far, as studies involving younger children are also the ones in which trained observers were the informants.

The studies reviewed in this section typify much of the psychosocial research on craniofacial anomalies over the past 30 years in their focus on the relative adjustment of CFA and normative groups, using measures of central tendency as the basis of comparison (e.g., mean scores on a behavior problem checklist). The group comparison approach has provided us with limited information about individual differences in psychosocial outcomes. It is not clear from these studies what percentages of the CFA samples have fallen into clinically significant problem status subgroups (e.g., scoring above the 90th percentile) or to what extent the mean group differences that have been found were influenced by the extreme scores of a few outliers. We know very little from this research about children with CFA who are functioning very well and how they might compare with their normative counterparts (e.g., do the best-functioning individuals in a CFA sample score as well as the best-functioning children in the "normal" group?). We believe that there has been an underemphasis thus far on individual subject and subgroup analyses, or—when sample sizes permit—correlational techniques, which would allow us to discover individual subject variables associated with "good" vs. "poor" adjustment *within* CFA samples.

Isolating the Effects of Facial Disfigurement on Adjustment

One exception to the preceding statement is the analysis of adjustment by CFA diagnosis. Several studies have used this strategy to determine the relative importance of overt facial impairment in explaining variations in psychosocial adjustment, in most cases by comparing cleft lip and palate with cleft palate only (e.g., Brantley & Clifford, 1979; Harper et al., 1980; Kapp, 1979; Richman, 1976; Richman & Harper, 1978; Simonds & Heimburger, 1978; Starr, 1978, 1980; Tobiason & Hiebert, 1984). None of these studies found differences in behavioral/emotional status as a function of CFA type. Although this finding may result in part from the very small sample sizes that have been involved in these analyses, we must remain open to the alternative explanation that facial disfigurement is *not* a critical factor—at least as a single variable—in accounting for the behavioral adjustment of CFA children. It is more likely that facial appearance is one of several factors associated with CFA (e.g., feeding difficulties and surgeries in early life) that are important in understanding the adjustment of these children.

Parent-Child Relationships Involving Children with CFA

More than a quarter-century ago, Clifford (1969) observed that "it is almost folklore to assume that giving birth to a child with a defect has a decided impact upon the family, particularly upon the mother" (p. 235). This assumption is still widely accepted today and is so intuitively appealing that there is a tendency to attribute much of the family's subsequent stress and conflict to the birth of the disabled or impaired child rather than to preexisting conditions or normative processes and events associated with the birth of any child. Among families with children having facial impairment, this belief is further supported by research on the negative social effects of unattractive facial appearance in normal children. In one review of this literature indicating consistent negative effects, Adams (1980) wondered "Can mother love overcome the effects of having an unattractive child?" (p. 30). Research on attractiveness (e.g., Langlois, this volume) has greatly influenced hypotheses about the impact of CFA on the development of the parent–child relationship. For example, Tobiason (1984, this volume) has proposed a model in which parental avoidance of a child, stemming primarily from reactions to the child's facial characteristics, plays an important role in the child's social adjustment and academic performance. Thus, both theory and common sense would lead us to expect stress and conflict and perhaps rejection and avoidance in parental/family relationships with CFA children, particularly those involving children with visible impairment. How adequate is the empirical evidence for this hypothesis? As before, we will review this research in relation to who is providing information about the relationship: parent, child, or trained observer.

Parent-Reported Aspects of the Relationship

Clifford (1969) was one of the first investigators systematically to examine clinical impressions of the extreme negative impact of infants with CFA on maternal well-being (Macgregor, Abel, Brut, Lauer, & Weissman, 1953; Tisza & Gumpertz, 1962). The reported reactions of mothers or fathers to more and less severely impaired infants (cleft lip *and* palate and cleft lip *or* palate, respectively) were recorded during a structured interview. Self-report measures of infant symptom severity, marital happiness, and infant behavior and temperament were also used. All data were gathered within two years of the children's birth. Mothers of the infants in the more severely impaired group rated their babies as more active and less cute, likable, and intelligent than did mothers of the less impaired infants. No such effect was obtained for fathers. Marital happiness was not related to either symptom status or sex of the infant.

In the only other study examining parental reports within close proximity to the child's birth, Barden et al. (1989) gave the Satisfaction with Parenting Scale, the Life Experience Survey, and a social support measure to five mothers of infants under six months of age with mixed CFA and five mothers of healthy infants. The mothers of the CFA babies reported significantly more parenting satisfaction and positive life experiences that the control mothers. The investigators interpreted this finding as an indication of mothers' denial of psychological distress.

One other study of maternal reactions to early parenting experiences used a retrospective questionnaire called the "When My Child Was

Born" test, given several years after the child's birth (Brantley & Clifford, 1979). This instrument contains four factor-derived dimensions that pertain to different aspects of mothers' recall of their infants' early years: 1) concern about the babies' health; 2) apprehension about showing or exhibiting the infants; 3) concern about caregiving responsibilities; and 4) self-evaluations of avoidance behavior in relation to the infants. In comparing 44 cleft children and 61 controls, maternal reports were significantly less favorable on three of the four factors (concern about health, apprehension about showing, worry about child care). No differences were found in subgroup analyses of cleft lip vs. cleft lip and palate children.

Two studies reviewed earlier on parental reports of child adjustment are relevant to the nature of the parent–child relationship. On one of the four items discriminating cleft children from matched controls in the Simonds and Heimburger (1978) study, the mothers of cleft children rated their children as more dependent than the mothers of typical children. In another study using a parent behavior checklist of concurrent child behavior (Tobiason & Hiebert, 1984), a significant difference was found between cleft and normal parents in the number of child externalizing behaviors identified by the parent as problematic. This finding resulted from the unique format of the behavior checklist used in this study (the Eyberg Child Behavior Checklist), in which the parent is asked both to rate the frequency of a specific externalizing behavior and to respond "yes" or "no" to the question, "Is this a problem for *you*?" Cleft parents endorsed an average of 4.7 behaviors as problems, while parents in the control group rated an average of 7.1 such behaviors. The investigators concluded that cleft parents were more tolerant and permissive of child misbehavior than were parents of typical children. It is also possible that this finding was the result of better behavior-management skills on the part of the cleft parents (perhaps due to contact with developmental/ pediatric specialists, service providers, health care professionals, and cleft management teams) or simply a contrast effect in which parental perceptions of the behavior problems of cleft children were minimized in the face of perceived medical problem importance.

Child-Reported Perceptions of Relationship with Parents

Only two studies have examined the child's perception of their relationship with their parents. Richman and Harper (1978) administered the Children's Report of Parental Behavior Inventory to 36 children with cleft palate only, 32 children with cleft lip and palate, 68 children with cerebral palsy, and 68 typical children, ages 9 to 18. This instrument has a 3-factor structure pertaining to: 1) the child's perceived acceptance/ rejection (of the child by the parent); 2) perceived psychological control of the child by the parent vs. parental support of autonomy; 3) parental firm vs. lax disciplinary control. Groups were matched for sex, age, SES, and IQ. Sex by diagnostic group analyses found significant differences on only one factor—psychological autonomy and control—with male cleft palate children reporting greater perceived psychological control or intrusiveness by their mothers than did children of either sex in the cerebral palsy and control groups.

Brantley and Clifford (1979) examined the parental perceptions of the 44 cleft and 61 typical children in their sample, using an instrument called the "When I Was Born" test. This measure contains four factors that parallel the factor structure of the parental instrument described earlier ("When My Child Was Born") including child perceptions of: 1) parental feelings about the child; 2) parental concern about the child's welfare; 3) parental desire to show/exhibit the child as an infant; and 4) parental attitudes about the care-giving requirements of the child as an infant. Two of these factors significantly discriminated cleft and typical children: Cleft children viewed their parents as having had more negative feelings and being more worried about them as infants than did the control children.

Observations of Trained Observers

In the Field and Vega-Lahr (1984) study reviewed earlier, mothers of the cleft lip and palate infants and mothers of control infants were videotaped during a 10-minute face-to-face play interaction. Differences between cleft and control mothers were found on several measures of maternal responsiveness. As compared to control mothers, cleft mothers showed less frequent game playing, contingent responsivity, imitation, vocalization, and facial expressiveness. Overall, the cleft mothers spent proportionately less time looking at and vocalizing to their infants (47%) than did the mothers of the typical babies (73%). Finally, in the Barden et al. (1989) study, six maternal behaviors similar to those in the Field and Vega-Lahr (1984) study (e.g., smiling, verbalization/vocalization) and three global ratings of the quality of maternal interaction (gratification, responsiveness, and affect) were used. These measures were taken during three situations (free play, instructions to the mother to elicit vocalizations from the infant, and instructions to imitate the infant's behavior), thus creating 27 possible comparisons between the CFA and normal groups. Of these, eight were statistically significant in a direction suggesting less responsiveness/activity on the part of mothers of CFA infants.

Summary of Parent–Child Relationship Research

Clifford's (1969) observation that very little was then known about the specifics of early parental reactions to CFA infants and how they might fluctuate over time is still largely true. To this day, few studies have evaluated maternal reactions in relatively close proximity to the birth of the infant. Most of our information is retrospective, tapping primarily mothers' and children's memories of earlier events or evaluations of their relationship as perceived currently during the child's grade school years and adolescence. Nevertheless, the available evidence suggests that, as compared to normative groups, the types of difficulties in the mother–child relationship that would be expected to occur are in fact present to some degree, at least as subjectively reported by both parties. That is, mothers do report greater concern and worry and perhaps overprotectiveness that correspond with reciprocal impressions on the part of their children. However, none of the findings suggested extreme stress or conflict in the relationship. Factor-derived dimensions of parent and child reports that might be expected to reveal the more dysfunctional extremes of relationship problems (e.g., the acceptance/rejection scale of the Children's Report of Parental Behavior Inventory; the avoidance scale of the "When My Child Was Born" test) did not show differences between CFA children and control subjects.

The studies that present the most worrisome picture of the parent–CFA child relationship are again those involving infants and dependent measures based upon the ratings of trained observers (Field & Vega-Lahr, 1984; Barden et al., 1989). These findings suggest that the mothers of CFA babies are less responsive than are mothers of healthy infants, perhaps "turned off" by the babies' appearance or other problems (e.g., feeding difficulties). However, several issues require careful consideration before reaching this conclusion. First, the possibility discussed earlier of trained observers being more susceptible to observer bias than other types of informants needs to be considered here as well. Further, although these studies have shown group differences in *absolute levels* of selected maternal behaviors, it is not clear whether maternal behaviors differed *in relation to* the lower levels of CFA infant responsiveness also found in these studies. Optimal levels of maternal behavior can only be understood in relation to infant behavior, such that mothers' behavior "matches" or accommodates to infant behavioral parameters (Brazelton, Koslowski, & Main, 1974). It is unclear from these studies whether the less active/engaged behavior of the infants led to similar behaviors on the part of the mothers or vice versa. Field and Vega-Lahr (1984) noted that the direction of the maternal differences in their study was inconsistent with research involving other high-risk infant samples, in which mothers of impaired infants are usualy *more* active and directive, presumably in a compensatory effort to elicit "normal" responsiveness in otherwise unresponsive babies. This is a maternal reaction that may not be the best strategy for facilitating the developmental progress of infants with developmental delays or disabilities, in that excessive directiveness may overwhelm the infants' capacity to respond (Mahoney, 1988). Thus, the meaning and implications of the differences found in these studies are unclear. We believe that it would be premature to conclude that these findings are evidence of less-than-optimal maternal responsiveness to CFA infants. Further research using cross-lag sequential analyses is needed to determine the degree of contingency in the mother–infant interactions of CFA vs. normal dyads.

Models and Research Strategies

As Tobiason (1984) has observed, the psychosocial study of CFA children has proceeded for many years without clear theoretical direction or purpose. There has been little integration between the study of CFA children and developmental psychology, with its multivariate emphasis on a broad range of child, family, and ecological variables that are seen as making interactive contributions to the child's psychosocial adjustment. "Adjustment" from a developmental perspective is viewed as a series of adaptations and transitions to changing, age-related tasks including, for example, the formation during infancy of effective attachment relationships, the need for increasing self-reliance during the preschool years, the development of same-sex friendships in the grade-school years, and family emancipation during adolescence (Sroufe, 1979).

In contrast, much of the previous research with children and infants with CFA has drawn far more on the social psychological study of facial attractiveness and its effects on cognitive attributions and interpersonal behavior (e.g., Adams, 1980; Langlois & Stephan, 1981). Tobiason (1984) reviewed this research in relation to its relevance for the conceptualization of CFA children's social and emotional development, concluding that there was strong support for a model in which facial appearance is the critical variable. Specifically, appearance is viewed as the primary stimulus in a causal chain in which disfigurement/unattractiveness leads to rejection/avoidance by caregivers and peers as the result of social expectancies and self-fulfilling prophecies. Eventually, such social responses are believed to produce withdrawal and low self-esteem in the disfigured or unattractive infant or child. Although Tobiason (1984) used the term "developmental" to describe this social expectancy model, it relies too extensively, we believe, on the "main effect" of facial appearance to the considered "developmental" in the way that this perspective has been applied to other high-risk groups (e.g., Cicchetti & Schneider-Rosen, 1981). Moreover, as indicated by the preceding literature review, empirical comparisons of CFA children with/without atypical facial features have not supported the notion that the presence of visible impairment is a critical factor in explaining variations in psychosocial outcomes among children with different types of CFA.

Although the social expectancy model of CFA has stimulated important research on the effects of CFA on social attributions (see Tobiason, this volume), it has limited application as a primary theoretical framework for the study of infants and young children. Implicit in this model is the questionable assumption that the research findings of negative social reactions to unattractive but morphologically *normal* facial characteristics can be generalized to *dysmorphic* facial features. Further, the assumption is made that social reactions to unattractive or dysmorphic characteristics are relatively pervasive and consistent; that is, little attention has been paid within the model to the host of variables that potentially mediate an observer's response to child appearance or other disabilities and impairments (e.g., the observer's emotional/psychological history and well-being; social support and satisfaction with other social relationships).

The model also does not address the possibility of "transactional" effects (Sameroff & Chandler, 1975) or the reciprocal and mutually influential effects of appearance on social response and, conversely, of social response on appearance. For example, adverse social reactions to appearance might affect subsequent facial movements, emotional responses, and other subtle behaviors that contribute to perceived attractiveness. Moreover, there has been little recognition of other variables associated with CFA that may have as much or more influence than appearance, such as feeding problems, hospitalizations, and language delays or other infant/child variables less directly associated with CFA (e.g., cognitive skills, temperament). Finally, social responses to disfigurement or other characteristics of the CFA child have not been considered within the context of specific age-related processes and transitions. For example, the transition from dependence on parents during infancy to autonomous functioning during the preschool years may mark a particularly critical period for the influence of child facial appearance on caregiver "attachment expectations" (i.e., caregiver expectations related to protection vs. support for child exploration and risk taking). To summarize, we believe that the social expectancy approach to the study of CFA children, while intuitively appealing, implies a somewhat direct, linear relationship between appearance and social response that belies the complexity of the many parent, child, and ecological variables that influence the course of any child's development.

A Developmental Model

Bates and Bayles (1988) have observed that the construct of attachment security is "somewhere close to the center of the social developmental process" (p. 294). In our formulation, we have also emphasized infants' early regulation of proximity and protective contact with primary caregivers. Also of central importance in our model are the affective and cognitive *representations* of attachment that influence children's subsequent expectations about the availability and responsiveness of others and perceptions of self-worth in this regard (Sroufe & Fleeson, 1986). Such representations—which Bowlby (1969) has called the "internal working model"—are believed to reflect primarily the quality and responsiveness of early caregiving environments, serving as a later "guide" for children's social behavior and a "filter" for new information about people and relationships (Sroufe & Fleeson, 1986). It is important, however, to view attachment not as a "main effect," producing child behavioral outcomes in a linear way, but, rather, as a risk factor that, in combination with subsequent environmental supports and stressors and developmental changes in parents and children, indicates a course of probable outcomes (Sroufe, 1988). Indeed, insecure attachment in the first two years of life—as measured by anxious, resistant, avoidant or disorganized patterns of reunion behavior in the Strange Situation (Ainsworth, Blehar, Waters, & Wall, 1978)—has been shown in longitudinal studies to predict poor behavioral and emotional adjustment in children between ages three and eight years (Bates & Bayles, 1988; Bates, Maslin, & Frankel, 1985; Erickson & Farber, 1983; Erickson, Sroufe, & Egeland, 1985; Lewis, Feiring, McGuffog, & Jaskir, 1984; Matas, Arend, & Sroufe, 1978; Sroufe, Fox, & Pancake, 1983).

An important antecedent of attachment is the parents' capability to monitor, correctly interpret, and respond promptly and sensitively to infant communications of need. Mothers rated as more sensitive and synchronous and showing more frequent behaviors such as verbalization/vocalization and quick response to infant crying are more likely to have securely attached infants than are mothers who are not as responsive (Bates et al., 1985; Egeland & Farber, 1984; Grossman, Grossman, Spangler, Suess, & Unzner, 1985). Biological limitations affecting the infant's capacity to signal needs are important as well (e.g., difficult temperament or physical disability), but such factors have not shown consistently strong associations with attachment (Belsky, Rovine, & Taylor, 1984) and their effect may be indirect, mediated by the parents' capacity to accommodate and adapt to variations in infant reactivity, orientation, and so on. The parents' potential to respond in such a manner is multiply determined, influenced by a broad range of factors, including parental emotional stability both before and after the infant's birth, the quality of the parents' past and current relationships, and the capacity of the marriage to withstand the transition to parenthood (Belsky & Isabella, 1988).

Research on the early reactions of family and social environment to birth defects and developmental disabilities (for a review, see Crnic, Friedrich, & Greenberg, 1983) suggests that there are strong affective and cognitive parental responses postnatally that potentially undermine mothers' ability to accommodate infant behavior. Case studies in these areas have suggested that initial reactions of parental grief, disbelief, and guilt are common (Lansdown, 1981), followed by considerable anxiousness about the survival and physical welfare of the infants (Spreisterbach,

1963). These affectual responses are believed to parallel or precede cognitive/attitudinal responses in which the parents struggle with attributions related to causality and responsibility for the birth defect (Affleck, Mcgrade, Allen, & McQueeny, 1985; Horan, 1982). These reactions may be compounded by a perceived or an actual decrease in the social support and availability of relatives and friends, who themselves may be upset or uncertain about their reaction to the birth of such children (Kazak & Marvin, 1984). The marriage may be similarly affected as each parent's personal affective reaction to the birth may hinder dyadic communication and sharing of affect at a time when such interaction is critical. Any or all of these factors have the potential to disrupt significantly the responsiveness of parents of children with developmental disabilities or other birth defects, increasing the probability of insecure attachment (Blacher & Myers, 1983; Emde & Brown, 1978).

The critical tasks of social and emotional development take on a new focus beyond infancy. Attachment relationships in toddlerhood and the preschool years become increasingly more organized in relation to internal models and affective processes (what attachment theorists have called "felt security") than in relation to physical dimensions of proximity seeking and contact maintenance (e.g., using mother as a "secure base"). This transition from primarily overt to primarily (but not exclusively) internalized regulation of attachment is facilitated in typical children by the children's newly acquired skills of locomotion, increased interest in exploration, the beginnings of both symbolic play and representation, the use of language, and the developing recognition of self (Greenberg & Speltz, 1988). Language development also helps the child to communicate and understand the emotions of others and to differentiate and discuss internal states, a process that is fundamental to the acquisition of self-control (Greenspan & Greenspan, 1985). All these factors play a role in children's efforts to individuate, becoming more autonomous and less dependent upon the physical care and proximity of caregivers. In young children with disabilities, many barriers stand in the way of this transition. Parents may become overprotective of the disabled child (Wallander & Hubert, 1987), discouraging children's efforts to individuate by becoming overcontrolling and intrusive in their parenting interactions (Mahoney, 1988). This may create a relationship that further impedes children's acquisition of new skills and their development of peer relationships. As suggested by Rubin and Wilkinson (this volume), such parental overprotection and control—reflecting parents' efforts to shield children from unpleasant social responses—may reduce the children's opportunities for self-guided explorations of novel social situations.

All the factors listed above can apply to children with wide-ranging types of birth defects or developmental disabilities. Infants and young children with CFA may be further affected by these variables in several specific ways. First, for infants with visible impairment, facial appearance may reduce maternal responsiveness—at least before corrective surgery—because of maternal aversion to the appearance of the infants' faces or because of infants' relative inability to display the expected range of facial movements and expressions in response to maternal elicitations of infant response. This may attentuate subsequent maternal efforts to elicit a social response from the infants. Second, the feeding problems associated with cleft palate may not only disrupt the synchronous "flow" and mutual gratification of mother–child interaction but may also begin to affect mothers' sense of parenting competence. That is, a mother may begin to attribute interactional difficulties during feeding not only to infant characteristics but also to her own incompetence, depending upon previous experience (e.g., with other infants) and individual differences in preexisting self-efficacy. For example, a first-time mother with a history of low self-confidence may begin to believe that she lacks the skills to feed her infant properly. A third factor affecting parental responsiveness to CFA infants, particularly those with visible impairment, is related to social network reactivity. Social support for the parents and family may unravel as a function of cultural factors associated with infant attractiveness ("All babies are cute") and related social interaction and amenities that are an expected part of social network response to the birth of a new infant (e.g., the expectation that others need to comment favorably on the infant's appearance or health during initial interactions with a new mother and baby). Awkwardness, embarrassment, or uncertainty about what to say/how to act in these situations—on the part both of parent and other—may disrupt the family's social support, which will, in turn, undermine the parents' adaptation to the infant's disability and, ultimately, their responsiveness to the infant.

Hospitalization and corrective surgery are additional factors that may have negative effects on maternal responsiveness and infants' security of attachment. The separation and interruption of caregiving routines brought about by the hospitalization itself is one obvious source of risk, particularly separations occurring during the first few months of life. Although surgical corrections of the lip and/or palate may eventually normalize parent–child interactions, the short-term effects related to parental anxiety about the infants' ability to survive the surgery, apprehension over the quality of the restoration, feelings of disappointment in the immediate or eventual results of the surgery, all may serve to disrupt the responsiveness of the parent.

Postinfancy for CFA children may be marked by two other factors of importance to psychosocial development. Expressive language delays associated with the cleft palate (decreased vocabulary, poor articulation, grammatical and syntactical errors) may hamper the children's use of language for emotional regulation as described earlier (i.e., for discriminating and talking about internal states, labeling affect in others). As with children with hearing impairment (see Greenberg & Kusche,

1989), the parents may need to make extraordinary accommodations in helping cleft children to acquire affect language. Finally, the transition from dependency to separation–individuation may be particularly difficult for the parents of CFA children to navigate successfully. On the one hand, cleft children by preschool age are nearly normal in all respects, including at least some degree of facial restoration and correction of the palate. Physical caretaking needs by this age will thus have become quite similar to the levels of care required by typical children. On the other hand, historical factors may greatly work against the parents' capacity to encourage autonomous functioning (e.g., the heightened need for physical care earlier, effects of early and worrisome hospital-related separations), as well as culturally driven fears regarding the reaction of the children's peers to appearance or language problems. In families in which separation/individuation problems do become significant and the children's initial adjustment to the peer group is poor, it is unclear to what extent peer problems reflect the children's enmeshment with parents vs. specific peer reactions to the children's impairment.

To summarize, then, we believe that individual differences in the developing behavioral competencies and problems of children with CFA can be best understood in relation to five factors, taken from the model that we have presented:

1. Parental responsiveness to infant and the factors that potentially enhance or undermine responsiveness, including personality and attachment history; marital and extrafamilial social support.
2. Infant security of attachment, reflecting in large part the responsiveness of care received during the first year.
3. The young child's internal representations of modal interactions within the context of early relationships (self-system) and the influence of this "internal working model" on the child's general expectations regarding the responsiveness and availability of others.
4. The child's acquisition of affect language and parental support and facilitation of the use of such language.
5. The parent–child dyad's ability to transition successfully from a relationship characterized by child proximity regulation and the use of parents as a secure base, to one in which parents encourage the child's independent functioning while at the same time establishing appropriate limits.

Our model thus adds to the formulations of Tobiason (1984), Barden et al. (1989), Bull and Rumsey (1988), and others by specifying variables that both mediate the response of caregivers to appearance and buffer or protect the children from whatever adverse social reactions might occur. The facial disfigurement of some CFA children is important in this model only insofar as it influences the major "building blocks" of social/

emotional development that we have specified previously. From this perspective, reactions to visible impairment may be of less importance in terms of relative predictive power than such variables as degree of feeding difficulty, speech delays, maternal attachment history, paternal involvement, parental attitudes and expectations about surgery, and so on. Of course, the relative weights of these different variables are unknown, thus indicating a major direction for further research.

Preliminary Research Within a Developmental Model

As a first step in the investigation of our model, we conducted a pilot study involving children ages one to three with various CFAs and a healthy control group matched for SES, sex, and family size (Speltz et al., 1990). We decided to focus on this age group both for practical reasons (infants are more difficult to recruit) and because of the fact that there is a significant gap in previous research with respect to postinfancy children with CFA prior to school entry. The study was designed in relation to three specific questions:

1. Are the dyadic interactional differences between clinic and control groups found in previous studies involving very young CFA infants (Barden et al., 1989; Field & Vega-Lahr, 1984) evident as well in children of this age?
2. What effect does CFA diagnostic status have on the types of distal influences that were addressed in our model (maternal personality and well-being, self-evaluations of parenting competence, marital adjustment, and social support)?
3. Among children with different types of CFA in this age group, is maternal functioning or child behavior influenced specifically by the presence of facial disfigurement?

To answer these questions, we recruited 33 mother–child dyads containing an infant or toddler with CFA (mean age = 20 months) from our Craniofacial Clinic at Children's Hospital in Seattle. The comparison group contained 22 mother–infant dyads with healthy infants recruited from a nearby pediatric practice. There were 12, 11, and 10 children in 3 clinical subgroups: cleft palate, cleft lip and palate, and sagittal synostosis, respectively. All mothers were given a battery of self-report measures, including the Parenting Stress Index, the General Well-Being Schedule and Social Health Inventory (Ware, Johnston, Davies-Avery, & Brook, 1979), and the Locke-Wallace Marital Adjustment Scale. Thirty-seven of the total sample were available for videotaping during a 5-minute structured teaching task (in which the mothers were asked to teach their children developmentally appropriate tasks) and a 5-minute free, play session. Observational measures for the free-play session were based on the Eyberg and Robinson (1981) Dyadic Parent-Child Interaction Coding System, which includes frequency measures of nine categories of maternal behavior (e.g., praising, giving directions, describing play activity). Teaching interactions were analyzed using the Nursing Child Assessment Teaching Scale, or NCATS (Barnard, Hammond, Booth, Bee, Mitchell, & Spieker, 1988). The NCATS is organized into six subscales, four of which describe mothers' behavior (sensitivity to cues, response to child distress, social/emotional growth fostering, and cognitive growth fostering) and two of which pertain to the infants' behavior (clarity of cues and responsiveness to mother).

Play interactions were also rated in terms of the more global aspects of the interaction (affective tone, maternal sensitivity to child, child responsiveness to mother, child level of play organization and focus) using an expanded version of a rating system developed by Crnic et al. (1983). This coding system is the same as used by Barden et al. (1989) in their study of 3-month-old infants.

Speltz et al. (1990) reported on the subgroup and group comparisons of dependent variables. First, there were no significant subgroup differences on any measure, a finding consistent with several previous studies involving CFA children in which measures of psychosocial variables failed to reveal differences (e.g., Brantley & Clifford, 1979; Harper et al., 1980; Kapp-Simon, 1986; Richman, 1976; Richman & Harper, 1978; Simonds & Heimburger, 1978; Starr, 1978, 1980; Tobiason & Hiebert, 1984). Although, as noted earlier, this may reflect in part the reduced power of such analyses (given a typically small cell size), the consistency of this null effect may also mean, as we have theorized, that risk factors common to various CFA diagnostic subgroups (and, indeed, to many different types of infant disability) have more influence on maternal and child psychosocial status than facial disfigurement specifically. Our remaining analyses thus combined the diagnostic subgroups into a single clinic group and comparisons were made with the nonimpaired control group. Clinic mothers reported higher stress associated with parenting activities, higher levels of negative affective states (e.g., anxiousness, despondency, concern about health), and greater dissatisfaction with their marital relationship. This difference in marital satisfaction may indicate a possible source of vulnerability for the infants, as attachment security at the end of the first year of life has been found to be associated with marital adjustment to the stress of having a new child (Belsky & Isabella, 1988).

The clinic mothers in our study were also more likely to report negative self-appraisals, seeing themselves as lacking competence as a parent, although their reports of *child* characteristics (e.g., temperament, difficulty of care) did not differ from those of the control group mothers. Thus, there appeared to be a tendency for the clinic mothers to attribute the caregiving difficulties of a CFA child to self, rather than to child limitations. The lack of group differences in mothers' reports of child characteristics would seem to be illogical in view of the obviously greater caregiving demands and problems associated with the CFA child. However, much like the clinic mothers in the Barden et al. (1989) study, who reported *greater* parenting satisfaction than controls, the clinic mothers in our study might have been making an effort via their self-reports of child to emphasize and selectively focus on the most positive aspects of the relationship. We might call this "denial" or defensive reporting, but this form of report bias may not necessarily be unhealthy. There is evidence that mothers who report generally positive perceptions of child behavior and temperament, despite objectively measured stressors, are more likely to have securely attached infants (see Spieker & Booth, 1988, for their discussion of negative and positive affectivity). Further, the combination of minimizing child problems while acknowledging self-doubts about parenting competence, might also be somewhat adaptive. Affleck et al. (1985) found that positive outcomes among children with disabilities were related to mothers' attributions of their own responsibility for problems, even those clearly linked to the disability.

Group differences between the clinic and control groups in interactive behavior were not found, as indicated by our observational measures of maternal and child behavior. Thus, mothers of the CFA and normal children were equally responsive during play and showed equivalent levels of skill during the teaching tasks. The children themselves were equally responsive to mothers in both situations. How would we interpret these "negative" findings, in light of the previous research finding clear mother and infant clinic control group differences during the first year (i.e., Barden et al., 1989; Field & Vega-Lahr, 1984)? One explanation is simply that the two previous studies involved a period of infancy in which mothers may have been in more of an acute stage of emotional reactivity to the infants' birth. Also, most of the rigorous caregiving demands of early infancy have subsided by the second year. Perhaps the most obvious explanation is that both the Barden et al. and Field and Vega-Lahr studies examined infants *before* corrective surgery, whereas, with only two exceptions, all our children were seen postsurgery (the two exceptions were cleft palate only children without palate repair). Thus, changes associated with improved appearance and/or resolution of feeding/breathing and perhaps early language problems may have led to "normalized" interactional characteristics in the dyads that we observed. Whatever the case, the primary hypothesis for future research resulting from this study is that CFA mothers and children go through stages of adaptation, characterized by atypical interactions during early infancy (although, as noted earlier, not necessarily less-than-optimal interactions) followed by "recovery" during the second and third years of life.

Implications for Research

Although, as indicated by our reviews earlier in this paper, CFA children would appear to be at elevated risk for adjustment problems, the majority would seem to be indistinguishable from typical children, at least by school age. Thus, it may be time within this field to move beyond the focus on group comparisons—and the corresponding goal of determining in what ways CFA children are different from typical children—to an emphasis on the individual differences among these children that are important predictors of risk. This is not to say that normative comparisons or "control" groups are not important, but only that our methodology in future studies should attend to both between- and within-group analyses of dependent variables. We believe that the most important question for future research is what variables, within the CFA population, are associated with particular vulnerability to normative and impairment-related stressors? Answers to this question will require prospective, longitudinal research of the type that is now standard practice in research on other high-risk samples (e.g., Beckman, 1984; Ramey, Bryant, Sparling, & Wasik, 1984; Vietze & Coates, 1986).

Ideally, this research would begin with the study of the infants and their families prior to the first surgical correction of the anomaly. Predictor variables during the period of early infancy should be far-ranging, including both proximal measures of the interactional "details" of the parent–child relationship (e.g., mother–infant interactions during feeding and play) as well as the more distal family, ecological, and medical treatment factors that we have identified in our model as being influential in determining the course of developing interactions throughout the first year (Speltz, Goodell, Endriga, & Clarren, 1994). As one measure of outcome at the end of the first year, observations of dyadic interaction during the separation/reunion paradigm would provide important information about the status of the mother–infant relationship with respect to attachment (Speltz, Greenberg, Endriga, & Galbreath, 1994). As suggested by research on the antecedents of secure attachment and the two studies finding differences between CFA and typical dyads before surgery (Barden et al., 1989; Field & Vega-Lahr, 1984), we would hypothesize that interactions associated with less secure forms of attachment (weak proximity seeking; avoidance during reunion) would be more frequently observed in dyads containing CFA infants than those with healthy infants. From the lack of interactional differences found in our pilot work at ages one to three, we would also hypothesize improving dyadic interaction by the end of the first year, with such change predicted most strongly by degree of parent-perceived surgical outcome. For this reason, it may be that by 24 months of age, a repeated observation of separation/reunion behavior would indicate less difference in attachment security between CFA and healthy infants. Looking ahead, we would expect that measures of preschool outcome (behavior problem checklist data; teacher and parent ratings of problem-solving skills, peer social skills, frustration tolerance) would be related to early attachment classifications, subsequent events related to surgical outcome, and the number and intensity of family stressors in the interim (Speltz, Morton, Goodell, & Clarren, 1993).

Implications for Treatment

If infancy risk factors could be identified in relation to child psychosocial functioning at preschool or school entry, clinic observations of dyadic or family interaction and parent self-report measures could be used to screen for such factors, and preventive interventions could be offered through hospital-based cleft/craniofacial teams. For example, if, as indicated by research on other samples of infants, maternal contingent and sensitive responding to the infant in the first six months is predictive of secure attachment, than specialized interaction training (e.g., Greenspan & Greenspan, 1985) could be offered to dyads that meet high-risk thresholds.

With respect to current clinical practice in advance of longitudinal research, a word of caution is in order: The differences found thus far in dyadic interactions and marital/family factors between CFA and typical samples may not necessarily be maladaptive or changeworthy; rather, such differences may represent adaptational adjustments to infant impairment or disability. Sroufe and Rutter (1984) have noted the powerful "self-righting" tendency in human development, and what is atypical may, in fact, serve some adaptive purpose that is only or most apparent at some later point in time. For example, the finding of greater self-rated parenting incompetence among the clinic mothers in our pilot study could represent a gross misattribution of responsibility for caregiving problems that will eventually tax the capacity of these mothers to respond sensitively. On the other hand, this could be a protective and self-righting cognitive strategy that helps some mothers to provide continuing sensitive care under conditions of enormous stress. Self-reported competence did not correlate significantly with any concurrent measure of observed child or maternal behavior in our study; thus, determining which of these interpretations is most correct may only be possible by doing the type of longitudinal research proposed herein. In the meantime, it would be unwise to intervene on the basis of such findings without long-term follow-up (e.g., convincing clinic mothers that they are, or can be, competent). It would seem, then, for both researchers and clinicians, that it is best to assume until proven otherwise that differences between CFA infants/families and normative groups represent adaptation rather than deviance.

Acknowledgments. Preparation of this article was supported in part by National Institute of Child Health and Human Development Grant HD25987 to Matthew Speltz.

References

Achenbach, T.M., & Edelbrock, C.S. (1981). Behavioral problems and competencies reported by parents of normal and disturbed children aged four through sixteen. *Monographs of the Society for Research in Child Development, 46,* Serial No. 188.

Adams, G. (1980). The effects of physical attractiveness on the socialization process. In G. Lucker, K. Ribbens, & J. McNamara (Eds.), *Psychological aspects of facial form.* Ann Arbor, MI: University of Michigan Press.

Affleck, G., McGrade, B., Allen, D., & McQueeney, M. (1985). Mothers' beliefs about behavioral causes for their developmentally disabled infant's condition: What do they signify? *Journal of Pediatric Psychology, 10,* 293–303.

Ainsworth, M.D.S., Blehar, M.C., Waters, E., & Wall, S. (1978). *Patterns of attachment: A psychological study of the Strange Situation.* Hillsdale, NJ: Erlbaum.

Barden, R., Ford, M., Jensen, A., Rogers-Salyer, M., & Salyer, K. (1989). Effects of craniofacial deformity in infancy on the quality of mother-infant interactions. *Child Development, 60,* 819–824.

Barnard, K., Hammond, M., Booth, C., Bee, H., Mitchell, S., & Spieker, S. (1988). Measurement and meaning of parent-child interactions. In F. Morrison, C. Lord, & D. Keating (Eds.), *Applied developmental psychology.* New York: Academic Press.

Bates, J.E., & Bayles, K. (1988). Attachment and the development of behavior problems. In J. Belsky & T. Nezworski (Eds.), *Clinical implications of attachment* (pp. 235–239). Hillsdale, NJ: Erlbaum.

Bates, J.E., Maslin, C.A., & Frankel, K.A. (1985). Attachment security, mother-child interaction, and temperament as predictors of behavior-problem ratings at age three years. In I. Bretherton & E. Waters (Eds.), *Growing points in attachment theory and research. Monographs of the Society for Research in Child Development, 50,* 167–193.

Beckman, P.J. (1984). A transactional view of stress in families of handicapped children. In M. Lewis (Ed.), *Beyond the dyad.* New Brunswick NJ: Plenum.

Belsky, J. (1984). The determinants of parenting: A process model. *Child Development, 58,* 83–96.

Belsky, J., & Isabella, R. (1988). Maternal, infant, and social-contextual determinants of attachment security. In J. Belsky & T. Nezworski (Eds.), *Clinical implications of attachment* (pp. 3–17). Hillsdale, NJ: Erlbaum.

Belsky, J., Rovine, M., & Taylor, D. (1984). The Pennsylvania Infant and Family Development Project: III. The origins of individual differences in infant-mother attachment: Maternal and infant contributions. *Child Development, 55,* 718–728.

Bjornsson, A., & Agustsdottir, S. (1987). A psychosocial study of Icelandic individuals with cleft lip or cleft lip and palate. *Cleft Lip Journal, 24,* 152–157.

Blacher, J., & Meyers, C.E. (1983). A review of attachment formation and disorder of handicapped children. *American Journal of Mental Deficiency, 4,* 359–371.

Bowlby, J. (1969). *Attachment and loss. Vol. 1: Attachment.* New York: Basic Books.

Brantley, H.T., & Clifford, E. (1979). Maternal and child locus of control and field-dependence in cleft palate children. *Cleft Palate Journal, 16,* 183–187.

Brazelton, B.T., Koslowski, B., & Main, M. (1974). The origins of reciprocity: The early mother-infant interaction. In M. Lewis & L.A. Rosenblum (Eds.), *The effect of the infant on its caregiver* (pp. 49–76). New York: John Wiley & Sons.

Bull, R., & Rumsey, N. (1988). *The social psychology of facial appearance.* New York. Springer-Verlag.

Cicchetti, D., & Schneider-Rosen, K. (1986). An organizational approach to childhood depression. In M. Rutter, C. Izard, & P. Read (Eds.), *Depression in young people: Clinical and developmental perspectives* (pp. 71–134). New York: Guilford.

Clifford, E. (1969). Parental ratings of cleft palate infants. *Cleft Palate Journal, 6,* 235–244.

Clifford, E. (1983). Why are they so normal? *Cleft Palate Journal, 20,* 83–84.

Crnic, K.A., Friedrich, W.N., & Greenberg, M.T. (1983). Adaptation of families with mentally retarded children: A model of stress, coping, and family ecology. *American Journal of Mental Deficiency, 88,* 125–138.

Crnic, K.A., Greenberg, M.T., Ragozin, A.S., Robinson, N.M., & Basham, R.B. (1983). Effects of stress and social support on mothers and premature and full-term infants. *Child Development, 54,* 209–217.

Egeland, B., & Farber, E.A. (1984). Infant-mother attachment: Factors related to its development and changes over time. *Child Development, 55,* 753–771.

Emde, R.N., & Brown, C. (1978). Adaptation to the birth of a Down's Syndrome infant: Grieving and maternal attachment. *Journal of the American Academy of Child Psychiatry, 17,* 299–323.

Erickson, M.F., Sroufe, L.A., & Egeland, B. (1985). The relationship between quality of attachment and behavior problems in preschool in a high-risk sample. In I. Bretherton & E. Waters (Eds.), *Growing points of attachment theory and research. Monographs of the Society for Research in Child Development, 50,* 147–166.

Erickson, M.F., & Farber, E.A. (1983). *Infancy to preschool: Continuity of adaptation in high-risk children.* Paper presented at the Society for Research in Child Development, Detroit, MI.

Eyberg, S.M., & Robinson, E.A. (1981). *Dyadic parent-child interaction coding system: A manual* (3rd rev.). Unpublished manuscript, Oregon Health Sciences University, Portland, OR.

Field, T.M., & Vega-Lahr, N. (1984). Early interactions between infants with craniofacial anomalies and their mothers. *Infant Behavior and Development, 7,* 527–530.

Fox, D., Lynch, J., & Brookshire, B. (1978). Selected developmental factors of cleft palate children between two and thirty-three months of age. *Cleft Palate Journal, 15,* 239–245.

Gluck, M.R., McWilliams, B.F., Wylie, H.L., & Conkwright, E.A. (1965). A comparison of clinical characteristics of children with cleft palates and children in a child guidance clinic. *Perceptual and Motor Skills, 21,* 806.

Greenberg, M.T., & Kusche, K.C. (1989). Cognitive, personal and social development in deaf children and adolescents. In M.C. Wang, H.J. Walberg, & M.C. Reynolds (Eds.), *The handbook of special education: Research and practice* (1–3). Oxford, England: Pergamon Press.

Greenberg, M.T., & Speltz, M.L. (1988). Attachment and the ontogeny of conduct problems. In J. Belsky & T. Nezworski (Eds.), *Clinical implications of attachment* (pp. 177–218). Hillsdale, NJ: Erlbaum.

Greenspan, S.I., & Greenspan, N.T. (1985). *First feelings: Milestones in the emotional development of your baby and child.* New York: Viking.

Grossmann, K., Grossmann, K.E., Spangler, G., Suess, G., & Unzner, L. (1985). Maternal sensitivity and newborns' orientation responses as related to quality of attachment in Northern Germany. In I. Bretherton & E. Waters (Eds.), *Growing points of attachment theory and research. Monographs of the Society for Research in Child Development, 50,* (1–2, Serial No. 209), 233–256.

Harper, D., Richman, L., & Snider, B. (1980). School adjustment and degree of physical impairment. *Journal of Pediatric Psychology, 5(4),* 377–383.

Heller, A., Tidmarsh, W., & Pless, I. (1981). The psychosocial functioning of young adults born with cleft lip or palate. *Clinical Pediatrics, 20,* 459–465.

Horan, M.L. (1982). Parental reaction to the birth of an infant with a defect: An attributional approach. *Advances in Nursing Science, 5,* 57–68.

Kapp, K. (1979). Self-concept of the cleft lip or palate child. *Cleft Palate Journal, 16,* 171–176.

Kapp-Simon, K. (1986). Self-concept of primary-school-age children with cleft lip, cleft palate, or both. *Cleft Palate Journal, 23,* 24–27.

Kazak, A.E., & Marvin, R.S. (1984). Differences, difficulties and adaptation: Stress and social networks in families with a handicapped child. *Family Relations: Journal of Applied Family and Child Studies, 33,* 67–77.

Langlois, J., & Stephan, C. (1981). Beauty and the beast: The role of physical attractiveness in the development of peer relations and social behavior. In S. Brehm, S. Kassin, & F. Gibbons (Eds.), *Developmental social psychology: Theory and research.* New York: Oxford University Press.

Lansdown, R. (1981). Cleft lip and palate: A prediction of psychological disfigurement? *British Journal of Orthodontics, 8,* 83–88.

Lewis, M., Feiring, C., McGuffog, C., & Jaskir, J. (1984). Predicting psychopathology in six-year-olds from early social relations. *Child Development, 55,* 123–136.

Long, N.V., & Dalston, R.M. (1982). Gestural communication in twelve-month-old cleft lip and palate children. *Cleft Palate Journal, 19,* 57–61.

Mahoney, G. (1988). Maternal communication style with mentally retarded children. *American Journal on Mental Retardation, 92,* 352–359.

MacGregor, F.C., Abel, T.M., Brut, A., Lauer, E., & Weissman, S. (1953). *Facial deformities and plastic surgery: A psychosocial study.* Springfield, IL: Charles C. Thomas.

Matas, L., Arend, R.A., & Sroufe, L.A. (1978). Continuity of adaptation in the second year: The relationship between quality of attachment and later competence. *Child Development, 49,* 547–556.

McWilliams, B.J., & Paradise, L.P. (1973). Educational, occupational and marital status of cleft palate adults. *Cleft Palate Journal, 10,* 223–229.

Quay, H.C. (1979). Classification. In H.C. Quay & J.S. Werry (Eds.), *Psychopathological disorders of childhood* (2nd ed.). New York: Wiley.

Quay, H., & Petersen, D. (1967). *Manual for the behavior problem checklist.* Champaign, IL: University of Illinois Press.

Ramey, C.T., Bryant, D.M., Sparling, J.J., & Lasik, B.H. (1984). A biosocial systems perspective on environmental interventions for low birth weight infants. *Clinical Obstetrics and Gynecology, 27,* 672–692.

Richman, L.C. (1976). Behavior and achievement of cleft palate children. *Cleft Palate Journal, 13,* 4–10.

Richman, L.C. (1978). The effects of facial disfigurement on teachers' perception of ability in cleft palate children. *Cleft Palate Journal, 15,* 155–160.

Richman, L.C., & Eliason, M. (1982). Psychological characteristics of children with cleft lip and palate: Intellectual, achievement, behavioral, and personality variables. *Cleft Palate Journal, 19,* 249–257.

Richman, L.C., & Harper, D.C. (1978). Observable stigmata and perceived maternal behaviors. *Cleft Palate Journal, 15,* 215–219.

Richman, L.C., & Harper, D.C. (1979). Self-identified personality patterns of children with facial or orthopedic disfigurement. *Cleft Palate Journal, 16,* 257–261.

Sameroff, A.J., & Chandler, M.J. (1975). Reproductive risk and the continuum of caretaking casualty. In F.D. Horowitz (Ed.), *Review of child development research* (Vol. 4) (pp. 187–244). Chicago: University of Chicago Press.

Simonds, J.F., & Heimburger, R.E. (1978). Psychiatric evaluation of youth with cleft lip-palate matched with a control group. *Cleft Palate Journal, 15,* 193–201.

Speltz, M.L., Armsden, G., & Clarren, S. (1990). Effects of craniofacial birth defects on maternal functioning post-infancy. *Journal of Pediatric Psychology, 15,* 177–196.

Speltz, M.L., Goodell, E.W., Endriga, M.C., & Clarren, S.K. (1994). Quality of early feeding interaction between infants with craniofacial anomalies and their mothers. *Infant Behavior and Development, 17,* 131–139.

Speltz, M.L., Greenberg, M.T., Endriga, M.C., & Galbreath, H. (1994). Developmental approach to the psychology of craniofacial anomalies. *Cleft Palate-Craniofacial Journal, 31,* 61–67.

Speltz, M.L., Morton, K., Goodell, E.W., & Clarren, S.K. (1993). Psychological functioning of children with craniofacial anomalies and their mothers: Follow-up from late infancy to school entry. *Cleft Palate-Craniofacial Journal, 30,* 482–489.

Spieker, S.J., & Booth, C.L. (1988). Maternal antecedents of attachment quality. In J. Belsky & T. Nezworski (Eds.), *Clinical implications of attachment* (pp. 95–135). Hillsdale, NJ: Erlbaum.

Spriesterbach, D. (1963). Psychosocial factors of cleft lip and palate rehabilitation. In B. Rogers (Ed.), *Facial disfigurement: A rehabilitation problem.* Washington, D.C.: Vocational Rehabilitation Administration.

Sroufe, L.A. (1979). The coherence of individual development: Early care, attachment, and subsequent developmental issues. *American Psychologist, 34,* 834–841.

Sroufe, L.A. (1988). The role of infant-caregiver attachment in development. In J. Belsky & T. Nezworski (Eds.), *Clinical implications of attachment* (pp. 18–38). Hillsdale, NJ: Erlbaum.

Sroufe, L.A., & Fleeson, J. (1986). Attachment and the construction of relationships. In W. Hartup & Z. Rubin (Eds.), *Relationships and development*. Hillsdale, NJ: Erlbaum.

Sroufe, L.A., Fox, N.E., & Pancake, V.R. (1983). Attachment and dependency in developmental perspective. *Child Development, 54,* 1615–1627.

Sroufe, L.A., & Rutter, M. (1984). The domain of developmental psychopathology. *Child Development, 55,* 17–29.

Starr, P. (1978). Self-esteem and behavioral functioning of teenagers with oral facial clefts. *Rehabilitation Literature, 39,* 233–235.

Starr, P. (1980). Facial attractiveness and behavior of patients with cleft lip and/or palate. *Psychology Reports, 46,* 579–582.

Starr, P., Chinsky, R., Canter, H., & Meier, J. (1977). Mental, motor and social behavior of infants with cleft lip and/or palate. *Cleft Palate Journal, 14,* 140–147.

Tisza, V.B., & Gumpertz, E. (1962). The parents' reaction to the birth and early care of children with cleft palate. *Pediatrics, 30,* 86–90.

Tobiasen, J. (1984). Psychosocial correlates of congenital facial clefts: Conceptualization and model. *Cleft Palate Journal, 21,* 131–139.

Tobiasen, J.M., & Hiebert, J.M. (1984). Parents' tolerance for the conduct problems of the child with cleft lip and palate. *Cleft Palate Journal, 21,* 82–85.

Ullmann, L.P., & Krasner, L. (1975). *A psychological approach to abnormal behavior*. Englewood Cliffs, NJ: Prentice-Hall.

Vietze, P., & Coates, D. (1986). Research with families of handicapped persons. Lessons from the past, plans for the future. In J. Gallagher & P. Vietze (Eds.), *Families of handicapped persons*. Baltimore, MD: Brookes.

Wallander, J.C., & Hubert, N.C. (1987). Peer social dysfunction in children with developmental disabilities: Empirical basis and a conceptual model. *Clinical Psychology Review, 7,* 205–221.

Ware, J., Johnston, S., Davies-Avery, A., & Brook, R. (1979). Conceptualization and measurement of health for adults: Vol 3. Mental Health (R-1987/3-HEW). Washington, D.C.: U.S. Government Printing Office.

Index

B

F

G

Q

R

T

MIX
Papier aus verantwortungsvollen Quellen
Paper from responsible sources
FSC® C105338

If you have any concerns about our products,
you can contact us on
ProductSafety@springernature.com

In case Publisher is established outside the EU,
the EU authorized representative is:
Springer Nature Customer Service Center GmbH
Europaplatz 3, 69115 Heidelberg, Germany

Printed by Libri Plureos GmbH
in Hamburg, Germany